MEDICAL
MICROBIOLOGY

Tony Hart MB BS BSc PhD FRCPath

Professor
Department of Medical Microbiology
University of Liverpool, UK

Paul Shears MD MRCPath

Senior Lecturer
Department of Medical Microbiology
University of Liverpool, and
Liverpool School of Tropical Medicine, UK

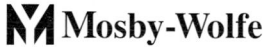

Mosby-Wolfe

London Baltimore Barcelona Bogotá Boston Buenos Aires Caracas Carlsbad, CA Chicago Madrid Mexico City Milan
Naples, FL New York Philadelphia St. Louis Seoul Singapore Sydney Taipei Tokyo Toronto Wiesbaden

Publisher:	Richard Furn
Development Editor:	Jennifer Prast
Project Manager:	Dave Burin
Production:	Jane Tozer
Layout:	Lindy van den Berghe
Illustration:	Lee Smith
Cover Design:	Lara Last
Index:	Jill Halliday

₦ Mosby-Wolfe

An imprint of Harcourt Publishers Limited

Copyright © 1996 Times Mirror International Publishers Limited
Copyright © 2000 Mosby International Limited
₦ is a registered trademark of Harcourt Publishers Limited
Printed in Spain by Grafos S.A. Arte sobre papel, Barcelona. Spain
ISBN 0 7234 2322 9

Published 1996. Reprinted 2000, 2001

A CIP catalogue record for this book is available from the British Library.

Library of Congress Catologing-in-Publication Data has been applied for.

Contents

Preface

Medical microbiology is the study of the micro-organisms pathogenic for man. It encompasses not just the specific diagnosis of infection but also the epidemiology, pathogenesis, treatment and prevention of microbial disease. Although the incidence of microbial disease is not now so great in the developed world, outbreaks of infection still have the capacity to elicit great public concern. In developing countries, microbial disease still exerts a great toll both in terms of morbidity and mortality. It is estimated that each year there are between 3 and 5 billion cases of diarrhoeal disease (which can be due to one of thirty or more pathogens) resulting in 5–10 million deaths (primarily in children). However, even diarrhoeal disease pales into insignificance compared with the 12 million deaths annually due to acute respiratory tract infection. Infections such as poliomyelitis, whooping cough and typhoid fever (which have largely been eliminated in developed countries) are still important in global terms. There are up to 10 billion cases of infection with polio virus resulting in 10 million cases of poliomyelitis and 10 thousand deaths each year. Tuberculosis was described as 'the captain of all the men of death' in nineteenth century Europe when it was responsible for an annual mortality rate of 500 per 100,000 population. With improved nutrition, social conditions, appropriate chemotherapy and immunization there was a dramatic decrease in the incidence of tuberculosis. For example in the 1960s and 1970s the incidence showed a decline of 5–10% each year. Unfortunately this plateaued at an incidence of infection in developed countries of 10 per 100,000 population but from 1985 to 1992 the incidence has increased, for example in the USA by 20%.

In addition to the re-emergence of 'old' pathogens, such as *Mycobacterium tuberculosis,* we are seeing the recognition (and even emergence) of 'new' pathogens alongside advanced technologies, altered life-styles and improved capacity for maintaining human life. We estimate that over the last 20 years two to three 'new' pathogens have been described each year. Examples include viruses such as Muerto canyon (causing hantavirus pulmonary syndrome), human immunodeficiency virus (causing AIDS) and astrovirus (causing diarrhoeal disease); bacteria such as *Bartonella henselae* (causing cat scratch fever), *Legionella pneumophila* (causing Legionnaires' disease) and *Tropheryma whippelii* (causing Whipple's disease); parasites such as *Cryptosporidium parvum* and

Cyclospora cayetanensis (both causing diarrhoeal disease) and *Strongyloides fullebornii* (causing neonatal death in Papua New Guinea).

It had been expected that with the onset of the antibiotic (and even antiviral) era, most infections would be amenable to treatment with 'magic-bullets'. Although our expectations were realized initially, of late bacteria resistant to many antibiotics have now emerged ('super-bugs'). Examples include strains of *Salmonella typhi* (the agent of typhoid fever) resistant to all first-line antibiotics (co-trimoxazole, ampicillin, chloramphenicol, tetracycline and ciprofloxacin). Most of the genes responsible for this antibiotic resistance are carried on plasmids (extrachromosomal DNA) which are readily transferred between bacterial species and genera. Currently, the emergence of antibiotic resistance is lagging only slightly behind the production of new antibiotics. This is due partly to misuse of antibiotics and partly to the infinite capacity of bacteria to replicate (under optimal conditions they have a doubling time of 20 min) and mutate under the selection pressure of antibiotics.

Finally, there has been an explosion of new technologies which have helped our understanding of how micro-organisms cause disease, of how best to diagnose infection and which have even defined 'new' pathogens. For example, hepatitis C virus has never been grown in artificial culture yet, by a mixture of cloning, insertion into vectors, amplification by polymerase chain reaction and expression of viral genome, diagnostic tools and typing methods have been devised.

The aim of this atlas is to provide a framework for understanding the pathogens (prions, viruses, bacteria, fungi, protozoa and multicellular parasites) that infect man. Their characteristics, disease associations and specific diagnoses are described in pictures, tables and flow charts. We hope that we can convey at least some of our enthusiasm for the subject to our readers.

C.A. Hart, P. Shears, April 1996

Acknowledgements

We gratefully acknowledge the help of Miss Carol Boutin in typing the manuscript, Mr Brian Getty for photography and electron microscopy, Mrs Norma Lowe for bacterial culture and photomicrography and Mr John McKeown for fungal cultures. We also thank members of the Department of Medical Microbiology for their willing help.

The following colleagues kindly contributed slides.

Dr R. Ashford
Dr W. Bailey
Mr B. Baker
Dr G. Barnish
Dr D. Baxby
Dr A. Carty
Dr A. Caunt
Mr J. Corkill
Dr D. Dance
Dr J. Fletcher
Dr C. Gilks
Mr M. Guy
Ms L. Hindle
Mr K. Jones
Prof. D. Kelly
Dr S. Lewis-Jones
Prof. K. McCarthy

Dr I. McDicken
Dr T. Makin
Dr I. Marshall
Dr J. Midgely
Dr R. Nevin
Dr J. Pennington
Prof. A. Percival
Prof. T. Rogers
Dr G. Sharpe
Dr D. Smith
Dr D. Theakstone
Dr W. Tong
Prof. H. Townson
Prof. S. Trees
Dr C. Valentine
Dr J. Varley
Dr C. Wray

To Jenny and Anne

1.
The Scope of, and on, Microbiology

THE SCOPE OF MICROBIOLOGY

The pathogens causing disease in man cover a large spectrum (1). At the smallest end are the small, self-replicating proteins called prions (*proteinaceous infectious agents*). These are responsible for the transmissible spongiform encephalopathies such as kuru, Creutzfeldt–Jakob disease and, in cattle, 'mad cow' disease (bovine spongiform encephalopathy, BSE). Next in ascending size are the viruses which are from 20 to 400 nm in diameter. These are obligate intracellular pathogens and are incapable of independent existence. They have various replicative strategies which utilize the host cell's biosynthetic pathways.

Bacteria vary in size from 500 nm to 10–15 µm and different genera have different shapes. For example *Escherichia coli* is rod shaped, *Staphylococcus aureus* is spherical and grows to form grape-like clusters, *Streptococcus pyogenes* is also spherical but grows to form long chains of cocci and *Vibrio cholerae* is comma-shaped. Bacteria are prokaryotes in that they have no nucleus but, in most cases, a single loop of chromosomal DNA. Although some bacteria, such as *Chlamydia trachomatis* are obligate intracellular pathogens, most are able to grow on simple cell-free culture media. Bacteria reproduce by binary fission. Most have a cell wall composed of peptidoglycan.

Fungi are eukaryotes; that is they have a nucleus, enclosed by a nuclear membrane, and a variety of membrane-bound organelles in their cytoplasm. They are larger than bacteria and may aggregate to produce much larger structures. They reproduce by binary fission and their cell walls are composed not of peptidoglycan but of chitin. Pathogens in this kingdom include yeasts such as *Candida albicans* and *Cryptococcus neoformans* and more complex mycelia-forming dermatophytes such as *Epidermophyton floccosum.*

For precise diagnosis of diseases due to protozoa and multi-cellular parasites the expertise of specialized centres such as Schools of Tropical or Geographical Medicine is often required. Nevertheless the diagnosis and management of some protozoal and parasitic infections are within the competence of medical microbiology. Protozoa are unicellular eukaryotic micro-organisms that reproduce by binary fission but may also have a complex life cycle involving various stages and sexual reproduction. They vary in size from 5 to 30 µm. Examples include *Entamoeba histolytica, Cryptosporidium parvum* and *Giardia intestinalis*, all of which cause diarrhoeal disease; *Trichomonas vaginalis*, a sexually transmitted pathogen; and *Plasmodium falciparum,* which causes malaria. The multicellular parasites or

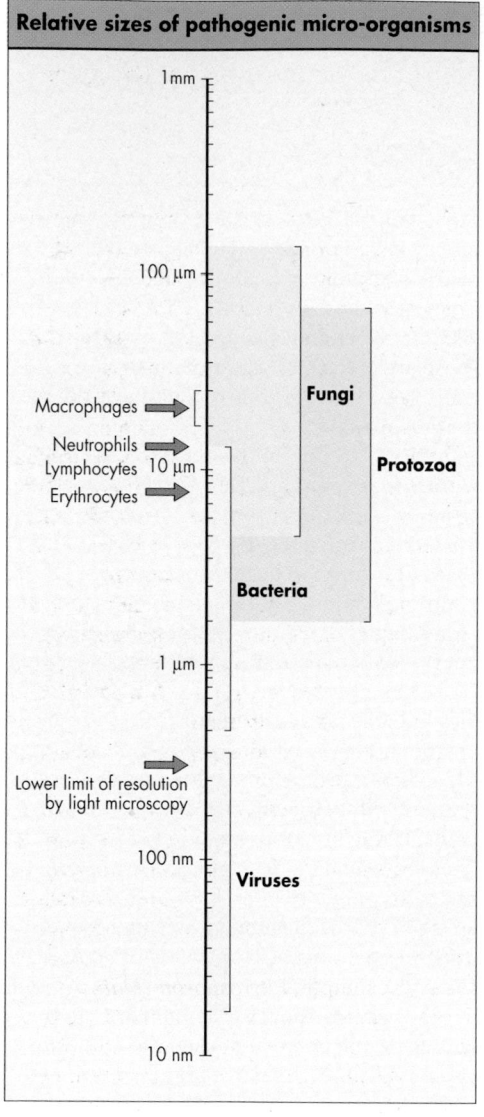

Relative sizes of pathogenic micro-organisms

1 Relative sizes of pathogenic micro-organisms.

The scale is logarithmic, running from 10 nm to 1 mm (10^6 nm). To the right of the scale are the ranges of sizes for viruses, bacteria, fungi and protozoa. The smallest helminths are just too large for this scale (*Enterobius vermicularis* 0.2 mm diameter, 2–5 mm long). To the left of the scale are the sizes of some cells involved in immunity to infection. The light microscope cannot resolve objects smaller than 300 nm; the minimum resolution of the electron microscope is about 0.5 nm.

helminths can vary in size from 5 mm to 3 m in length. Some (such as the beef tapeworm, *Taenia saginata*) produce asymptomatic infection; others (such as the threadworm, *Enterobius vermicularis*) are mere irritants, whereas *Strongyloides stercoralis* can cause a fatal hyperinfection syndrome.

WHAT IS NORMAL?

Although viruses, bacteria and fungi often are thought of as aggressive micro-organisms invading the human body, this does not present the whole picture. In fact the human body is normally colonized by very large numbers of micro-organisms that constitute the 'normal flora'. It has been estimated that the adult male or female is only 10% human. There are approximately one hundred million million (10^{14}) cells in the human adult but only ten million million (10^{13}) are human. The remaining 9×10^{13} cells are the bacteria, fungi, protozoa and even arthropods that comprise the normal flora. In addition to this, certain viruses persistently infect humans, following primary infection, and are excreted for life. Examples include the herpesviruses such as cytomegalovirus, Epstein–Barr virus and human herpesvirus-6, as well as human immunodeficiency virus (HIV). Whether these should also be included as normal flora is a moot point.

In utero, the fetus remains microbiologically sterile. It will acquire micro-organisms during passage through the birth-canal and from its mother during feeding. The establishment of a stable normal flora takes 2–3 weeks for term breast-fed babies. For premature babies or for those who are bottle-fed the process is longer and colonization with aberrant flora can occur.

The normal flora is not distributed uniformly and some areas are not normally colonized (2). In these areas detection of a micro-organism implies infection. Bacteria make up the major part of the normal flora and anaerobic bacteria tend to predominate at most sites. Potentially pathogenic bacteria may also be part of the normal flora. For example, *Streptococcus pneumoniae, Haemophilus influenzae* and *Neisseria meningitidis,* each of which can cause bacterial meningitis, are found in the throats of a proportion of subjects. Disease occurs when these micro-organisms gain access to normally sterile areas.

Fungi are found less commonly but, for example, *Pityrosporon (Malassezia) ovale* is found on skin and *Candida albicans* in the mouth and vagina. Protozoa such as *Entamoeba coli* and *Endolimax nana,* and even some zymodemes of *Ent. histolytica,* can be found in the intestine in the absence of disease. Infection with cestodes such as *Taenia solium* or *T. saginata* is rarely symptomatic as is that with the whipworm (*Trichuris trichiura*). The arthropod *Demodex follicularum,* as its name implies, can be found in the hair follicles and sebaceous glands of the face.

The normal microbial flora of humans

Areas normally colonized		Areas normally sterile
Density of colonization	**Predominant micro-organisms**	
Skin: varies from 10/cm^2 on hands to 10^5/cm^2 in perineum or on face	*S. epidermidis*, *S. aureus*, peptococci, fungi such as *Pityrosporon* (*Malassezia*) *ovale*	**Respiratory tract** (below the vocal cords)
Naso-oropharynx: up to 10^9/ml depending on site	Anaerobes outnumber aerobes up to 1000:1 but 20–40% of population carry *S. pneumoniae*, 40–80% *H. influenzae*, 10–20% *S. aureus*, 5–20% *N. meningitidis* and 5–10% *S. pyogenes*	**Sinuses and middle ear**
Oesophagus and stomach: 10^2–10^3/ml	Usually transients taken in with food. A proportion of adults may have *Helicobacter pylori* asymptomatically present in the stomach	**Pleura and peritoneum**
Small intestine: 10^2–10^3/ml	Usually transients but some *Lactobacillus* spp. may be present	**Liver and gall bladder**
Large intestine: 10^{10}–10^{12}/ml	Predominantly anaerobes such as *Bacteroides*, *Clostridium*, *Eubacteria* and *Veillonella* spp. *E. coli* (10^7/ml) is the commonest aerobic Gram-negative bacterium	**Urinary tract above anterior urethra**
Vagina: 10^8/ml	Predominantly anaerobes and *Lactobacillus* spp. May also contain faecal flora	**Bone, joint, muscle, blood**
Anterior urethra: (about 2.5 cm) 10^2/cm^2	*S. epidermidis*, *Lactobacilli*, anaerobes, *E. coli*	**Cerebrospinal fluid**

2   The normal microbial flora of humans.

THE SCOPE ON MICROBIOLOGY

From as early as 1546, it was suggested by Fracastoro that invisible organisms caused infection but until the development of the microscope by van Leeuwenhoek in the seventeenth century it was not possible to see these 'invisible' organisms. In 1676 van Leeuwenhoek described seeing animalcules, which were probably protozoa, and even bacteria. However, it was not until 1876 that a direct link between human infection (anthrax) and bacteria (*Bacillus anthracis*) was proved by Koch. Microbiology developed very rapidly over subsequent years but there is no doubt that being able to see the bacteria that cause disease was a key event. Viruses were detected and their dimensions estimated indirectly by using very small pore-sized filters but until 1933, when Ruska developed the electron microscope, it was not possible to visualize them.

LIGHT MICROSCOPY

The resolving power of a microscope is dependent upon the wavelength of the incident radiation. Thus the smallest object visible by light microscopy is 200–300 nm. Modern microscopes are all compound microscopes; that is they employ two or more lenses. At its simplest, the image is formed by the objective lens and then further magnified by the eyepiece lens (**3a**). The original light microscopes are called bright-field microscopes because the object is a dark image against a bright background (**3b**). Because the numerical aperture of lenses working in air cannot be greater than 1, the highest objective lens magnification is around ×40. For magnifications above this, the lens cannot collect sufficient light. To circumvent this, colourless liquid (immersion oil) with a greater refractive index than air (in fact similar to that of glass) is placed between the object and the objective lens. This allows objective lenses with a magnification of ×100 to be used. This, together with a ×15 eyepiece, provides a maximum practical magnification for bright-field microscopy of ×1500. Most often bright-field microscopy is used for examining fixed and stained micro-organisms (**3b**).

Living, unstained micro-organisms can be visualized using either dark-field or phase-contrast microscopy. In dark-field microscopy, a dark-field stop and condenser are used to focus a hollow cone of light on the specimen (**4a**). This is arranged so that only the light that is reflected off, or refracted by, the specimen is collected by the objective lens. Thus the micro-organism appears as a bright object against a black background (**4b**).

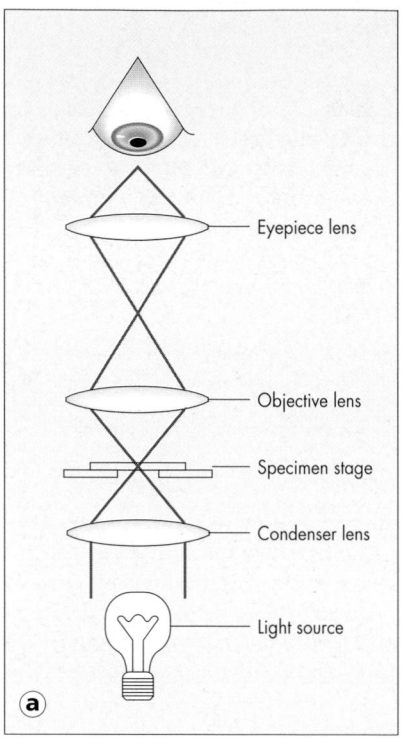

3 a Showing the light path of a bright-field microscope. b Silver stained *Salmonella typhi* showing flagella. In the bright-field microscope the light (mirror or electric light) is concentrated at the plane of the specimen by means of a substage condenser. The objective lens magnifies the object forming an enlarged primary real image. This is further magnified by the eyepiece. The total magnification is the magnification of the eyepiece lens multiplied by the magnification of the objective lens. Thus if the objective lens has a x40 magnification and the eyepiece x10 the total magnification is 400-fold.

Eyepiece lens

Objective lens

Specimen stage

Condenser lens

Light source

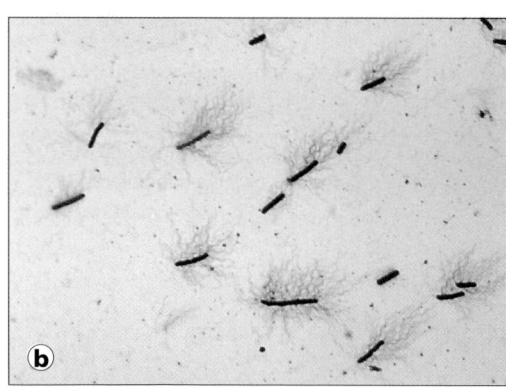

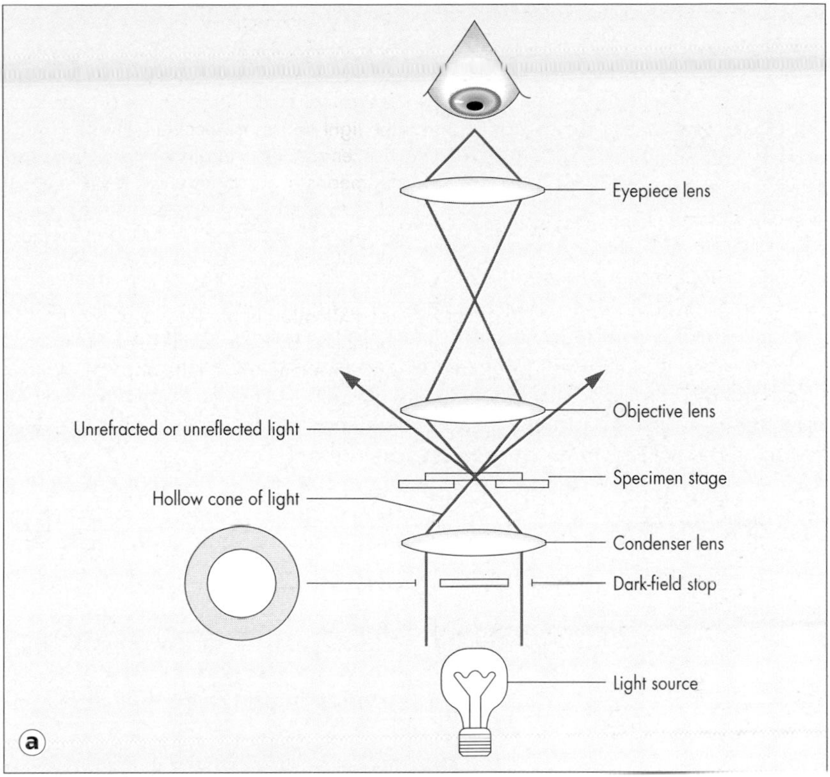

Eyepiece lens

Objective lens

Unrefracted or unreflected light

Specimen stage

Hollow cone of light

Condenser lens

Dark-field stop

Light source

(a)

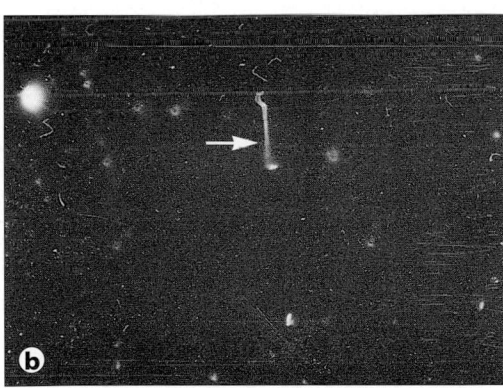

(b)

4 a Showing the light path of a dark-field microscope. b *Leptospira canicola*, a tightly coiled spiral bacterium. In dark-field microscopy only the incident light that is reflected or refracted by the micro-organism is collected by the objective lens. The micro-organism (arrow) shines out like a beacon against a black background.

In phase-contrast microscopy (**5a**) the condenser has an annular stop which also produces a hollow cone of light. This is focused to the plane of the specimen. As the cone passes through the cell some rays are deviated and retarded by about one quarter wavelength. The deviated light is focused to form an image. The undeviated rays pass through a phase ring in a phase plate. The phase ring is constructed such that it advances the wavelength by about one quarter wavelength. Thus the deviated and undeviated rays are approximately one half wavelength apart and when brought together cancel each other out. Therefore the image of the specimen, viewed through the eyepiece, will be of varying dark tones against a bright background. As phase-contrast microscopy can be used on unfixed material, it is particularly useful for visualizing internal structures and organelles of bacteria, fungi and protozoa (**5b**).

In fluorescence microscopy, the micro-organism is stained directly or indirectly (via antibody or lectin) with a fluorochrome. The fluorochrome absorbs ultraviolet light and re-emits it at a higher wavelength in the visible spectrum (**6a**). The colour of the emitted light varies according to the fluorochrome used. For example, fluorescein absorbs UV light at a wavelength of 495 nm and re-emits it as yellow-green light (wavelength 525 nm). Direct fluorochrome staining with auramine–phenol is used, for example, in the diagnosis of tuberculosis (**6b**).

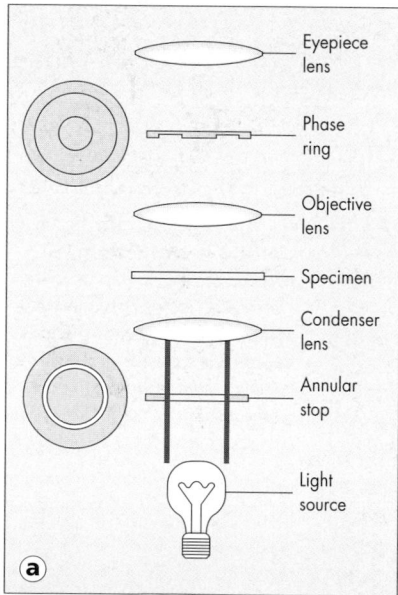

Eyepiece lens

Phase ring

Objective lens

Specimen

Condenser lens

Annular stop

Light source

(a)

5 a Showing the light path of a phase-contrast microscope. b An oocyst of *Isospora belli* by Nomarski phase-contrast. (Note the two sporocysts inside the oocyst). The phase-contrast microscope converts small differences in refractive index into differences in light intensity. Nomarski phase-contrast is a more sophisticated method that provides a three-dimensional image.

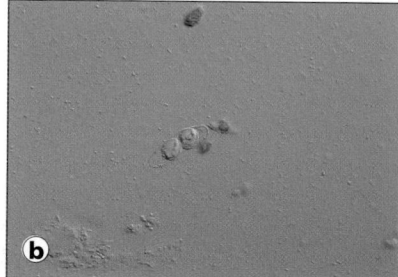

(b)

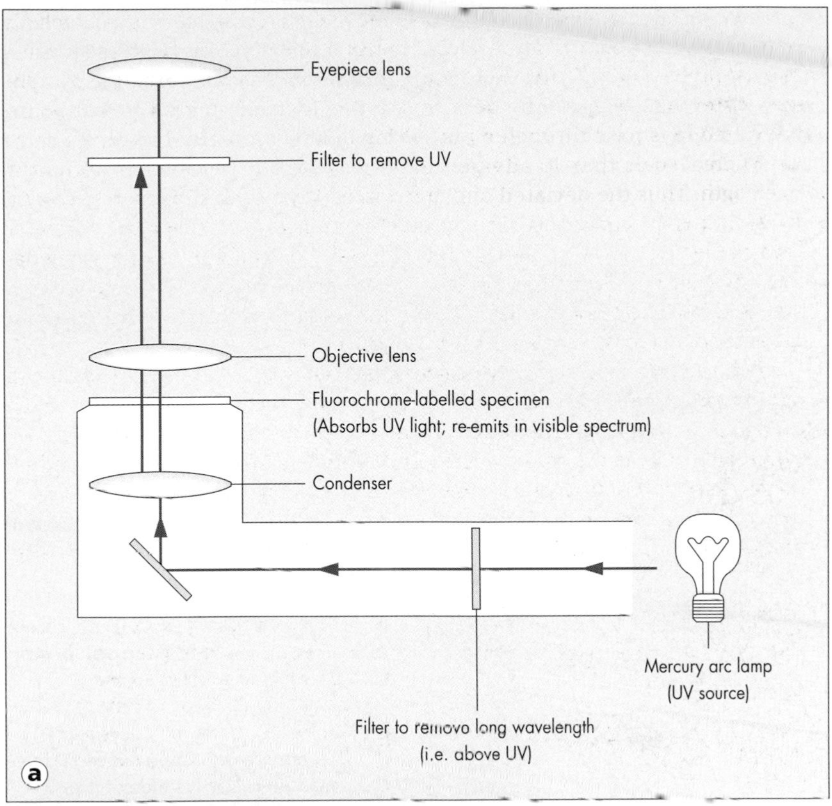

Eyepiece lens

Filter to remove UV

Objective lens

Fluorochrome-labelled specimen
(Absorbs UV light; re-emits in visible spectrum)

Condenser

Mercury arc lamp
(UV source)

Filter to remove long wavelength
(i.e. above UV)

(a)

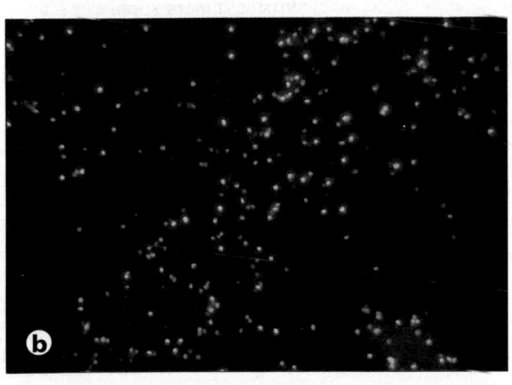

(b)

**6 a The fluorescence microscope.
b *Mycobacterium tuberculosis* stained with auramine–phenol and viewed down a fluorescence microscope.**

Immunofluorescence employs antibodies to which fluorochromes are covalently attached. The fluorochrome is attached to the Fc portion of the antibody rather than the antigen-binding (Fab) end; thus the antibody is still able to bind to its epitope. In direct immunofluorescence (**7a**), the fluorochrome is attached to the antibody that binds to the micro-organism. In indirect immunofluorescence, the fluorochrome is attached to an antibody raised against, for example, human

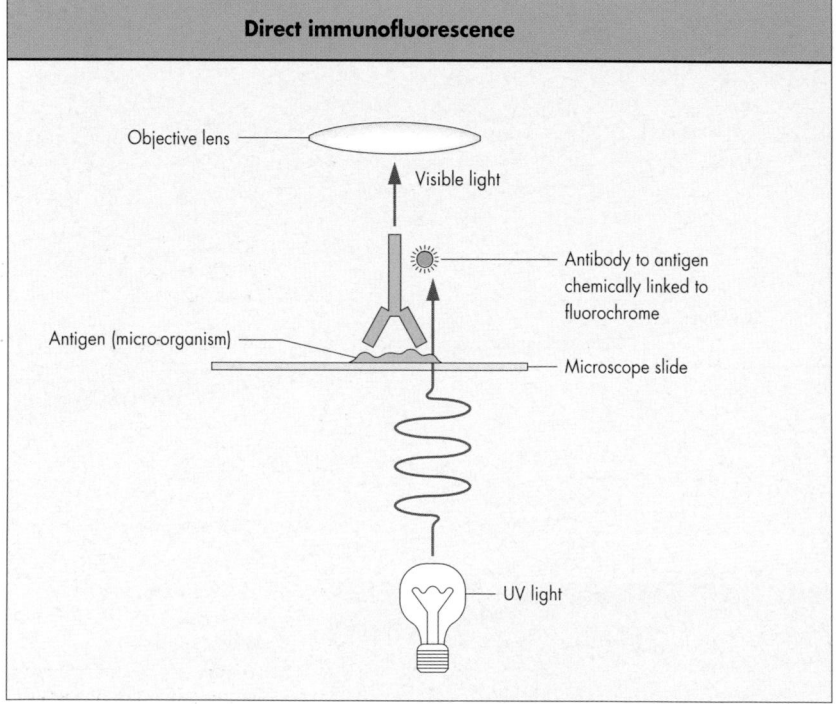

7 a Direct immunofluorescence. In direct immunofluorescence the object is visualized using a fluorescein-tagged antibody directed against epitopes on the micro-organism.

antibody (**7b**). Direct immunofluorescence is used to detect specific micro-organisms; the specificity is imparted by the antibody. Indirect immuno-fluorescence can be employed to detect specific micro-organisms but is most often used to detect antibodies to a particular micro-organism present in a patient's serum.

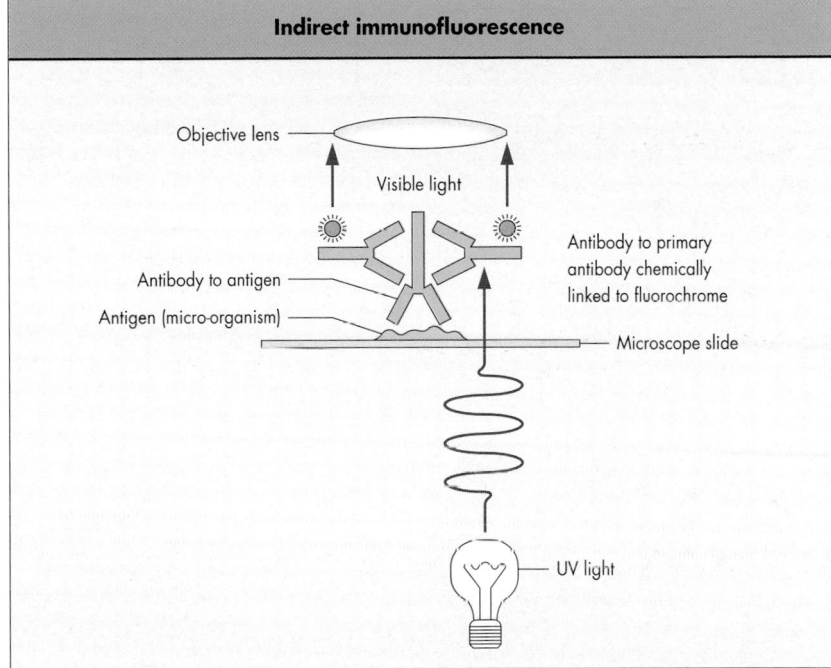

Indirect immunofluorescence

Objective lens

Visible light

Antibody to antigen

Antibody to primary antibody chemically linked to fluorochrome

Antigen (micro-organism)

Microscope slide

UV light

7 b Indirect immunofluorescence. In indirect immunofluorescence the antiserum directed against the micro-organism is added and the slide washed. Then a fluorescent-labelled antibody directed against the first antibody is added. This technique can be used to detect either micro-organisms or antibodies to the micro-organism in a patient's serum.

Much information has been obtained by light-microscopic examination of micro-organisms. However, it soon became apparent that some transmissible agents were too small to be seen by light microscopy (i.e. <0.2 μm). Electrons behave as light rays and can be focused, not by glass lenses but by annular (doughnut-shaped) electromagnets (**8**). The wavelength of electrons is approximately 10^5 times shorter than that of visible light. This means that the conventional electron microscope can resolve objects as close as 0.5 nm. With

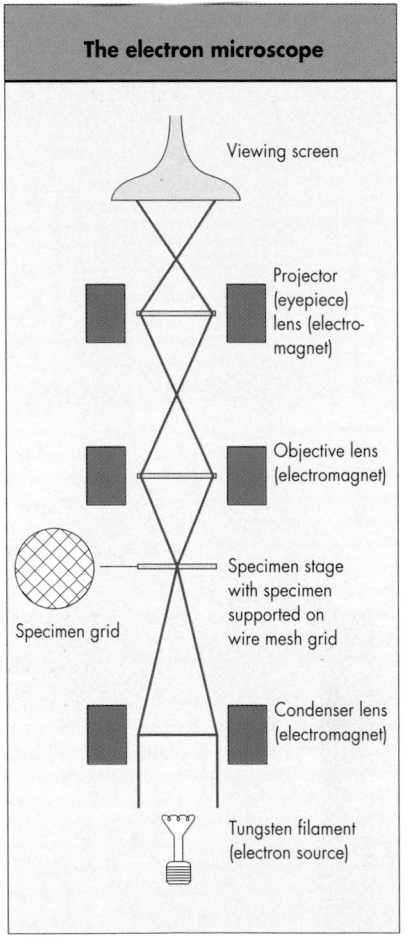

The electron microscope

Viewing screen

Projector (eyepiece) lens (electro-magnet)

Objective lens (electromagnet)

Specimen grid

Specimen stage with specimen supported on wire mesh grid

Condenser lens (electromagnet)

Tungsten filament (electron source)

8   The path of the electron beam in an electron microscope. The electron beam is generated from a tungsten filament. The beam is focused on the specimen by a condenser magnet. It is magnified by further objective and projector lens magnets. The electrons impinge on a fluorescent screen to produce the image, or onto a photo-graphic plate for a more permanent record. Because electrons are absorbed by air, the column containing the lenses and the specimen is under a high vacuum.

the electron microscope, the image is seen when electrons impinge on a cathode ray screen (9). In the transmission electron microscope, the specimen is supported on a small copper grid (10) and is viewed through the interstices of the grid. The specimen must be no more than 100 nm thick and sufficiently well supported and tough to withstand being bombarded by electrons in a high vacuum. Micro-organisms may be visualized in a specimen directly, following negative-staining using phosphotungstic acid. With this technique the negative

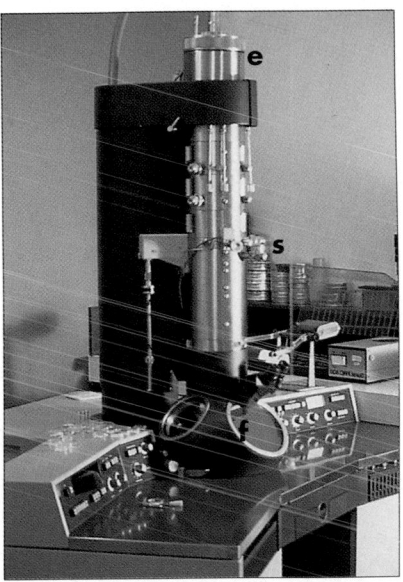

9 The electron microscope. An electron microscope showing the electron gun (**e**) at the top of the column, the specimen stage (**s**) and fluorescent screen (**f**).

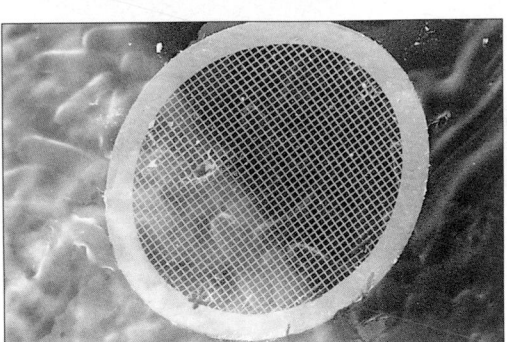

10 Electron microscope grid. This is approximately 4 mm in diameter. The specimen is supported by the grid and the micro-organisms are viewed through the holes of the grid.

stain sticks around the edge of the bacterium or virus and absorbs the electron beam. The micro-organism is thus highlighted against a light background (**11**). Another technique is to coat the specimen with a thin film of platinum or other heavy metal. The heavy metal is evaporated from a source and impinges on the specimen, at an angle of about 45°, so that a shadow is cast. This technique is particularly useful for studying bacterial surface appendages such as fimbriae (pili) or flagella (**12**). Micro-organisms or their appendages can also be immunologically labelled for the electron microscope in a manner analogous to immunofluorescence. In this case the antibody is coupled not to a fluorescent dye but to small electron-dense gold particles (**13**). A three-dimensional image can be obtained using a scanning electron microscope (**14**), although this is rarely used in diagnostic microbiology.

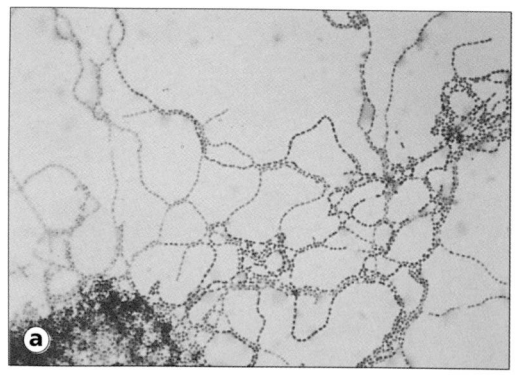

11 a A light micrograph of a chain of Gram-positive *Streptococcus pyogenes*. b A negative stain electron micrograph of a chain of *Streptococcus pyogenes (bar = 2.0 µm).

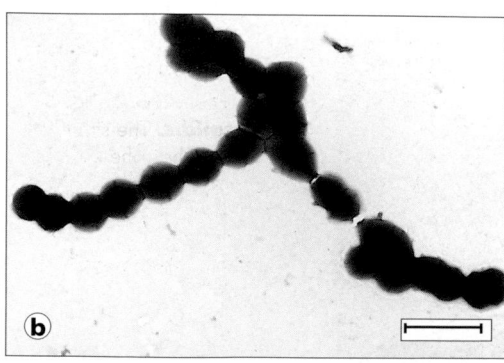

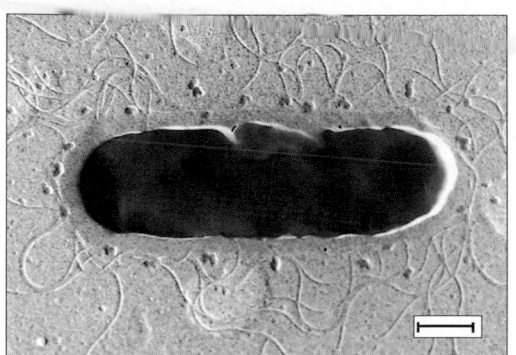

12 A shadow-cast electron micrograph of *Escherichia coli* showing flagella. These are protein spikes used by the bacterium to move in liquid media. *(bar = 0.5 µm)*

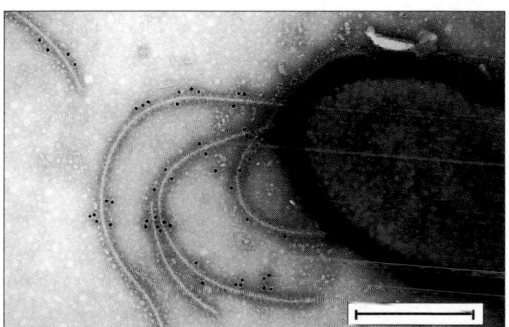

13 An immuno-gold electron micrograph showing *Pseudomonas aeruginosa* flagella. Antibody to flagellin coupled to small gold particles has bound to the flagella. *(bar = 0.5 µm)*

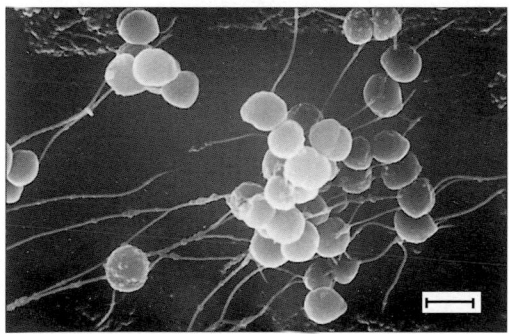

14 A scanning electron micrograph of *Staphylococcus epidermidis*. The strands connecting the spheres or cocci are the condensed remnants of an extracellular matrix that rejoices in the scientific name of slime. *(bar = 1.0 µm)*

2.
Prions and Transmissible Spongiform Encephalopathies

The transmissible spongiform encephalopathies (TSEs) are a group of diseases affecting a variety of animal species. These include man (kuru, Creutzfeldt–Jakob disease (CJD) and Gerstmann–Straüssler disease); cattle (bovine spongiform encephalopathy); sheep (scrapie); and cats (feline spongiform encephalopathy). All are characterized by subacute degeneration of the brain. Post-mortem examination of the brain reveals microcystosis of the neurones and neuropil in the grey matter. This results in a sponge-like (spongiform) appearance of the brain (**15**). There is a gradual loss of neurones and proliferation of astrocytes but no evidence of inflammation of the brain (hence encephalopathy). This is accompanied by an accumulation of a fibrillar protein called prion protein (PrP) (**16**). Although some reports have implicated small (10–12 nm diameter) virus-like

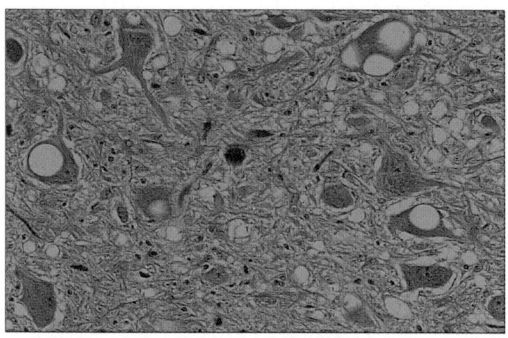

15 A section of brain from a patient with Creutzfeldt–Jakob disease. Showing vacuolation of neurones and neuropil, resulting in a spongiform appearance.

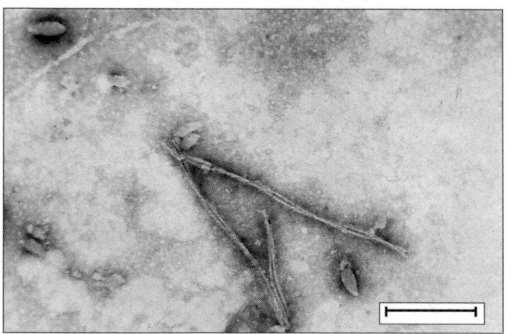

16 A negative-stain electron micrograph of fibrillar prion protein. This accumulates in the brains of subjects with transmissible spongiform encephalopathy. (bar = 50 nm).

structures as agents of TSE, the hypothesis that PrP is a self-replicating protein and the aetiological agent of TSEs has gained wide acceptance. PrP has the same amino acid sequence as part of a protein occurring normally in the brain. It has been post-translationally modified so that it can no longer be digested by proteolytic enzymes. It thus accumulates in the brains of affected individuals.

Kuru was transmitted by ritual cannibalism but was limited to one tribal area in Papua New Guinea (the Fore language group). No new cases have occurred in those born after a ban on ritual cannibalism.

In contrast, CJD has a world-wide distribution. It is a rare disease affecting about $1/10^6$ population. Transmission has occurred via stereotactic surgery, corneal transplants and injections of growth hormone derived from human pituitaries. The incubation period is long (1–30 years). The disease progresses inexorably through dementia to death. There is no specific treatment. There are no non-invasive diagnostic tests. Diagnosis is most often made by brain biopsy or at autopsy.

3.
Viruses and Disease

Although it had been known for some time that very small 'filterable' agents were responsible for some infections in man, the 'virus era' did not begin until after 1950. Over the next 40 years our knowledge increased exponentially. This has been made possible by cell and virus culture techniques, by serological characterization and by ever-improving molecular biological techniques.

Viruses are the smallest and most primitive of the conventional infective agents. They differ from most bacteria, fungi and protozoa in being obligate intracellular pathogens. Viruses do not possess the full complement of enzymes (i.e. the 'machinery') necessary for their replication. They must, therefore, 'hijack' the host cell's energy stores, nucleotides, amino acids, lipids and biosynthetic systems to reproduce themselves. In fact most viruses possess factors that switch off the host cell's own biosynthetic processes and divert them into producing new virus particles. This in part leads to death of host cells and contributes to the clinical manifestations of the infection. The other major differences between viruses and higher micro-organisms are:

- the viral genome is RNA or DNA, never both
- bacteria, fungi and protozoa reproduce by binary fission whereas viruses have a complex mode of disassembly, replication and re-assembly within the host cell
- viruses have no cell wall, no cellular organization and are much smaller than the other micro-organisms.

Two major consequences of these differences are that, once excreted from the host the numbers of virus particles can only decrease. They are unable to multiply in the inanimate environment unlike bacteria and fungi. Secondly, because viruses replicate using host cell systems, designing effective non-toxic antiviral drugs is much more difficult than for antibacterial agents.

VIRUS CLASSIFICATION

Originally viruses were classified by disease causation and epidemiological and ecological considerations. Now classification is largely on biophysical, antigenic and molecular biological considerations.

Viruses are subdivided into families, subfamilies and genera on the basis of genome structure and organization, capsid symmetry, viral size, site of assembly and presence and site of acquisition of lipid envelope. Within the genus, different members are defined by possession of different antigens (e.g. subdivisions of

ECHO and Coxsackie viruses) by differences within the genome (e.g. human papillomaviruses) or even differences in disease manifestations and vectors (e.g. Flaviviridae).

GENOME

The first major subdivision is by whether the genome is RNA or DNA (**17,18**). For RNA viruses the genome can be single stranded (e.g. Picornaviridae) or double-stranded (e.g. rotavirus). In some the genome may be circular (e.g. Arenaviridae) but in most it is linear (**17**). The genome may consist of one long strand (e.g. Retroviridae) or several segments (e.g. Orthomyxoviridae or rotavirus). Finally, the single-stranded genome may be positive sense (can be translated directly to produce viral polypeptides, e.g. Coronaviridae), negative sense (must be transcribed to mRNA, e.g. Myxoviridae or Rhabdoviridae), or even ambisense (e.g. Bunyaviridae).

For DNA viruses (**18**) the genome can be double-stranded linear (e.g. Herpesviridae) or circular (e.g. Adenoviridae). The only single-stranded DNA virus is parvovirus and its genome is mostly negative sense.

CAPSID SYMMETRY

The capsid is a protein shell that surrounds and protects the viral genome. The individual protein subunits making up the capsid are called capsomers and the genome plus capsomers is called the nucleocapsid. The capsid can be arranged either in the form of a helix (**19**) or as a three-dimensional structure with three axes of symmetry (cuboidal). In fact, most cuboidal capsids have twenty facets, termed an eicosahedron (from Greek *eicosa*: twenty, *hedron*: side). Finally some viruses have a symmetry which is undefined (e.g. Flaviviridae) or complex (e.g. Poxviridae) .

LIPID ENVELOPE

In general those viruses that are unenveloped (e.g. rotavirus, Picornaviridae, Adenoviridae) are able to survive for longer in the inanimate environment than those with a lipid envelope (e.g. Myxoviridae, Retroviridae, Herpesviridae). For enveloped viruses, except Poxviridae, loss of the lipid envelope is associated with loss of infectivity. Thus enveloped viruses can be inactivated by ether or detergents. Enveloped viruses have glycoprotein spikes on their outer surface which mediate attachment to and penetration into the host cell. The envelope can be acquired by virus budding through the nuclear membrane (**20**), into the golgi (e.g. hantavirus) or through the plasma membrane (**21**).

RNA viruses of medical importance

	Size (nm)	Envelope	Symmetry*	Strand	Sense	Genome Segmented	Size (kb)	Site of Assembly†
Picornaviridae Enterovirus (Polio, Coxsackie, ECHO) Heparnavirus Rhinovirus	28–30	No	E	Single linear	Positive	No	7.2–8.4	C
Astrovirus	27–30	No	E	Single linear	Positive	No	7.8	C
Caliciviridae	35–40	No	E	Single linear	Positive	No	8.0	C
Hepatitis E	35–40	No	E	Single linear	Positive	No	7.8–8.0	C
Hepatitis D virus	36	No	E	Single circular	Negative	No	1.2	C
Reoviridae Rotavirus	70–80	No	E (double shell)	Double linear	—	Yes (11)	16–21	C
Flaviviridae Yellow Fever Hepatitis C virus	40–50	Yes	?	Single linear	Positive	No	10	C, G
Togaviridae Alphavirus Rubella	60–70	Yes	E	Single linear	Positive	No	12	C, M
Coronaviridae	50–160	Yes	H	Single linear	Positive	No	16–21	C, M
Rhabdoviridae	75 × 180	Yes	H	Single linear	Negative	No	13–16	C, M
Retroviridae Oncornavirinae (HTLV) Spumavirinae Lentivirinae (HIV 1 & 2)	80 × 130	Yes	E	Single linear	Positive	No	3.5–9	C, M

* H = helical; E = eicosahedral. † C = cytoplasm; G = Golgi; M = plasma membrane.

RNA viruses of medical importance (cont.)

	Size (nm)	Envelope	Symmetry*	Strand	Sense	Segmented	Size (kb)	Site of Assembly†
						Genome		
Arenaviridae Lymphocytic choriomeningitis (LCM) Lassa, Machupo, Junin, Sabia	50–300	Yes	H	Single linear	Negative and Ambisense	Yes (2)	10–14	C, G
Bunyaviridae Bunyavirus Nairovirus Phlebovirus Hantavirus	90–120	Yes	H	Single linear	Negative	Yes (3)	13.5–21	C, G
Orthomyxoviridae Influenza A, B & C	90–120	Yes	H	Single linear	Negative	Yes (7 or 8)	16–20	C, M
Paramyxoviridae Paramyxovirus (1–4, mumps) Pneumovirus (RSV) Morbillivirus (measles)	150–300	Yes	H	Single linear	Negative	No	16–20	C, M
Filoviridae Marburg, Ebola	80 x 1000	Yes	H	Single linear	Negative	No	12.7	C, M

*H = helical; E = eicosahedral.   †C = cytoplasm; G = Golgi; M = plasma membrane.

17 RNA viruses of medical importance.

DNA viruses of medical importance

| | Size (nm) | Envelope | Symmetry | Genome | | | | |
				Strand	Sense	Segmented	Size	Site of Capsid Assembly
Parvoviridae B19	18–21	No	E	Single linear	Mostly negative	No	5 kb	N
Papovaviridae Polyoma (JC, BK) Papilloma (1–75)	45–55	No	E	Double circular	—	No	5–8 kbp	N
Hepadnaviridae	42	Yes	E	Double circular	—	No	3.2 kbp	N
Adenoviridae (1–49)	70–90	No	E	Double linear	—	No	36–38 kbp	N
Herpesviridae HHV-1* (herpes simplex I) HHV-2 (herpes simplex II) HHV-3 (varicella zoster) HHV-4 (Epstein–Barr) HHV-5 (Cytomegalovirus) HHV-6 HHV-7 HHV-8 (Kaposi's sarcoma)	150–200	Yes	E	Double linear	—	No	120–200 kbp	N
Poxviridae Orthopox (smallpox, cowpox) Parapox (orf) Molluscum contagiosum Yabapox, Tanapox	350 × 400	Yes†	Complex	Double linear		No	130–280 kbp	C

* HHV = human herpesvirus.
† Envelope present but not necessary for infectivity.

18 DNA viruses of medical importance.

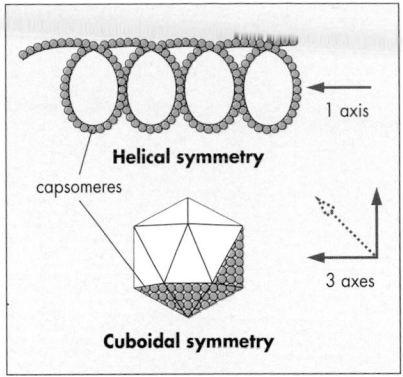

19 Helical and cuboidal symmetry of the virus nucleocapsid.

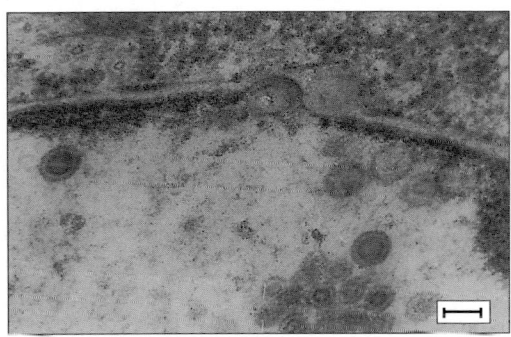

20 A thin-section electron micrograph showing varicella-zoster virus acquiring its lipid envelope by buddings through the nuclear membrane *(bar = 0.1 μm).*

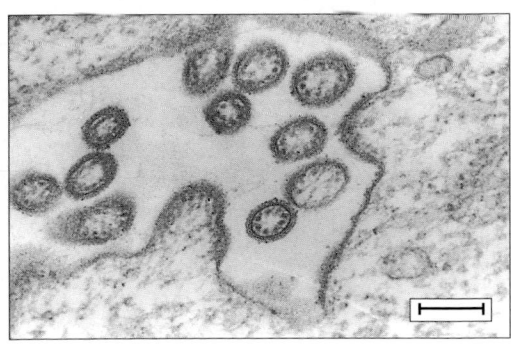

21 A thin-section electron micrograph showing parainfluenza virus acquiring its lipid envelope by budding through the plasma membrane. *(bar = 0.1 μm)*

UNENVELOPED RNA VIRUSES

The infections caused by unenveloped RNA viruses are shown in **22**.

Infections with unenveloped RNA viruses					
	Major infections	Less common infections	Vaccine preventable	Incubation period	Period of infectivity
Picornaviridae Poliovirus	Poliomyelitis, encephalitis	Asymptomatic (90–95%)	Yes	1–35 days	>5 weeks
ECHO	Exanthems, enanthems, meningo-encephalitis, respiratory tract infection (RTI), carditis	Asymptomatic (90–95%)	No	1–35 days	1–3 weeks
Coxsackie A	Exanthem, enanthems, conjunctivitis, carditis, RTI, meningo-encephalitis	Asymptomatic (90–95%)	No	1–20 days	3–5 weeks
Coxsackie B	Meningo-encephalitis, exanthem, pleurodynia, carditis, RTI	Asymptomatic (90–95%)	No	1–20 days	3–5 weeks
Heparna	Acute hepatitis	Asymptomatic (50–80%)	Yes	2–6 weeks	1 week before to 1 week after jaundice
Astrovirus	Diarrhoea, vomiting		No	2–5 days	7–10 days
Calicivirus	Diarrhoea, vomiting		No	2–5 days	6–8 days
Hepatitis E	Acute hepatitis	Asymptomatic	No	25–50 days	7–10 days
Hepatitis D	Fulminant hepatitis (only with HBV co-infection)		No	2–6 months	Lifetime
Rotavirus	Diarrhoea, vomiting		No	3–5 days	6–14 days

22 Infections with unenveloped RNA viruses.

PICORNAVIRIDAE

These are the smallest (20–30 nm) of the RNA viruses (**23**). The name is an acronym for *p*oliovirus, *i*nsensitivity to ether (they have no lipid envelope), *c*oxsackievirus, *o*rphan virus, *r*hinovirus and RNA. Fortuitously pico is also a very small unit of measurement (10^{-12}). There are five genera (cardiovirus, aphthovirus, heparnavirus, rhinovirus, enterovirus) but only three (heparnavirus, rhinovirus and enterovirus) are pathogenic for man.

The optimal temperature for primary isolation of rhinoviruses is $33°C$, which is similar to temperatures in the upper respiratory tract. Rhinoviruses are a cause of the common cold, sore throats and coryza. There are over 118 different serotypes and infection with one does not necessarily confer immunity to others. Rhinoviruses are responsible for approximately half of the cases of common cold.

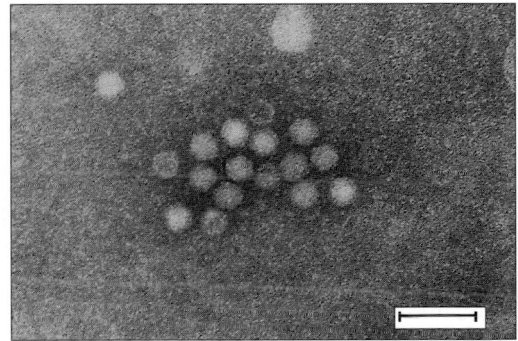

23 Negative stain electron micrograph of a picornavirus. The virus is unenveloped, has cuboidal symmetry and a single-stranded positive sense RNA genome (MW about 2.5×10^6). *(bar = 100 nm)*.

Enteroviruses are subdivided into poliovirus, echoviruses and coxsackie viruses. More recently discovered members of the genus are all termed enterovirus (from enterovirus 68 onwards). Infections with enteroviruses are generally asymptomatic and in outbreaks an 'iceberg' phenomenon is apparent. For example, only between 1 and 10% of cases of infection with poliovirus are clinically apparent. The remainder is a silent reservoir to infect others.

There are three poliovirus serotypes (1, 2 and 3) as defined by neutralization tests and there is little cross-protection between serotypes. Man is the only natural host but viruses will grow readily in human and simian cell-lines.

Coxsackieviruses are named after a village in New York State. They are divided into groups A (24 serotypes) and B (15 serotypes) on the basis of their pathogenicity for mice. Group A viruses are difficult to grow in tissue culture but will infect suckling mice. Group A viruses are associated with a variety of exanthems (e.g. hand, foot and mouth disease) and enanthems (e.g. herpangina), neurological infections and conjunctivitis (A24). Group B viruses are associated with epidemic myalgia (Bornholm disease), meningitis and myocarditis.

Echo is an acronym for *e*nteric *c*ytopathic *h*uman *o*rphan (the latter meaning that there was no specific disease association). Most echoviruses grow readily in human and primate cell-lines. Aseptic meningitis, neonatal infections and exanthems are the major disease associations. Enterovirus 68 is associated with respiratory tract infection, enterovirus 70 with acute haemorrhagic conjunctivitis and enterovirus 71 with meningoencephalitis and a polio-like illness.

Hepatitis A virus which causes epidemics or sporadic cases of hepatitis (**24**) was classified as enterovirus 72 but is now allocated to a separate genus the Heparnaviridae.

Sources and modes of spread of picorna and other viruses are shown in **25**.

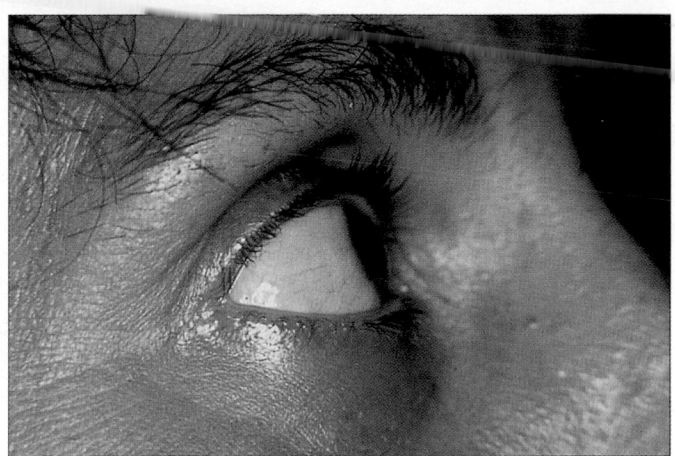

24 A patient with acute infective hepatitis due to hepatitis A virus. Note the yellow sclera.

Sources and transmission of viruses

	Man	Other animals	Insect vector	Faeco-oral spread	Droplet inhalation	Direct or indirect inoculation into — mucosa	Direct or indirect inoculation into — skin	Nosocomial	Blood to blood	Transplacental spread	Sexual transmission
RNA viruses											
Enteroviruses	+	−	−	+	(+)	(+)	−	+	−	?	(+)
Heparnavirus	+	−	−	+	−	(+)	−	+	(+)	−	+
Rhinovirus	+	−	−	−	(+)	+	−	+	−	−	−
Astrovirus	+	−	−	+	?	−	−	+	−	−	−
Calicivirus	+	−	−	+	?	−	−	+	−	−	−
Hepatitis D	+	−	−	−	−	−	−	(+)	+	−	+
Rotavirus	+	−	−	+	+	−	−	+	−	−	−
Flaviviruses	(+)	+	+	−	−	−	−	−	+	?	−
Hepatitis C	+	−	−	−	−	−	−	(+)	+	?	?
Togaviruses	(+)	+	+	−	−	−	−	−	−	−	−
Rubellavirus	+	−	−	−	+	+	−	(+)	−	+	−
Coronavirus	+	−	−	−	(+)	+	−	(+)	−	−	−
Rabies virus	−	+	−	−	−	+	+*	−	−	−	−
Retroviruses	+	−	−	−	−	+	−	(+)	+	+	+
Arenaviruses	(+)	+	−	−	+	−	−	(+)	−	?	(+)
Bunyavirus	−	+	+	−	−	−	−	+	−	−	−
Hantavirus	−	+	−	−	+	−	+*	−	−	?	−
Influenza	+	(+)	−	−	+	+	−	+	−	?	−
Parainfluenza and mumps	+	−	−	−	+	+	−	+	−	−	−
Measles	+	−	−	−	+	+	−	+	−	−	−
Respiratory syncytial virus	+	−	−	−	+	+	−	+	−	−	−
Filovirus	(+)	+	−	−	+	−	−	(+)	−	−	−

+ = Major source or route. (+) = Less common source or route. − = Not a source or route. * = Through skin via animal bite. ? = Possible, anecdotal or speculative.

Sources and transmission of viruses (cont.)

	Man	Other animals	Insect vector	Faeco-oral spread	Droplet inhalation	Direct or indirect inoculation into		Nosocomial	Blood to blood	Transplacental spread	Sexual transmission
						mucosa	skin				
DNA viruses											
Parvovirus	+	–	–	(+)	+	+	–	–	(+)	+	–
Polyomavirus	+	–	–	–	+	+	–	–	–	–	?
Papillomavirus	+	–	–	–	–	+	+	(+)	–	–	+
Adenovirus	+	–	–	+	+	+	–	+	?	–	–
Hepadnavirus	+	–	–	–	–	(+)	–	+	+	–	+
HHV-1 & 2	+	–	–	–	–	+	+	(+)	–	(+)	+
HHV-3	+	–	–	–	+	+	–	(+)	+	+	–
HHV-4	+	–	–	–	–	+	–	(+)	+	(+)	+
HHV-5	+	–	–	–	–	+	–	(+)	+	+	+
HHV-6	+	–	–	–	–	+	–	–	?	–	+
HHV-7	+	–	–	–	?	?	–	–	?	?	?
Poxvirus	+	+	–	–	+	+	+	–	–	(+)	–

+ = Major source or route. (+) = Less common source or route. – = Not a source or route. * = Through skin via animal bite. ? = Possible, anecdotal or speculative.

25 Sources and transmission of viruses.

ASTROVIRIDAE

These are small (about 27–30 nm) round, non-enveloped viruses with a distinctive star shape to their surface (**26**). There are at least five serotypes though serotype 1 predominates in UK. It is a cause of infantile diarrhoea and vomiting (about 10–12% of cases) and predominates in the winter time in temperate countries. Diagnosis is by electron microscopy, antigen detection or reverse transcriptase–polymerase chain reaction (RT–PCR).

CALICIVIRIDAE

These are also small (35–40 nm) round, non-enveloped viruses. They have a Star of David configuration on the capsid (**27**). This leads to the appearance of 'cup-shaped' depressions on the surface of the virus. (The name derives from the Greek

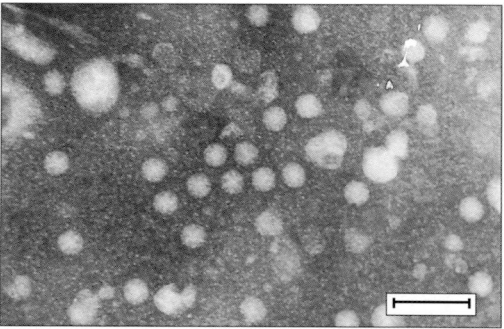

26 Negative stain electron micrograph of astrovirus. Note the characteristic six-pointed star. The astrovirus is positive strand RNA (7.8 kb) which is monocistronic. The protopolypeptide is then cleaved by protease to produce the individual structural proteins. *(bar = 100 nm)*

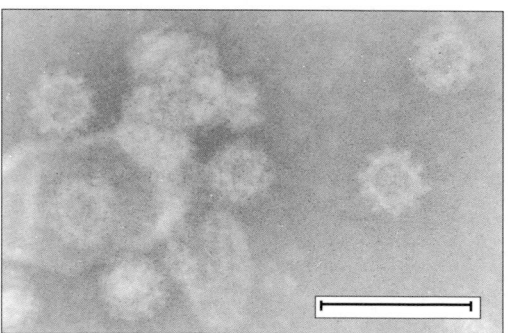

27 Negative stain electron micrograph of calicivirus. Note the cup-shaped depressions in the virus surface. The genome is positive strand RNA (8 kb). *(bar = 100 nm)*

calyx meaning cup). Caliciviruses are responsible for outbreaks of diarrhoea and vomiting affecting most age groups. Norwalk agent, another calicivirus, causes winter vomiting disease. Finally, it is thought that hepatitis E virus (HEV) is also a calicivirus. HEV is a cause of epidemic hepatitis and is spread faeco-orally. Diagnosis is by electron microscopy, antigen detection, RT–PCR, or, for HEV, by antibody detection.

REOVIRIDAE

Of the three genera (Orbiviridae, Reoviridae and Rotaviridae) in the family, only rotavirus is an important human pathogen. Rotavirus is a moderate-sized (70 nm) virus with a double-shelled capsid which gives the characteristic wheel-shape observed on electron microscopy (**28**). (In Latin, *rota* means wheel). The genome is double-stranded RNA in eleven segments (**29**) and this can be directly detected

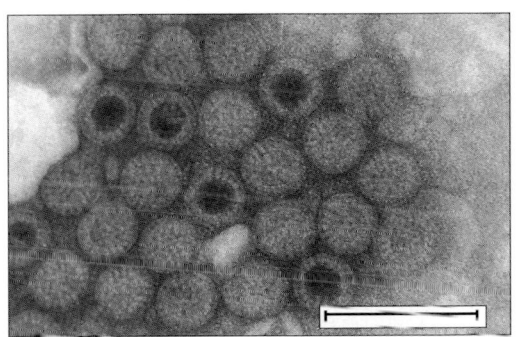

28 Negative stain electron micrograph of rotavirus. The double shelled capsid gives the typical wheel shape to the virus. *(bar = 200 nm)*

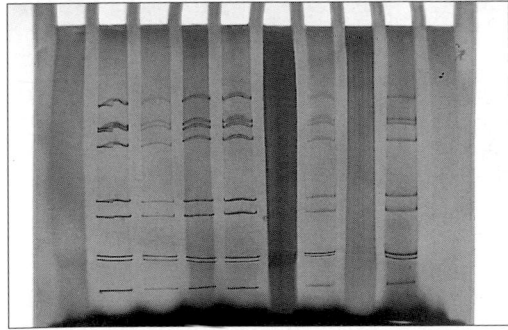

29 Poly-acrylamide gel electrophoresis of rotavirus RNA extracted directly from faeces. The RNA has been visualized using a silver stain. The migration pattern of the dsRNA provides useful epidemiological information.

in faeces of infected individuals. The pattern of migration of the dsRNA segments varies between viruses and can provide epidemiological information. There are seven rotavirus serogroups (A to G) but only group A and, to a lesser extent, B and C infect man. There are nine serotypes and antibody to the serotype antigen neutralizes infectivity. Unfortunately antibody to one serotype does not protect against others. Rotavirus is the major cause of diarrhoeal disease in children under 5 years (20–60% of cases). It, too, predominates in the winter months in temperate countries. Diagnosis is by electron microscopy, antigen detection or genome detection by RNA electrophoresis or RT–PCR.

ENVELOPED RNA VIRUSES

The medically important enveloped RNA viruses and their disease associations are shown in **30**. The term arboviruses was a classification used for those viruses that were transmitted to man by biting insects (*ar*thropod-*bo*rne). Such viruses multiply in the insect vector and are injected into man when it next feeds. This grouping was based on ecological considerations. In fact arboviruses comprise several virus families including Togaviridae, Flaviviridae and Bunyaviridae.

FLAVIVIRIDAE

These are small (40–50 nm) enveloped viruses with a single-stranded, positive sense RNA genome (about 10 kb). The symmetry of their capsid is undefined. Many have the mosquito as the vector and cause viral haemorrhagic fever (yellow fever and dengue viruses) and meningoencephalitis (Japanese B and St Louis viruses). Diagnosis is by virus isolation (which requires special containment facilities) or detection of antibody response.

Hepatitis C virus is probably a flavivirus but has no insect vector. It is an important cause of parenterally acquired non-A non-B hepatitis (about 90% of cases). Infection is transmitted blood-to-blood by transfusion, transplantation, needle-stick and needle sharing by intravenous drug abusers. It produces chronic hepatitis and virus may persist in the liver for life. Diagnosis is by detection of specific antibody or RT–PCR detection of viral genome.

TOGAVIRIDAE

The alphaviruses, rubiviruses and possibly pestiviruses are the genera that are pathogenic for man (**31**). The alphaviruses are transmitted principally via mosquitos and cause encephalitis (e.g. Eastern equine encephalitis virus) or a febrile exanthem with polyarthritis (e.g. chikungunya). All have a single-stranded linear positive sense RNA genome (about 12 kb). Viruses replicate within the cytoplasm and release by budding. Diagnosis is by serology, virus isolation or both.

Rubellavirus is the only member of the genus rubivirus. It is transmitted by both contact and the airborne route, and causes a febrile childhood exanthem but in many cases the infection is asymptomatic. It causes most problems if infection occurs in pregnancy. Rubellavirus can cross the placenta to infect the fetus causing intrauterine death or congenital malformations.

The pestiviruses cause diarrhoeal disease in cattle (bovine diarrhoeal virus) and pigs (European swine fever). There are recent reports linking a pestivirus to human diarrhoeal disease.

ARENAVIRIDAE

These are pleomorphic enveloped RNA viruses varying in size from 50 to 300 nm in diameter. The virus contains electron dense granules, rich in RNA, that resemble ribosomes (**32**) and give the appearance of grains of sand. (In Greek, *arena* means grain of sand.) The genome consists of two single strands of positive or ambisense RNA. They can be linear or join to form a loop. Infections are zoonotic. The various arenaviruses asymptomatically and persistently infect different rodent species and man is infected through contact with their excreta. Lymphocytic choriomeningitis virus is the only arenavirus found in Europe. It is excreted in mouse (*Mus musculus*) urine and is a rare cause of aseptic meningitis. The remaining arenaviruses are causes of viral haemorrhagic fever. In West Africa, Lassa fever virus persistently infects the multimammate rat (*Mastomys natalensis*) and is excreted in its urine. Inhalation or ingestion of urine can result in infection which can range from the asymptomatic through pharyngitis and fever to full blown haemorrhagic fever with bleeding into skin and viscera. Person-to-person transmission cannot be ruled out. The South American haemorrhagic fever viruses, Junin (in Argentina), Machupo (in Bolivia) and Sabia (in Venezuala) persistently infect *Calomys* spp. (vesper mouse). They produce a similar clinical picture to Lassa fever.

BUNYAVIRIDAE

This is a large family of viruses, some of which are transmitted by insects (Bunyamwera, Nairo and Phleboviruses); some infect plants (Tospovirus) and some are zoonotic (Hantaviruses). However, all are spherical (95 nm), enveloped

Infections by enveloped RNA viruses

	Major diseases	Less common diseases	Vaccine preventable	Incubation period	Transmission and period of infectivity
Flaviviridae					
Yellow Fever	Viral haemorrhagic fever	Meningoencephalitis	Yes	3–6 days	Mosquito borne (Aedes)
Dengue	Viral haemorrhagic fever	Febrile illness (in children)	No	2–7 days	Mosquito borne (Aedes)
Japanese B	Encephalitis	Asymptomatic (96–99% of cases)	Yes	4–14 days	Mosquito borne (Culex)
St Louis	Encephalitis	Asymptomatic (94–99% of cases)	No	5–21 days	Mosquito borne (Culex)
Hepatitis C	Acute & chronic hepatitis	Asymptomatic (20–40%)	No	40 days	6 months to lifetime
Togaviridae					
Eastern Equine	Encephalitis	Asymptomatic (88–97%)	No	5–15 days	Mosquito borne (Aedes)
Chikungunya	Fever, rash, polyarthritis	—	No	1–6 days	Mosquito borne (Aedes)
Rubella	German measles	Asymptomatic (80–90%)	Yes	16–21 days	1 week before, 3 weeks after rash
Coronavirus	Common cold	Pneumonia, diarrhoea	No	3 days	1 week
Rabies	Encephalitis (>99% mortality)		Yes	9 days to years depending on site of inoculation	Until death, but no case of human-to-human transmission
Retroviridae					
HTLV1	Tropical spastic paresis	Adult T-cell leukaemia, asymptomatic (90–99%)	No	3 weeks to 15 years	Lifetime
HIV	AIDS	Meningoencephalitis, asymptomatic	No	2–6 months (infants) 4–15 years (adults)	Lifetime

Infections by enveloped RNA viruses (cont.)

	Major diseases	Less common diseases	Vaccine preventable	Incubation period	Transmission and period of infectivity
Arenaviridae					
LCM	Febrile illness	Aseptic meningitis, Asymptomatic (95%)	No	7–21 days	?
Lassa, Junin, Machupo, Sabia	Haemorrhagic fever	'Flu-like' illness, Asymptomatic (20–30%)	No	10–11 days	?
Bunyaviridae					
Bunyamwera	Encephalitis	Myalgia, fever	No	3–7 days	Mosquito borne
Phlebovirus	Sandfly fever, encephalitis	Asymptomatic (25%)	No	3–7 days	Mosquito or sandfly borne
Nairovirus	Haemorrhagic fever	'Flu-like' illness	No	3–12 days	Tick borne
Hantavirus	Haemorrhagic fever/pneumonia	Asymptomatic (30–95%)	No	1–6 weeks	No person-to-person spread
Influenza	Influenza	Encephalitis	Yes	1–3 days	1–2 weeks
Paramyxoviridae					
Parainfluenza	Laryngo-tracheobronchitis	Croup in infants	No	1–3 days	1–2 weeks
Mumps	Parotitis	Aseptic meningitis	Yes	12–25 days	7 days pre and 15 days post parotitis
Measles	Acute exanthem	Pneumonia, encephalitis	Yes	10–14 days	4 days pre-rash until desquamation
Respiratory syncytial virus	Bronchiolitis	Pneumonia	No	3–7 days	2–3 weeks
Filoviridae					
Marburg, Ebola	Haemorrhagic fever (90% mortality)	—	No	7–9 days	4–5 weeks

30 Infections by enveloped RNA viruses.

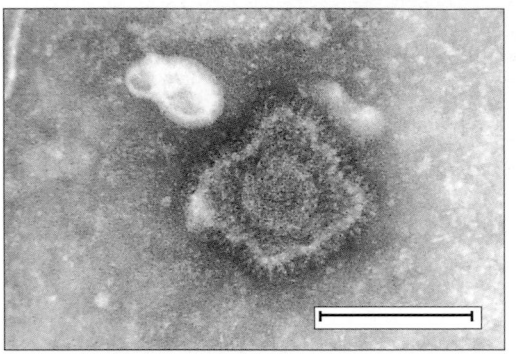

31 Negative stain electron micrograph of a togavirus. The spherical, enveloped virion has a diameter of 60–70 nm with glycoprotein spikes on the surface and an eicosahedral nucleocapsid (c. 25–35 nm diameter). It has a single linear positive sense genome (12 kb). *(bar = 70 nm)*

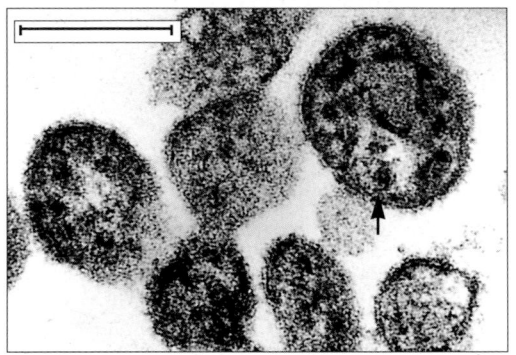

32 Thin-section electron micrograph of an arenavirus. The virus is a spherical, enveloped RNA virus with a largely positive sense genome. The electron dense granules (arrow) are ribosomes. *(bar = 200 nm)*

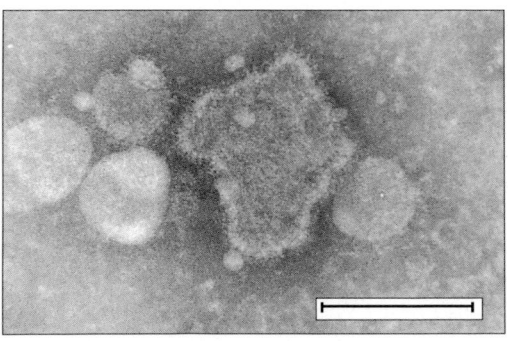

33 Negative stain electron micrograph of Puumala virus. This is a hantavirus in the family Bunyaviridae. They are enveloped viruses with a cuboidal ambisense RNA genome. The envelope has a tessellated appearance. *(bar = 100 nm)*

viruses (**33**) with a cuboidal nucleocapsid. Their RNA genome is linear in three segments and is mostly negative sense although some are ambisense. The Bunyamwera viruses are found world-wide and are transmitted by mosquitoes and may cause encephalitis (e.g. La Crosse) fever with myalgia (e.g. Guama) or undifferentiated febrile illness (e.g. Tahnya). There are approximately 45 phleboviruses but not all cause disease in man. Sandfly fever is transmitted by phlebotamine flies and is a febrile illness with headache, photophobia and joint pains. The disease is self-limiting and recovery complete with no deaths recorded. Nairoviruses are transmitted by ticks and the most important disease is Crimean-Congo haemorrhagic fever. It may also be transmitted person-to-person. Finally, the hantaviruses persistently infect a variety of animal species (predominantly rodents) and are excreted in their urine and saliva. Two distinct clinical syndromes occur. Haemorrhagic fever with renal syndrome (HFRS) occurs throughout the world. Severe HFRS occurs in the Far East (Hantaan) and the Balkans (Fojnica, Porogia), moderate HFRS (Seoul) occurs throughout the world and mild HFRS (nephropathia epidemica) due to Puumala virus occurs in northern Europe. The recently described hantavirus pulmonary syndrome is due to Muerto Canyon virus and cases have occurred with high mortality (about 60%) throughout North America.

Diagnosis of all of the above infections is by serology, antigen detection, culture or RT–PCR. They require special containment facilities.

FILOVIRIDAE

These are enveloped viruses with a helical nucleocapsid. They form rod-like or even branching structures (**34**) up to 14 mm long and 80 nm in diameter. They

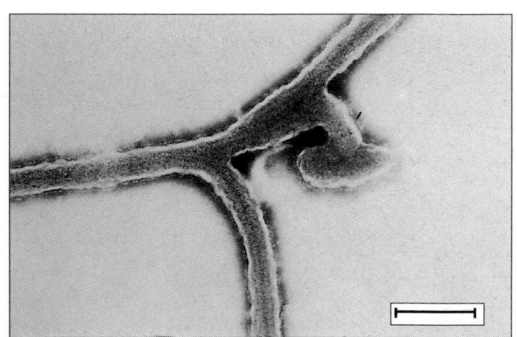

34 Negative stain electron micrograph of Ebola virus, a member of the Filoviridae. This is a filamentous, occasionally branching, enveloped virus with a helical RNA genome. (bar = 200 nm)

cause haemorrhagic fever with a high case-fatality rate (90%). They are zoonotic but person-to-person spread also occurs either through body secretions (saliva, sputum) or blood. Monkeys can transmit infection to man and the first human cases in Germany (Marburg) in 1967 were acquired in this fashion. However, the primary reservoir of infection is unclear. Since 1976 three outbreaks of infection have occurred, in northern Zaire (Ebola), southern Sudan and most recently (1995) in central Zaire.

RHABDOVIRIDAE

Rabies virus is the major human pathogen. It is a bullet-shaped, enveloped virus with a helical nucleocapsid (**35**). It has a single-stranded, negative sense genome (13–16 kb). The genus is called Lyssavirus. (In Greek, *lyssa* means rage.) Rabies is a zoonotic infection. The greatest risk of transmission is from adult unvaccinated dogs. Infection has also been transmitted from vampire bats, foxes, cats, raccoons and jackals. Infection is usually acquired by bites but can also be by inoculation of saliva into open cuts or even onto mucous membranes. Virus ascends via the peripheral nerves to the brain. The incubation period varies according to the distance of the site of inoculation to the brain. It can be as short as 9 days and as long as 3 years.

CORONAVIRIDAE

Coronaviruses are pleomorphic, enveloped, helical viruses with club-shaped glycoprotein spikes on the surface (**36**). There are two groups of antigenically

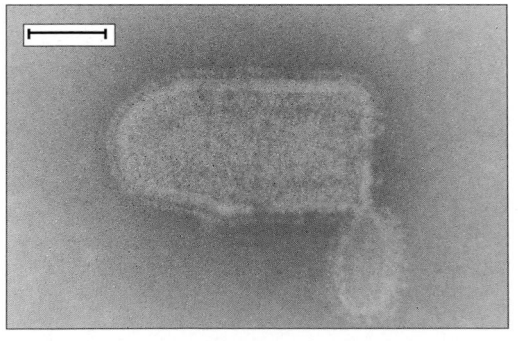

35 Negative stain electron micrograph of rabies virus. This is a bullet-shaped, enveloped, virus with a helical, negative sense RNA genome. *(bar = 50 nm)*

related strains of human coronavirus. Coronaviruses are a cause of the common cold and are responsible for 5–15% of cases of upper respiratory tract infection in children and adults. They may also be a cause of diarrhoeal disease.

ORTHOMYXOVIRIDAE

The influenza viruses are enveloped RNA viruses with a helical nucleocapsid and a segmented, single-stranded, negative sense linear genome (**37**). There are three distinct influenza viruses (A, B and C) based on antigens on the nucleoprotein.

There is a fringe of glycoprotein spikes on the surface of the virus which mediate attachment and penetration into host cell (haemagglutinin) and release of progeny virus (neuraminidase). Antibodies to these spikes provide protective

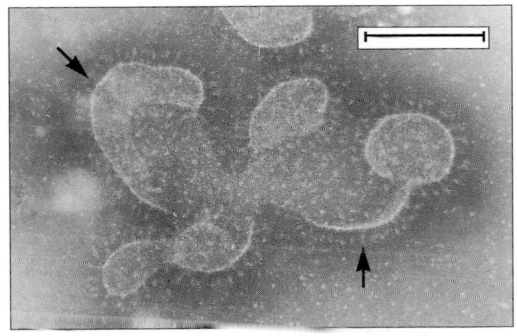

36 Negative stain electron micrograph of coronavirus. This is an enveloped, pleomorphic, helical RNA virus. Note the characteristic club-shaped glycoprotein spikes (arrowed). (bar = 50 nm)

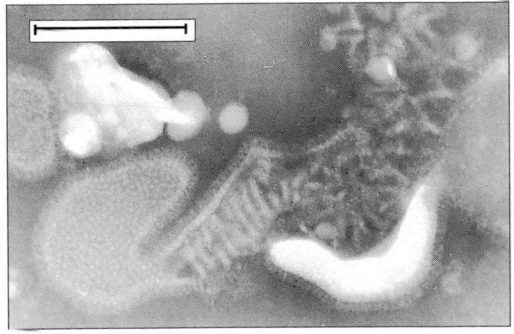

37 Negative stain electron micrograph of influenza virus. This is an enveloped, helical virus with a linear, segmented, negative sense RNA genome. There are two types of glycoprotein spike on the surface that mediate haemagglutinin (HA) and neuraminidase (NA) activities. (bar = 100 nm)

immunity and sub-unit vaccines, employing purified haemagglutinin and neuraminidase spikes, are used to induce immunity (**38**). Unfortunately the antigenic structure of haemagglutinins (HA) and to a lesser extent neuraminidase (NA) of group A influenza viruses can vary. This occurs in two ways: antigenic drift and antigenic shift. Antigenic drift is a slow change due to a gradual accumulation of nucleotide substitutions in the HA gene, resulting in an approximate annual change in amino acid composition of 1%. This is responsible for the epidemics of influenza that affect a proportion of the population each winter. Antigenic shift is a major change resulting from recombinations between different influenza viruses. This results in a virus with a 'new' antigenic HA and a pandemic that affects populations throughout the world.

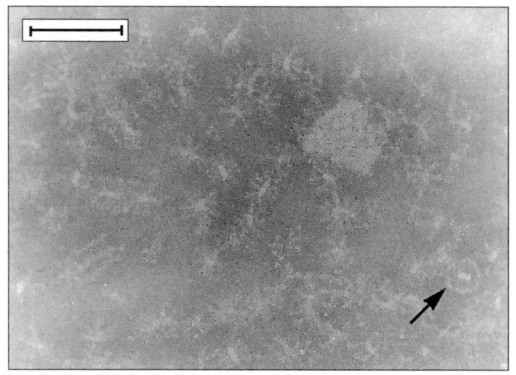

38 Negative stain electron micrograph of haemagglutinin (HA) and neuraminidase (NA) glycoproteins. These have been prepared from whole influenza virus by detergent solubilization of the envelope and separated from the nucleocapsid by centrifugation. The HA assume star-shaped figures and NA, cartwheels (arrow). They are used in a subunit vaccine to prevent influenza. *(bar = 50 nm)*

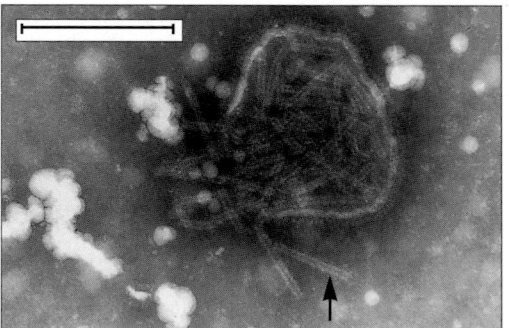

39 Negative stain electron micrograph of measles virus (a paramyxovirus). The lipid envelope has burst and the typical 'herring-bone' (arrow) appearance of the helical nucleocapsid can be seen. *(bar = 100 nm)*

PARAMYXOVIRIDAE

The Paramyxoviridae are also enveloped viruses with a helical nucleocapsid (**39**). They differ from orthomyxoviruses in having an unsegmented RNA genome. There are three major genera that are pathogenic for man, namely *Parainfluenza*, *Morbillivirus* and *Pneumovirus*. The parainfluenza viruses (1, 2, 3, 4a, 4b) cause respiratory tract infections, including croup in infants. The other member of the genus, mumps virus, causes the acute childhood infectious disease, characterized by parotitis and, occasionally, oophoritis, orchitis, pancreatitis and aseptic meningitis.

Measles virus is the human morbillivirus; canine distemper virus infects dogs and rinderpest, cattle. Measles is an acute febrile exanthematous disease of childhood, which in developing countries has a dire effect. Diagnosis of ortho- and paramyxoviruses can be by immunofluorescent antigen test (IFAT), virus culture, RT–PCR or serology.

RETROVIRIDAE

This is a large family of enveloped viruses with a cuboidal nucleocapsid (**40**). Each nucleocapsid contains two copies of a linear, positive sense, single-stranded RNA genome (3.5–9 kb). These viruses have the ability to turn the RNA genome back (in Greek *retros* means backwards) to a double-stranded DNA provirus which then becomes integrated into the genome of host cell. This is mediated by gene products in the *pol* region (**41**) including reverse transcriptase, endonuclease and integrase.

There are three major subfamilies of the Retroviridae. The spumaviruses induce intense vacuolation of the infected cell resembling foam (from Greek

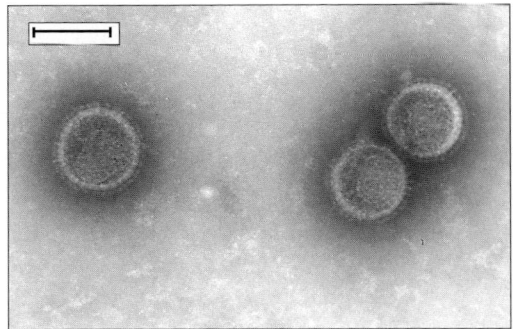

40 Negative stain electron micrograph of human immunodeficiency virus (a retrovirus). The glycoprotein spikes (composed of three molecules each of gp120 and gp41) can be seen on the surface. The virus has a cuboidal nucleocapsid with two copies of a positive sense, single-stranded RNA genome. (bar = 100 nm)

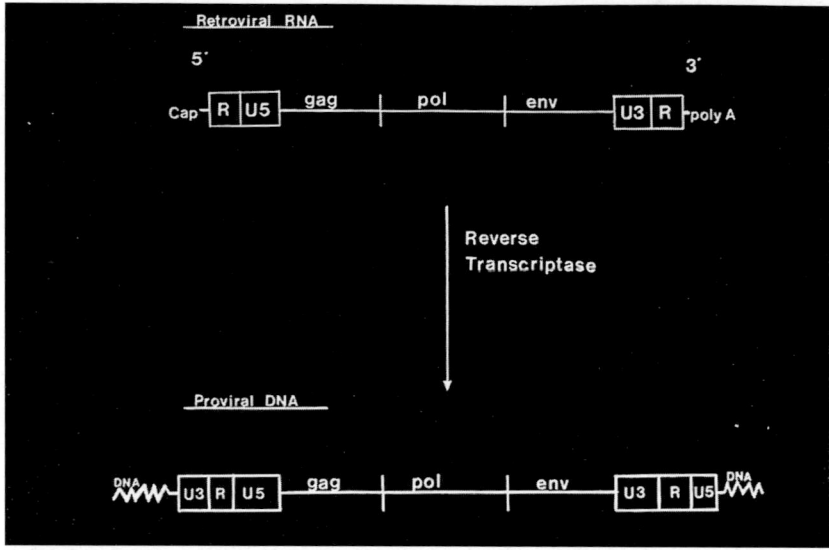

41 Reverse transcription of the HIV genome to proviral DNA which is inserted into the chromosome of the host cell.

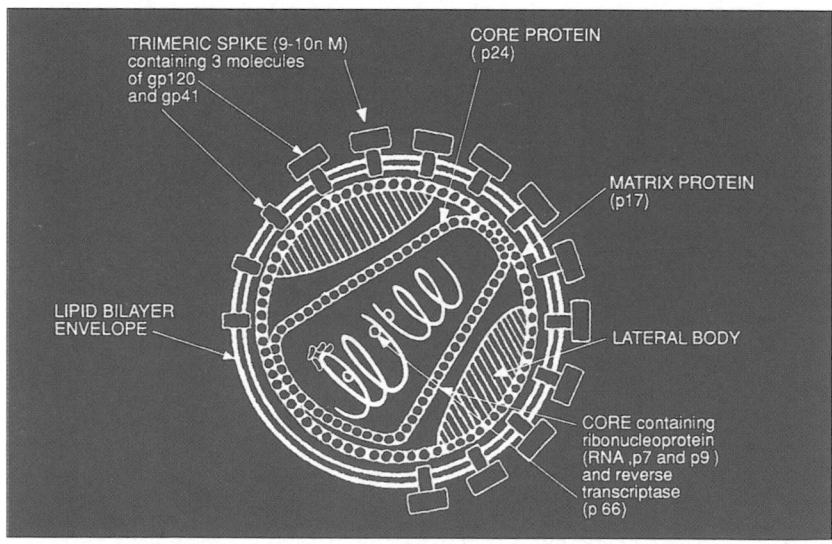

42 A diagram of the structure and polypeptides of HIV.

spuma foam). There are no proven disease associations. The lentiviruses have a long incubation period (Latin *lentus*, slow). The major human pathogens are human immunodeficiency viruses (HIV) 1 and 2, both of which can result in the development of AIDS. HIV-1 attaches to cells bearing its receptor (the CD4 antigen) and penetrates them using glycoprotein spikes on the viral surface (**42**). These spikes are composed of two glycoproteins (gp41 and gp120) encoded by the *env* region of the genome. The capsid and matrix proteins (e.g. p24 and p17, respectively) are encoded by the *gag* (group specific *antigen*) region.

The oncornaviruses are not a definitive sub-family and comprise four distinct morphological subgroups. This classification is based largely on their electron microscopic appearance on examination of thin sections of cells (**43**). Type A particles are 60–90 nm in diameter and occur intracellularly. Type B particles are seen following budding of a preformed capsid through the cell surface. They are 125–130 nm in diameter with an eccentrically sited electron-dense core. Murine mammary tumour virus is characteristic of the group. Type C particles have a nucleocapsid that assembles at the plasma membrane at the time of budding, are 80–120 nm in diameter and contain a central electron-dense core. C-type retroviruses include the murine, feline and simian leukaemia viruses. Type D particles have a characteristic bar-shaped core within the envelope which does not have a surface fringe. Human T-cell leukaemia virus 1 (HTLV-1) is a C-type virus which causes tropical spastic paresis and adult T-cell leukaemia in man.

DNA VIRUSES

The infections caused by DNA viruses are shown in Table **44**.

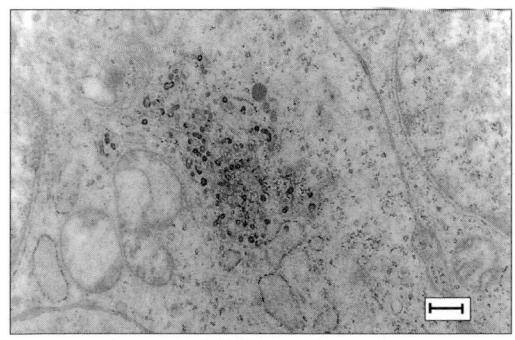

43 Thin-section electron micrograph of intra-cellular nucleocapsids of B-type oncornaviruses. *(bar = 200 nm)*

Infections by DNA viruses

	Major infections	Less common infections	Vaccine preventable	Incubation period	Period of infectivity
Parvovirus	Erythema infectiosum (5th disease)	Arthralgia, aplastic crises, hydrops fetalis	No	18–21 days	5 days (in blood 8–14 days post infection)
Papovaviridae					
Polyomavirus (JC, BK)	Asymptomatic	Progressive multifocal leuko-encephalopathy (JC)	No	?	Lifetime
Papillomavirus	Warts (cutaneous, mucosal), carcinoma of cervix, anus and rectum	—	No	1–20 months	Until resolution of wart
Hepatitis B	Acute or chronic hepatitis, hepatocellular carcinoma	Asymptomatic (50–60%)	Yes	2–6 months	Can be for life
Adenoviridae	URTI/LRTI (serotypes 1–5, 7, 14, 21) Pneumonia (serotypes 3, 4, 7b,14,21) Keratoconjunctivitis (serotypes 18, 19) Pharyngoconjunctival fever (serotypes 3, 7) Diarrhoeal disease (serotypes 40, 41)	Pertussis (1, 2, 3, 5) Cystitis (1, 4, 7, 11, 21) Asymptomatic (up to 50%)	No	5–10 days	Up to 900 days
Herpesviridae					
HHV-1	'Cold sores'	Encephalitis	No		Until lesions crust and then for life
HHV-2	Genital herpes	Encephalitis	No		Until lesions crust and then for life
HHV-3	Chickenpox, shingles	Pneumonia, encephalitis	Yes	14–21 days	4 days prior to chickenpox and until lesions crust
HHV-4	Glandular fever	Asymptomatic (80–90%)	No	14–28 days	For life
HHV-5	URTI	Asymptomatic (90–95%) pneumonia, congenital disease	No	14–28 days	For life
HHV-6	Exanthem subitum	Asymptomatic (80–90%)	No	5–15 days	For life
HHV-7	Exanthem subitum	?	No	?	?
HHV-8	?	Kaposi's sarcoma	No	?	?
Poxviridae*					
Cowpox	Skin lesions	Encephalitis	No	6–10 days	Until lesion crusts
Orf	'Milkers nodes'	-	No	3–7 days	Until lesion crusts
Molluscum contagiosum	Skin lesions	-	No	2–7 weeks	Until lesion heals

44 Infections by DNA viruses.

PARVOVIRIDAE

These are the smallest of the viruses (18–21 nm). They are unenveloped viruses with a single-stranded linear genome (5 kb) that is mostly negative sense (**45**). Parvovirus B19 is the human pathogen. In children it causes an acute febrile illness called erythema infectiosum, fifth disease or 'slapped cheek' syndrome. In adults it may also cause a prolonged arthritis. The virus infects, in particular, erythroid precursor cells in the bone marrow. (The P-blood group antigen is the receptor). In patients with haemolytic anaemia (e.g. hereditary spherocytosis or thalassaemia) infection can result in aplastic crises where the blood haemoglobin can drop precipitately. Parvovirus may also cross the placenta to infect the fetus resulting in still-birth, abortion or hydrops fetalis in 5–7% of cases. Diagnosis is by detection of genome or of IgM anti-parvovirus.

PAPOVAVIRIDAE

There are two sub-families in the Papovaviridae. The polyomaviruses (JC and BK) rarely cause disease in man. Both are persistently excreted, principally in urine, following initial infection. JC virus can cause a severe neurological infection (progressive multifocal leukoencephalopathy) in the immune compromised patient. The human papillomaviruses (HPV) form a large grouping of unenveloped cuboidal DNA viruses (**46**). They have a circular, double-stranded genome (c. 8 kbp). They are difficult to grow since they require differentiated skin to support replication. They are subdivided into genotypes (of which there are over 60) on the relatedness

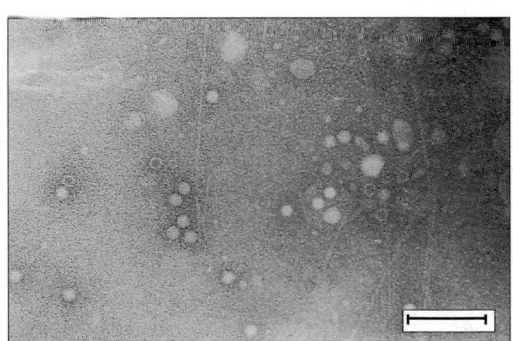

45 Negative stain electron micrograph of human parvovirus B19. This is an unenveloped, cuboidal virus with a single-stranded DNA genome. It causes 'slapped cheek' syndrome. *(bar = 100 nm)*

of DNA sequences. They are responsible for cutaneous (e.g. HPV1) and genital (e.g. HPV12) warts. There is a very strong association between certain HPV types (e.g. HPV16, HPV18 and HPV 33) and carcinoma of the cervix.

ADENOVIRIDAE

These are eicosahedral unenveloped viruses (**47**) with a linear, double-stranded DNA genome (36–38 kbp). There are approximately 42 adenovirus serotypes. Different serotypes have different disease associations and, like enteroviruses, infection can be asymptomatic. Up to 10% of cases of pneumonia in children may

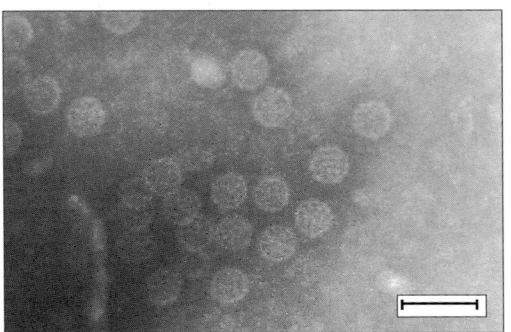

46 Negative stain electron micrograph of a papillomavirus. This is an unenveloped, cuboidal virus with a circular, double-stranded DNA genome. There are over 60 human papillomavirus genotypes. *(bar = 100 nm)*

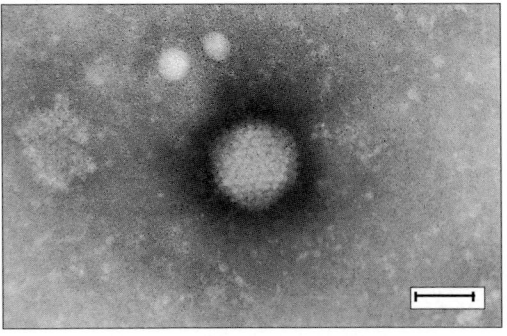

47 Negative stain electron micrograph of an adenovirus. This is an unenveloped virus with a double-stranded DNA genome. The capsid is made up of 20 triangular facets and each facet is made up of globular capsomers. *(bar = 50 nm)*

be due to adenovirus types 1, 2, 3, 5 and 7 and some serotypes can also cause a pertussis-like syndrome. Serotypes 40 and 41 cause acute diarrhoeal disease and types 1–5 have been associated with intussusception. Pharyngoconjunctival fever is due to serotypes 3 and 7a and epidemic keratoconjunctivitis to serotypes 3, 4, 7 and 8. Diagnosis is by viral culture, detection of viral antigen (for Ad40/41) or serology.

HEPADNAVIRIDAE

Hepatitis B virus (HBV) is a small (42 nm) enveloped virus with an eicosahedral nucleocapsid (**48**). Its DNA genome (3.2 kbp) is double-stranded with one strand forming a complete loop and the complementary strand a partial loop. HBV is a cause of parenterally acquired hepatitis and has a long (2–6 month) incubation period.

In a proportion of patients (especially when infection in neonatally acquired) the infection is not cleared by the immune system but persists in the hepatocytes. Persistent infection may ultimately result in chronic hepatic disease or even hepatocellular carcinoma. Patients with persistent HBV infection may have whole virus particles (Dane particles) with or without tubular and vesicular surface antigen (HBsAg) particles in their bloodstream (**49**). Detection of HBsAg in the blood of a patient without acute hepatitis indicates persistent infection. Detection of HBeAg indicates that they are high-risk carriers who could transmit infection by transfer of a small volume of blood, e.g. from a needlestick injury. If the donor is e-antigen negative it is likely that a large amount of blood (e.g. blood transfusion) would need to be transferred to transmit infection.

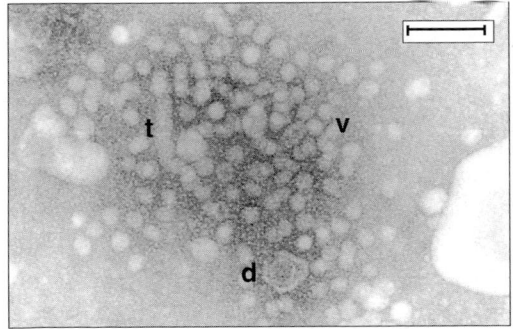

48 Negative stain electron micrograph of plasma from a patient with acute hepatitis B virus infection. The complete virus (Dane) particles (d) have a lipid envelope with a loop of double-stranded DNA genome in a cuboidal nucleocapsid. The tubular (t) and vesicular (v) particles are comprised of viral lipid envelope only. *(bar = 100 nm)*

HERPESVIRIDAE

The herpesviruses are a large family of enveloped viruses with an eicosahedral nucleocapsid (**50**). They have a double-stranded, linear, genome (120–200 kbp). There are currently eight human herpesviruses (HHV-1 to HHV-8) and following initial transmission each becomes established in latent or persistent infection. Herpes simplex virus type 1 (HHV-1) remains latent in the trigeminal ganglion and can reactivate and recrudesce to produce cold-sores. Herpes simplex virus type 2 (HHV-2) causes genital herpes. Varicella-zoster virus (HHV-3) causes chicken-

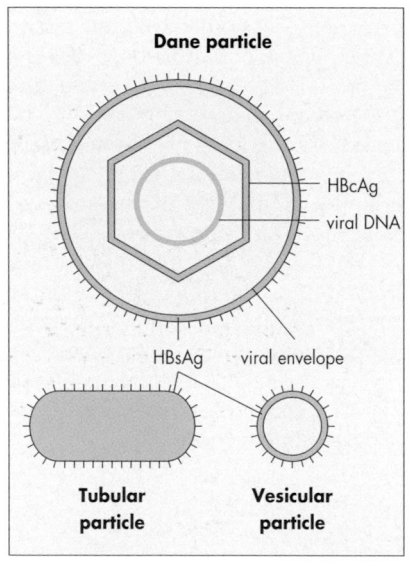

Dane particle

HBcAg

viral DNA

HBsAg · viral envelope

Tubular particle

Vesicular particle

49 A diagram showing the antigens of hepatitis B virus.

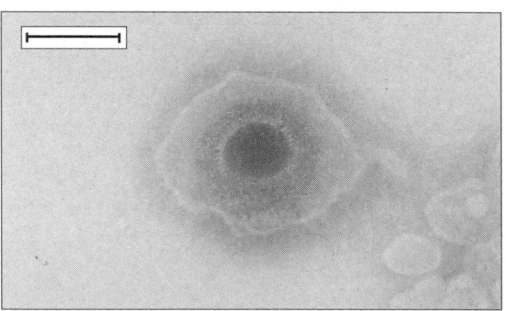

50 Negative stain electron micrograph of herpes simplex virus. This is an enveloped virus with a cuboidal capsid and a linear, double-stranded DNA genome. There are eight different human herpesviruses. (*bar = 100 nm*)

pox and subsequently reactivates to produce shingles. Epstein–Barr virus (EBV) is also known as HHV-4 and causes glandular fever. The infection is also known as infectious mononucleosis, since examination of a peripheral blood film reveals the presence of large, irregular, mononuclear cells (**51**). These are T-lymphocytes which have become activated in an attempt to kill the EBV-infected B-lymphocytes. Cytomegalovirus (HHV-5) infection is usually asymptomatic but can cross the placenta to infect the fetus. Under such circumstances it is the commonest infective cause of mental retardation. HHV-6, and to a certain extent HHV-7, cause exanthem subitum in young children. The recently described HHV-8 is probably the cause of Kaposi's sarcoma in both HIV-infected and HIV-uninfected individuals.

POXVIRIDAE

These are the largest (350 × 400 nm) and most complex of the viruses. They can have a lipid envelope (**52**) but this is not an absolute necessity for infectivity.

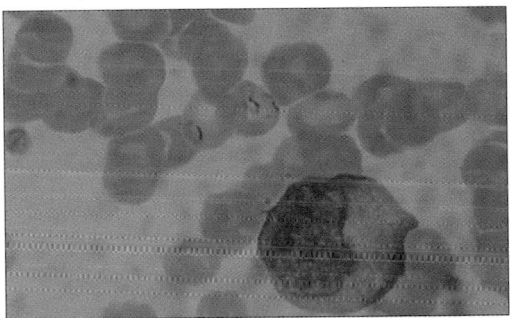

51 Peripheral blood film from a patient with glandular fever (infectious mononucleosis) due to Epstein–Barr virus (HHV-4). The large, irregular, mononuclear cells are activated T-lymphocytes.

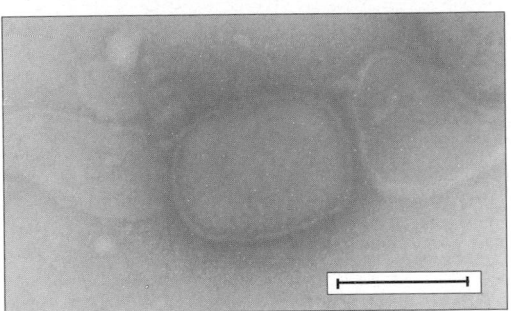

52 Negative stain electron micrograph of smallpox virus. Although a lipid envelope is visible, this is not necessary for infectivity. (bar = 300 nm)

Their capsid symmetry is complex and they have a double-stranded, linear DNA genome (130–280 kbp). The orthpoxviruses include smallpox (which has been eliminated) monkeypox and cowpox. Of the parapoxviruses only one, orf, is of importance in human infections (**53**). Molluscum contagiosum is an, as yet, unclassified poxvirus which has not been maintained in artificial culture. On electron microscopy it has been described as resembling a ball of string (**54**).

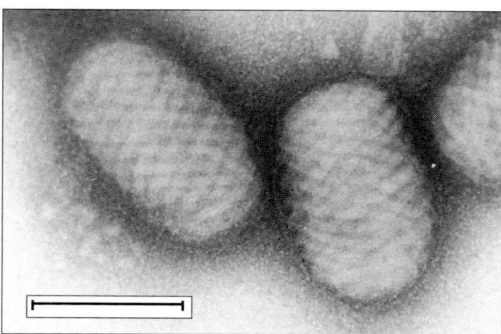

53 Negative stain electron micrograph of orf, a parapox virus. This complex DNA virus has a double-stranded, linear genome. The regular surface structure is characteristic of parapoxviruses. *(bar = 300 nm)*

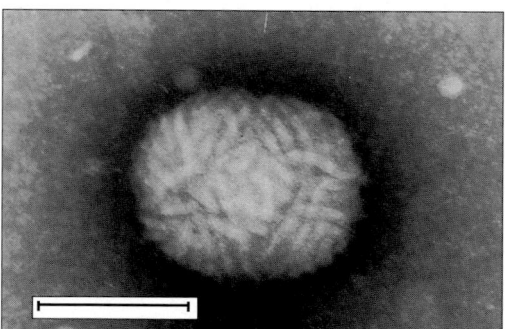

54 Negative stain electron micrograph of molluscum contagiosium virus. This virus has not been maintained in artificial culture. It is described as resembling a ball of string. *(bar = 300 nm)*

DIAGNOSTIC VIROLOGY

Although the presence of a virus infection can, on occasion, be inferred from non-specific measurements, such as presence of lymphocytosis (e.g. in CSF or blood) the precise diagnosis depends upon detection of virus, detection of viral antigens, detection of viral genome or detection of a serological response to the virus (**55**).

Diagnostic methods in virology		
Method	Rapidity of method	Sensitivity/specificity
Detection of virus		
Electron microscopy	Rapid	High
Culture (a)	Moderate (1–7 days)	High
Histology (inclusions) (a)	Moderate (1–14 days)	Low
Detection of viral antigens (a)		
ELISA	Rapid	High
Latex particle agglutination (LPA)	Rapid	Moderate
Radio-immunoassay (RIA)	Moderate (1–5 days)	High
Immunofluorescence	Rapid	High
Detection of viral genome		
RNA-polyacrylamide gel electrophoresis (b)	Moderate (24–36 h)	High
Genome hybridization	Moderate (1–5 days)	Moderate
Genome amplification by polymerase chain reaction (PCR)	Moderate (24–72 h)	High
Detection of serological response		
IgM response, e.g. for hepatitis A virus by ELISA	Rapid	High
Rising titre by:		
complement fixation	Slow (c)	High/moderate
haemagglutination inhibition	Slow	High
neutralization	Slow	High
LPA	Slow	Moderate
ELISA	Slow	High
RIA	Slow	High
immunofluorescence	Slow	High
(a) not available for all viruses (b) for rotavirus and picobirnavirus (c) requires acute and convalescent sera (at least 2 weeks between)		

55 Diagnostic methods in virology.

DETECTION OF VIRUS

Negative stain electron microscopy

This provides a rapid and specific diagnosis of most viral diarrhoeas but has also been used to detect respiratory viral infection (**56**). For virus to be seen the sample needs to contain at least 10^6 particles per ml. The sensitivity and specificity can be improved by the addition of specific antisera (immuno-electron microscopy).

Culture

Virus culture can be in whole animals (e.g. suckling mice for Coxsackie B viruses), in embryonated eggs (e.g. influenza or pox viruses) or in cultured cells. Animals are used rarely now for virus isolation.

Embryonated hens' eggs can be used for isolation of many different viruses. Different viruses require different inoculation sites (**57**). For example, influenza viruses are cultured in the amniotic cavity, parainfluenza viruses in the allantoic cavity, St Louis encephalitis virus in the yolk sac and poxviruses on the chorio-allantoic membrane (**58**). However, cell-lines are available for culture of most viruses and embryonated eggs are used less and less frequently. In fact, the major use of embryonated eggs is in the large-scale culture of influenza and measles viruses for vaccine production.

The ability to culture human and other mammalian cells led to great advances in animal virology since they provided a ready substrate for viral culture. Mammalian cells can be grown readily in plastic flasks containing appropriate growth medium (**59**) either attached to the plastic surfaces or in suspension. Cells may be derived directly from living normal tissue and are then called primary cell cultures. These tend to have a limited life-span. Transformed cells, derived either from malignant tumours or even cells transformed *in vitro*, provide rapidly

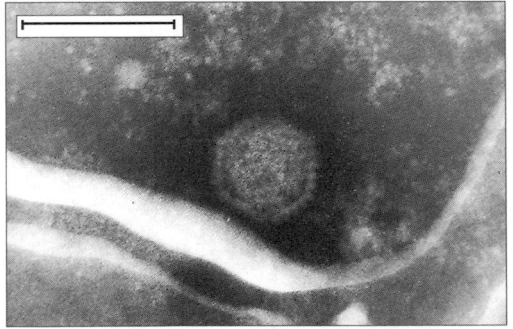

56 Direct negative stain electron micrograph of bronchial secretions from a child with bronchiolitis obliterans. Adenovirus was grown from the secretions. *(bar = 200 nm)*

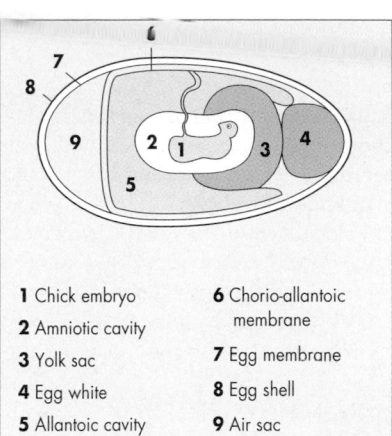

57 Diagram of a fertile hen's egg approximately 10 days old.

1 Chick embryo	**6** Chorio-allantoic membrane
2 Amniotic cavity	**7** Egg membrane
3 Yolk sac	**8** Egg shell
4 Egg white	**9** Air sac
5 Allantoic cavity	

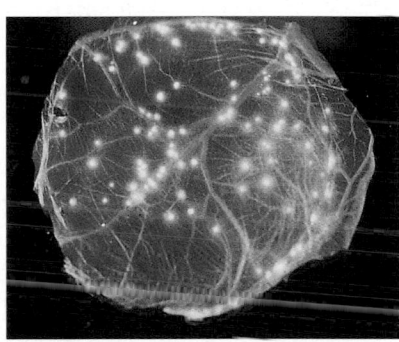

58 A chorio-allantoic membrane showing characteristic poxvirus lesions.

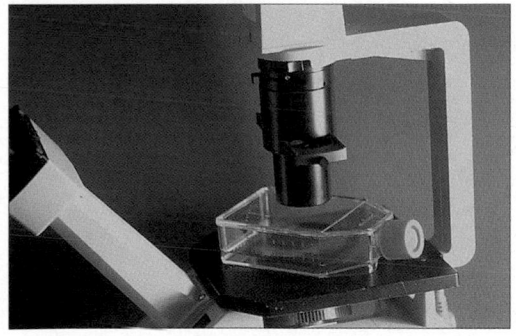

59 Disposable plastic flasks containing monolayers of cells bathed in growth medium.

growing immortal cell-lines. Some cells are fibroblastic (**60**) in appearance (e.g. MRC-5) some resemble epithelial cells (e.g. Vero, **61**) and some grow only in suspension and are derived from lymphoblastic (e.g. Raji) or macrophage/ monocyte (e.g. U937) precursors. No one cell-line will support the growth of all viruses; thus viral diagnostic laboratories maintain a range of cell-lines. Following inoculation and growth, viruses can be detected by their cytopathic effect (cpe). The time taken for cpe to appear varies with different viruses. For example that due to herpes simplex (**62**) takes under 24 h whereas cytomegaloviruses can take up to 5 days (**63**). For some viruses the cytopathic effect provides specific diagnosis (e.g. **62**, **63**) for others (e.g. enteroviruses) it is less clear-cut (**64**). In some cases little or no cytopathic effect is produced and virus is detected by other biological activities such as haemadsorption, interference, or antigen

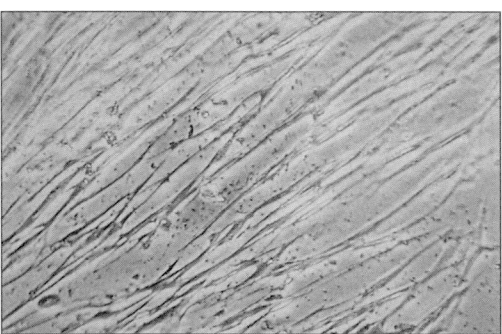

60 A monolayer of human embryo lung fibroblasts (MRC-5). The cells are spindle-shaped.

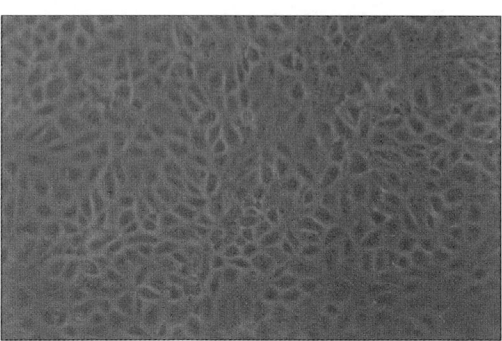

61 A monolayer of African green monkey kidney (Vero) cells.

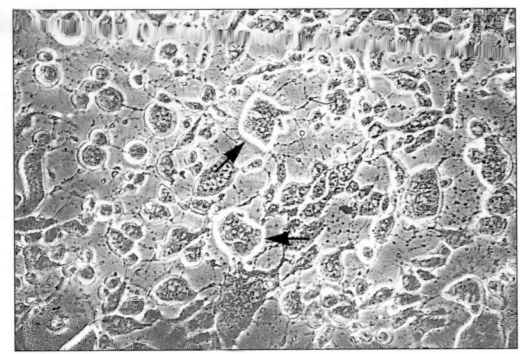

62 Typical cytopathic effect of herpes simplex virus on African green monkey kidney (Vero) cells . The plaques (arrows) consist of fused cells.

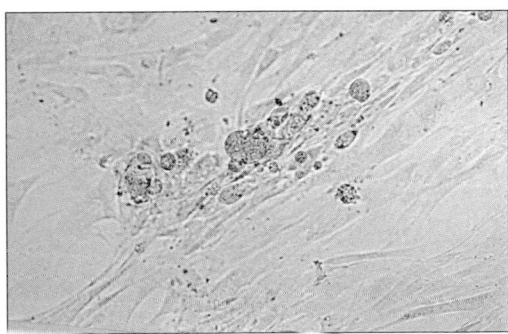

63 Typical cytopathic effect of cytomegalovirus on MRC-5 cells. The large refractile cells are infected by the virus.

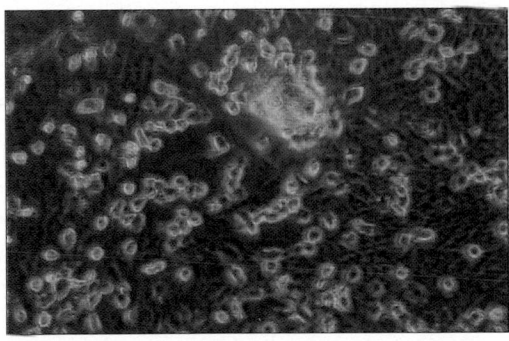

64 Cytopathic effect induced by poliovirus on Vero cells. The cells are killed but a similar picture can be induced by other viruses and some toxins.

production. Haemadsorption (**65**) occurs, for example, when the haemagglutinin spikes of influenza virus are expressed on the surface of infected cells. When erythrocytes are added they adhere focally to the infected cell. A variety of immuno-assays are used to detect viral growth either for rapid diagnosis prior to development of cpe (**66**) or for viruses that do not produce cpe. In most cases confirmation of virus growth and identity can be obtained by negative stain electron microscopy of the tissue culture fluid.

Inclusions

Finally, it is possible to detect viruses in tissue, or even peripheral blood cells, either by the presence of inclusions or by detection of viral antigens. Viral inclusions are aggregates of viral particles (**67**) and can be intranuclear or intracytoplasmic, depending upon the site of viral replication and assembly. Rabies virus produces intracytoplasmic inclusions in brain cells called Negri bodies (**68**). Herpesviruses such as varicella-zoster (**69**) and cytomegalovirus (**70**)

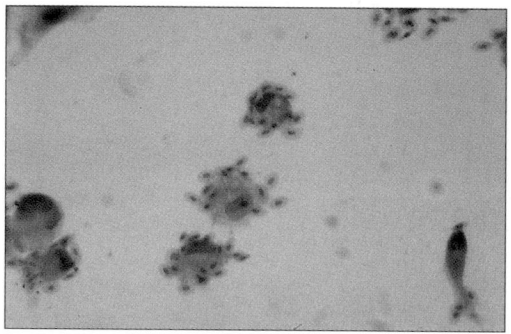

65 Haemadsorption of chicken erythrocytes to influenza virus infected cells.

66 The DEAFF (direct early antigen fluorescent focus) assay. The MRC-5 cells infected with cytomegalovirus are stained with fluorescein-conjugated antibody to CMV early antigen. This antigen appears within 24–36 h of addition of virus to cells.

produce intranuclear inclusions. (Indeed, perinatal infection with cytomegalovirus is also called cytomegalic inclusion disease.) Infected cells are large and show characteristic 'owl's eye' intranuclear inclusions (**70**). Simple histological stains are used to demonstrate such inclusions but their sensitivity and specificity is not high. The sensitivity and specificity can be increased by using specific antiviral antisera to stain the inclusions by, for example, immunoperoxidase or immuno-alkaline phosphatase (**71**).

DETECTION OF VIRAL ANTIGENS

In these assays antisera (mono- or polyclonal) are used to detect viral antigen, either free in body fluids or on exfoliated cells or white blood cells. Such assays can be highly sensitive since they can also detect antigens of disrupted virus particles which would not be cultivable or visible by electron microscopy. They

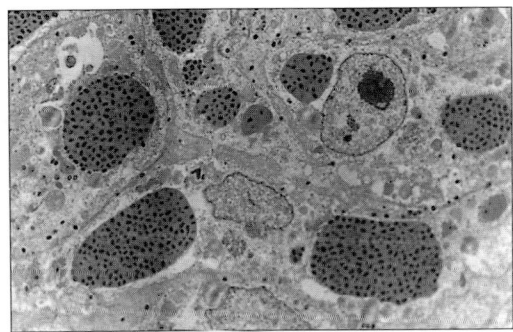

67 Thin-section electron micrograph of cowpox inclusions. They form intracytoplasmic inclusions which can also be stained by Giemsa for light microscopy.

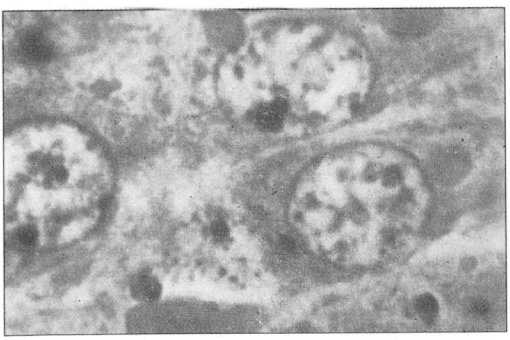

68 The pink cytoplasmic inclusions are characteristic of rabies virus infection. They are found in brain cells and are called Negri bodies.

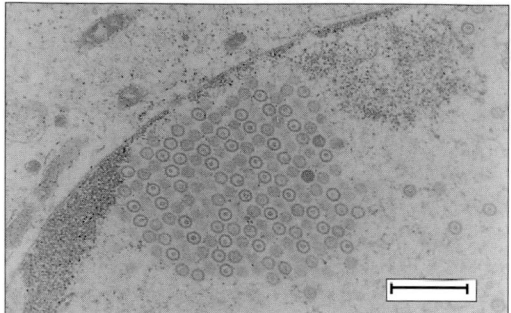

69 Intranuclear inclusions of cytomegalovirus which can also be visualized by Giemsa staining and light microscopy (see **70**). *(bar = 400 nm).*

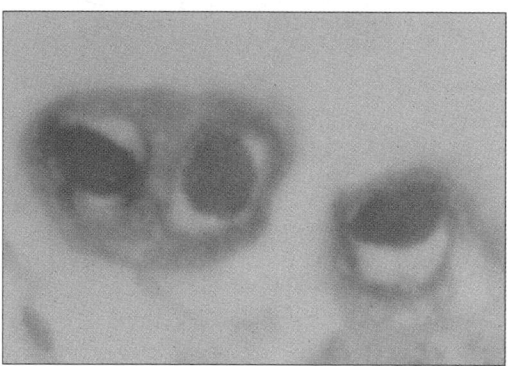

70 Typical 'owls-eye' intranuclear inclusions of cytomegalovirus infected cells.

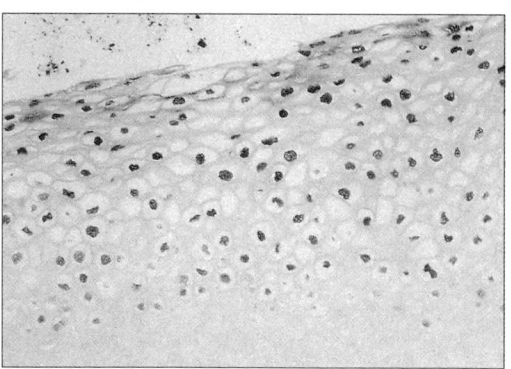

71 Cervical intra-epithelial neoplasia grade 1 (CIN-1) stained with alkaline phosphatase coupled to a monoclonal anti-human papillo-mavirus (HPV) antibody. The cells expressing HPV antigens are stained blue.

are, however, 'pathogen specific', i.e. a separate immunoassay must be employed for each pathogen, in contrast with electron microscopy and culture which are 'catch-all' techniques. The immunoassays vary according to the method used for detection of antigen–antibody binding.

Enzyme linked immunosorbent assay (ELISA)

These are antigen capture ELISAs (**72**). Such assays are available for a variety of viral enteropathogens (rotavirus, astrovirus, adenovirus 40/41, Norwalk agent),

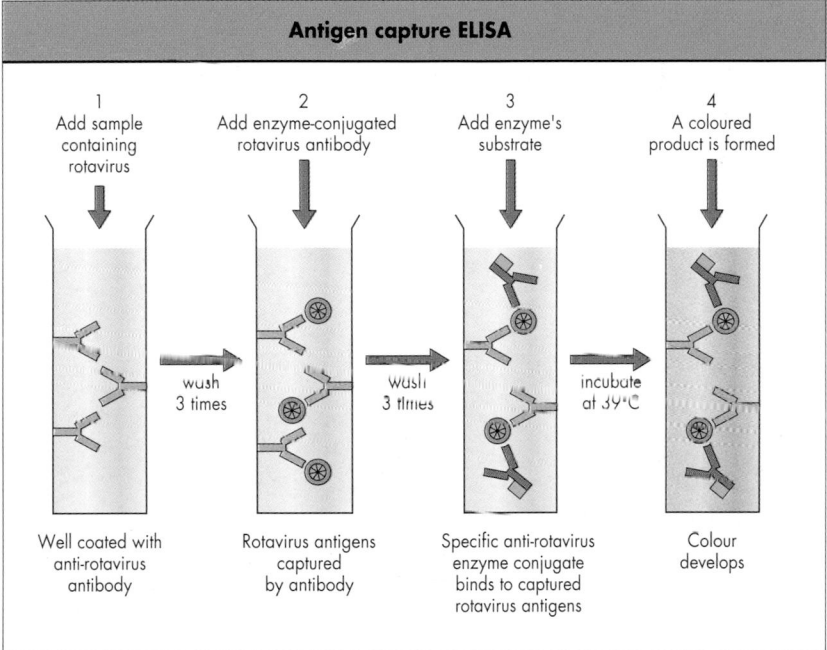

Antigen capture ELISA

1 Add sample containing rotavirus	2 Add enzyme-conjugated rotavirus antibody	3 Add enzyme's substrate	4 A coloured product is formed
wash 3 times	wash 3 times	incubate at 39°C	
Well coated with anti-rotavirus antibody	Rotavirus antigens captured by antibody	Specific anti-rotavirus enzyme conjugate binds to captured rotavirus antigens	Colour develops

72 Antigen capture ELISA. With antigen capture ELISA, the wells are coated with antibody to the virus. The sample containing virus (1) is added and, after washing several times, enzyme conjugated to an antibody to the virus in added (2). Finally, after a further cycle of washing, the enzyme's substrate (3) is added. A coloured product is formed if the viral antigen is present in the sample (4).

hepatitis B virus (HBsAg, HBeAg, HBcAg) and HIV (p24). In each case a coloured product is produced, the intensity of which is proportional to the amount of antigen present (**73**).

Latex particle agglutination (LPA)

In this system small latex particles are coated with specific antisera to a particular virus (**74**). If the virus is present in the sample, it cross-links the antibody-coated latex particles, causing the milky latex solution to curdle (**75**). LPA is available for the diagnosis of infection due to rotavirus or to respiratory syncytial virus. In general, the sensitivity and specificity of such assays is less than for ELISA.

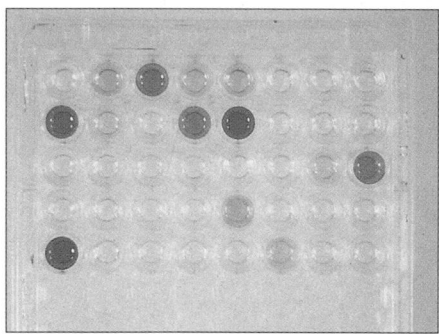

73 An ELISA plate showing positive (yellow/brown) and negative wells. In this case the enzyme used was alkaline phosphatase and antibody to hepatitis C virus was being detected.

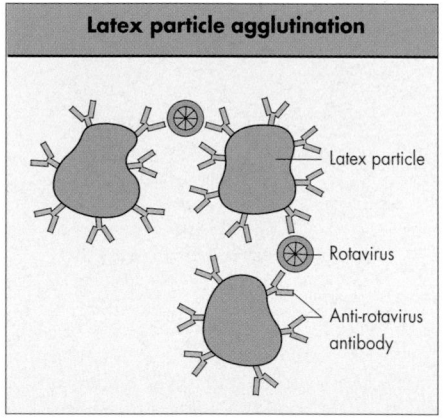

Latex particle agglutination

Latex particle

Rotavirus

Anti-rotavirus antibody

74 Latex particles coated with virus-specific antisera are clumped together by their antigen.

Immunofluorescence

Immunofluorescence either direct or indirect, is used to detect viral antigens on or in cells. It provides a rapid, sensitive diagnosis of respiratory tract infection (e.g. respiratory syncytial, parainfluenza, influenza and measles viruses). These viruses infect cells throughout the respiratory tract. Thus desquamated cells, obtained by nasopharyngeal aspiration, are fixed on microscope slides and separately stained with fluorescein-tagged specific antisera to each of the viruses (**76**). The technique is also used for the rapid detection of cytomegalovirus viraemia. CMV p66 antigen can be demonstrated in peripheral blood neutrophils (**77**).

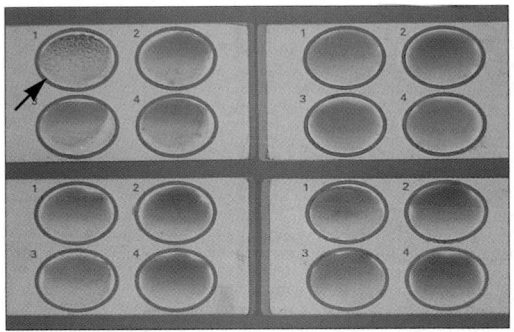

75 A rotavirus latex particle agglutination test. The curdled latex suspensions indicate the presence of rotavirus antigen (arrow).

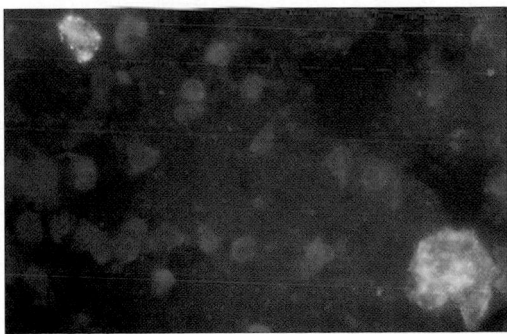

76 Direct immuno-fluorescence of nasopharyngeal cells from a child with bronchiolitis due to respiratory syncytial virus.

DETECTION OF VIRAL GENOME

RNA Polyacrylamide gel electrophoresis (RNA–PAGE)
This is only appropriate for the direct detection of rotavirus (**29**) or picobirnavirus and is only possible because their genomes are double-stranded RNA and they are excreted in large quantities in faeces.

Genome hybridization
This depends upon the ability of viral DNA or RNA to bind specifically (hybridize) with complementary strands of DNA generated either artificially (usually oligonucleotides) or from cloned virus genome (**78**). The binding is detected by

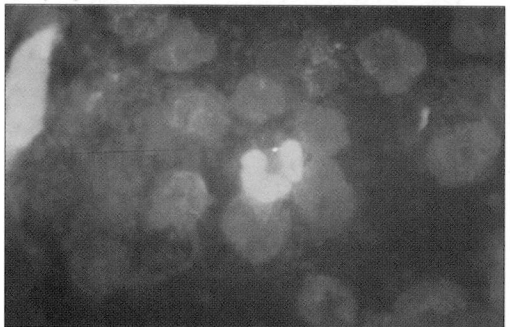

77 Direct immuno-fluorescence of peripheral blood neutrophils from a patient with acute cytomegalovirus infection. Antibody to CMV p66 protein conjugated to fluorescein is used to detect neutrophils containing CMV.

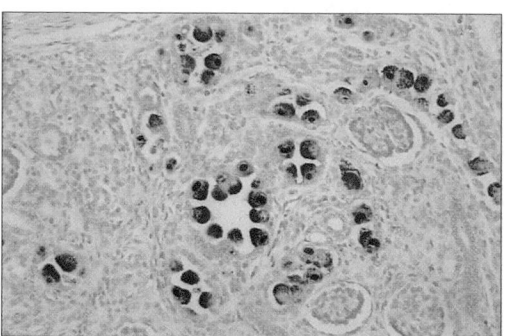

78 A section of kidney from a renal transplant patient with cytomegalovirus infection. The section has been stained with a CMV-DNA probe linked to alkaline phosphatase. The infected nuclei are stained red.

incorporation of a radiolabel or an enzyme system into the probe nucleic acid. Radioactive labels are detected using X-ray film usually as a dot blot. This is the most sensitive detection system, but it takes several days for the X-ray film to fog and radiolabels are not universally available. Incorporating an enzyme such as peroxidase or alkaline phosphatase (usually via biotinylated nucleotides) allows detection using an ELISA format. Genome hybridization can also be used for the direct detection of virus infection in histological section (**78**, **79**).

Genome amplification

With recent developments in molecular biology it has become possible to amplify fragments of the viral genome in patient's samples. A variety of methods has been developed including ligase chain reaction and the Q–β system. However, the first method developed and that most frequently employed is the polymerase chain reaction (PCR). In this, double-stranded DNA is first melted to separate the strands. The sample is mixed with primers which are complementary to sequences of nucleotides (c. 20) on the two DNA strands. Thus primers are chosen so that they are at either end of a sequence of 50 to 1000 bases (**80**). As the DNA cools, the excess of primers bind to their complementary sequences on the target DNA and nucleotides are added sequentially by the thermostable *taq* DNA polymerase. This generates two copies of the target DNA.

The mixture is reheated to separate the double-stranded DNA and allowed to cool so that the primers can bind and nucleotides be added. The *taq* (from *Thermus aquaticus*) enzyme is used since it is not denatured by the repeated heating and cooling. After 30–80 cycles of heating and cooling, carried out

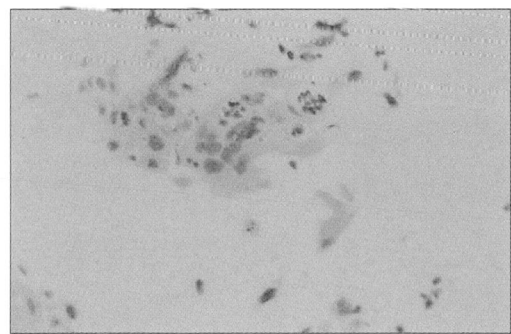

79 A section of oesophagus from an AIDS patient with herpes simplex (HSV) oesophagitis. The section has been stained with HSV-DNA linked to peroxidase. The infected cells are stained brown.

automatically using a thermal cycler (**81**) the amplified DNA can then be detected by electrophoresis on an agarose gel (**82**). However, it is important to show that the amplified DNA is of the expected target, either by restriction endonuclease

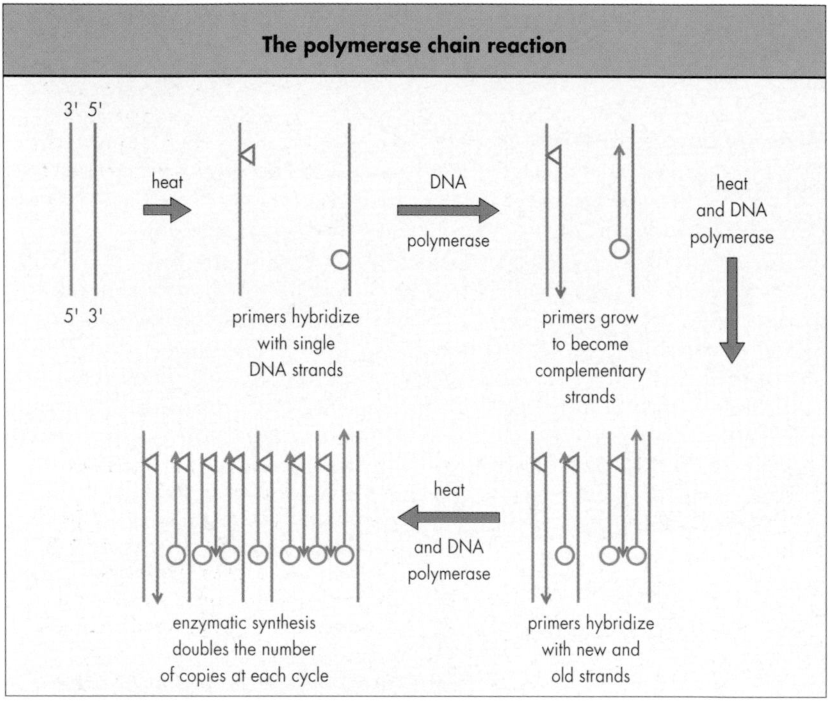

The polymerase chain reaction

3' 5'

heat

5' 3'

primers hybridize
with single
DNA strands

DNA
polymerase

primers grow
to become
complementary
strands

heat
and DNA
polymerase

enzymatic synthesis
doubles the number
of copies at each cycle

heat
and DNA
polymerase

primers hybridize
with new and
old strands

---

80 The polymerase chain reaction.

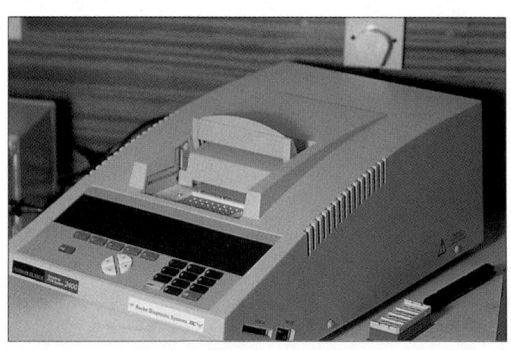

81 A thermal cycler used in the polymerase chain reaction.

digestion (**83**) or by DNA hybridization. The method can be modified to detect RNA viruses by incorporating a reverse transcriptase step before starting PCR. Theoretically, just one copy of the viral genome can be detected in a sample.

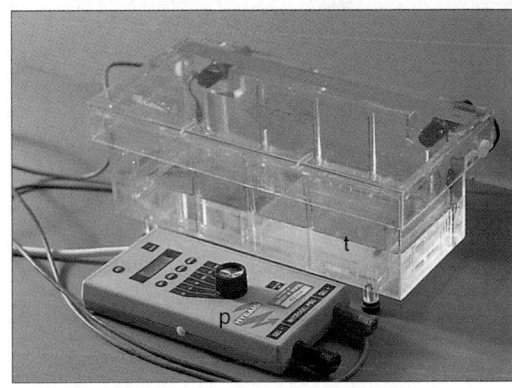

82 Equipment needed for agarose gel electrophoresis of PCR products, includes a power pack (p) and an electrophoresis tank (t).

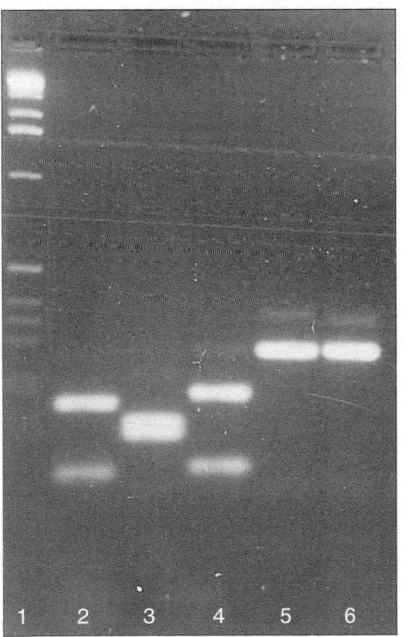

83 Ethidium bromide stained agarose gels of restriction endonuclease digested RT-PCR products amplified from the NP protein gene of respiratory syncytial virus. Lane 1 contains an 'λ-ladder' of molecular weight markers. Lanes 2 and 4, lanes 5 and 6, and lane 3 show three separate NP-types, respectively.

However, in practice larger amounts are needed. The sample may also contain inhibitors of the reaction which may cause false negative results. The method is exquisitely sensitive and false positives can occur due to contamination of the sample by exogenous target. It is thus advisable to have well-separated areas for preparation of samples, thermal cycling and detection of amplified product. The sensitivity and specificity of PCR can be improved by using 'nested' primers (**84**).

DETECTION OF SEROLOGICAL RESPONSE

Following initial challenge with an antigen (such as a viral or bacterial pathogen) a primary antibody response is mounted (**85**). This takes approximately 2 weeks to reach maximal levels and the antibody produced is principally of the IgM class. On subsequent challenge a secondary response is elicited which is much more rapid (of the order of 24–48 h) and produces higher levels of high affinity antibody, principally of the IgG class (**85**). This is, of course, the aim of immunization. However, from the above it follows that serological diagnosis of viral infection will most often not provide answers until the patient has recovered. Acute (taken on

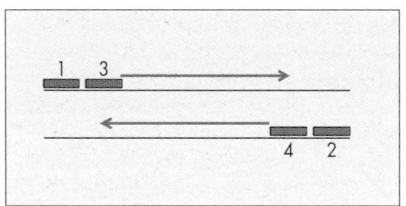

84 Nested primers increase the sensitivity and specificity of PCR.

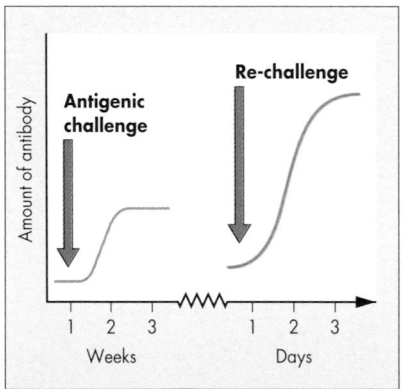

85 Primary and secondary immune responses. On first exposure to an antigen (vaccine or pathogen) peak antibody production takes 2–3 weeks and the antibody produced is primarily of IgM and low affinity. On second exposure the peak response is higher and more rapid (2–3 days). The antibody produced is of much higher affinity and predominantly IgG and IgA.

presentation) and convalescent (taken 10–14 days later) serum samples are required and, in general, a four-fold rise in titre is deemed to indicate infection.

IgM detection

IgM is the first class of antibody to be produced and its detection can provide early evidence of infection. It is used, for example, in the early diagnosis of EBV or *Mycoplasma pneumoniae* infections. However, they are usually negative until the fifth or sixth day of illness. Detection of IgM to hepatitis A virus (HAVIgM) does provide rapid diagnosis (**86**) since this antibody appears at the time the patient becomes jaundiced.

Detection of rising titre

A variety of techniques is available to detect specific antiviral antibodies. Complement fixation (**87**) is a tried and tested method. However, it suffers from somewhat lower sensitivity, it is technically challenging and, of course, detects

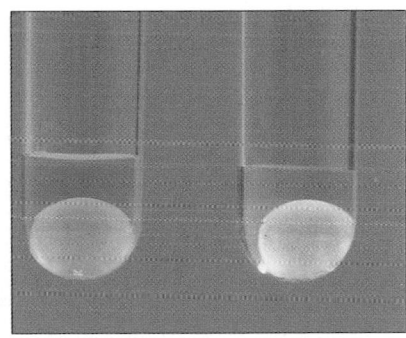

86 Detection of hepatitis A virus IgM. The bead is coated with anti-IgM. It is placed in the patient's serum, where it traps IgM. The bead is then placed in a solution containing enzyme-linked HAV antigen. If the patient has HAV IgM then the bead will trap the antigen–enzyme complex. Finally, the complex is placed in a solution of the appropriate substrate. A positive result in seen by the development of a coloured product.

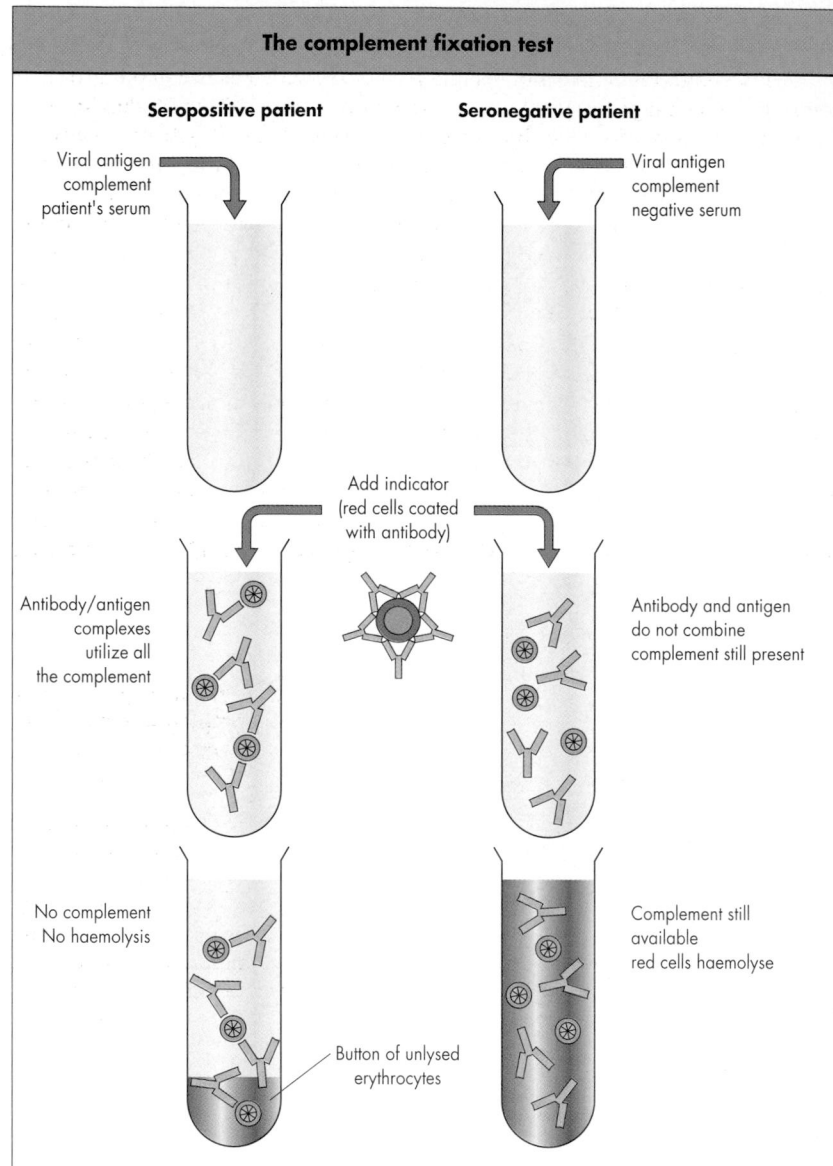

The complement fixation test

Seropositive patient **Seronegative patient**

Viral antigen
complement
patient's serum

Viral antigen
complement
negative serum

Add indicator
(red cells coated
with antibody)

Antibody/antigen
complexes
utilize all
the complement

Antibody and antigen
do not combine
complement still present

No complement
No haemolysis

Complement still
available
red cells haemolyse

Button of unlysed
erythrocytes

87 The complement fixation test.

IgG and IgM antibodies combined. It is less and less used as a diagnostic tool but can still be of value (00).

Antibodies to influenza, mumps and parainfluenza viruses can bind to their respective haemagglutinin spikes and prevent the viruses from binding to their receptors (sialic acid) on erythrocytes. Thus levels of antibody to these viruses can be estimated by haemagglutination inhibition (**89**). For estimation of neutralizing antibodies their ability to prevent viral replication is measured. Not all antibodies produced in response to infection are neutralizing and the technique is primarily used for virus typing (e.g. differentiating ECHO viruses). ELISA is perhaps the most versatile and sensitive of the techniques. Two formats are available (**90**). In the first, viral antigen is coated onto the wells, to which dilutions of the sera are added. To detect binding of patient's serum to the antigen, anti-human antibody coupled to an appropriate enzyme is added. By using anti-human IgG-, IgA-, IgM- or even IgE- enzyme conjugates, the different classes of anti-viral antibody can be detected. In the second format, the wells are coated with anti-human IgA or IgM or IgG, which captures all the antibody of that class in the sample. The specific viral antigen is then added followed by an enzyme–antibody conjugate against the viral antigen. This method is most useful when antibody levels are relatively low, for example for detecting specific IgA, IgM, or IgG in saliva.

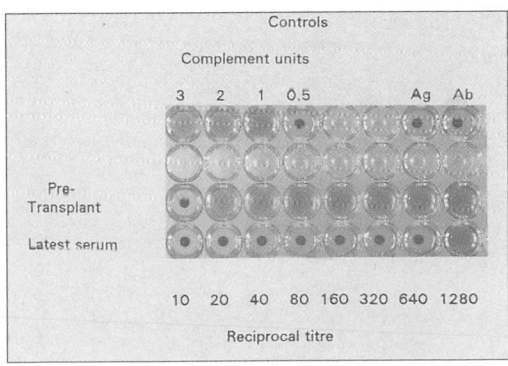

88 A WHO tray showing the complement fixation test. Haemolysis equals no antiviral antibody, lack of haemolysis indicates that antiviral antibody is present. The serum taken from the patient pre-transplant shows anti-CMV at a dilution of 1:10. The sample taken eight weeks post-transplant, during a rejection episode, shows the titre has risen to 1:640.

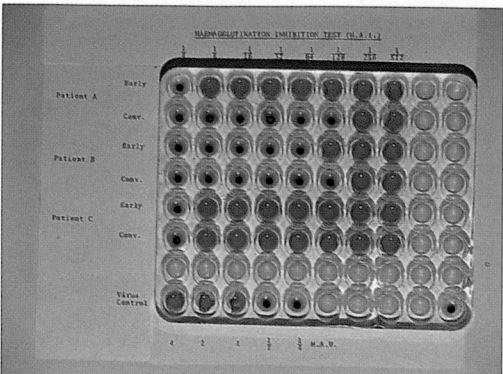

89 A haemagglutination inhibition test. A button of cells in the well indicates that the erythrocytes have not been agglutinated by influenza virus because specific antibody is present. Patient A shows an HAI titre of 1: 4 during the early part of his illness but three weeks later the titre has risen to 1:128.

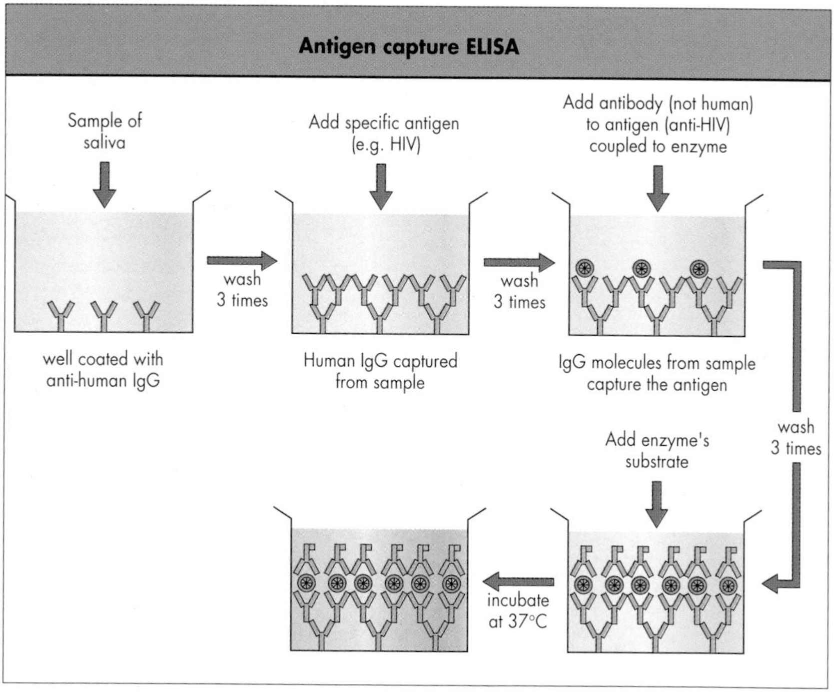

Antigen capture ELISA

Sample of saliva

Add specific antigen (e.g. HIV)

Add antibody (not human) to antigen (anti-HIV) coupled to enzyme

wash 3 times

wash 3 times

well coated with anti-human IgG

Human IgG captured from sample

IgG molecules from sample capture the antigen

wash 3 times

Add enzyme's substrate

incubate at 37°C

90 ELISA for detection of antiviral antibody. The antibody capture format provides a more sensitive assay for IgG, IgM or IgA in saliva.

4.
Bacteria and Disease

Infections due to bacteria are responsible for diseases ranging from a mild tonsillitis to epidemics of cholera and plague. Bacteria are remarkably adaptable micro-organisms. They may cause severe disease or innocently colonize the skin. They may survive and multiply in the environment and they may form spores which can survive for decades. Some bacteria are primarily parasites of animals, only infecting humans as a chance event. Others can only survive by intimate contact with their human host. While most bacteria replicate in hours or days, some are much slower growers, leading to chronic infections and difficulties in treatment. As well as diversity in their ecology, bacteria have the potential for variation in their genetic composition. Many bacteria contain plasmid DNA, which enables the transfer of genetic material both within and between species. This genetic adaptability can enhance both pathogenic mechanisms and resistance to antimicrobial agents.

BACTERIAL STRUCTURE

Bacteria are prokaryocytes, their DNA not being localized within a nucleus (**91**). Many bacteria contain extrachromosomal DNA circles termed plasmids. Within the cytoplasm there are no organelles other than ribosomes, which are smaller in size than in eukaryotic cells. Bacteria, other than mycoplasma, are surrounded by a complex cell wall, which differs between Gram-positive and Gram-negative bacteria. Many bacteria have flagella, pili or capsules external to the cell wall.

Both Gram-positive and Gram-negative bacteria have a plasma membrane formed by a lipid bilayer together with proteins. In both, the principal structural component of the cell wall is a three-dimensional framework of the polysaccharides N-acetylglucosamine and N-acetylmuramic acid and amino acids termed peptidoglycan.

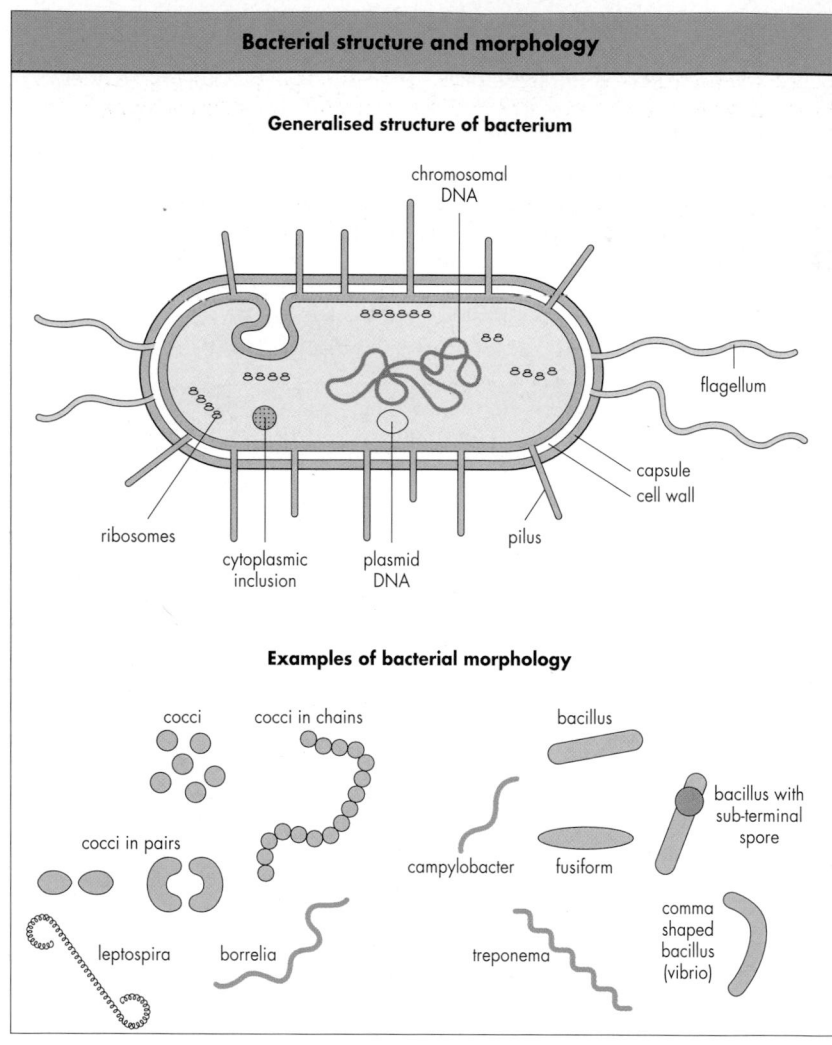

Bacterial structure and morphology

Generalised structure of bacterium

chromosomal DNA

flagellum

capsule
cell wall

pilus

ribosomes

cytoplasmic inclusion

plasmid DNA

Examples of bacterial morphology

cocci

cocci in chains

bacillus

bacillus with sub-terminal spore

cocci in pairs

campylobacter

fusiform

comma shaped bacillus (vibrio)

leptospira

borrelia

treponema

91 Bacterial structure and morphology.

In Gram-positive bacteria, the cell wall consists almost exclusively of this peptidoglycan layer with attached teichoic acid polymers (**92**). Gram-negative bacteria have a more complex cell wall. The peptidoglycan layer is thinner than in Gram-positives and is surrounded by an outer membrane comprised of

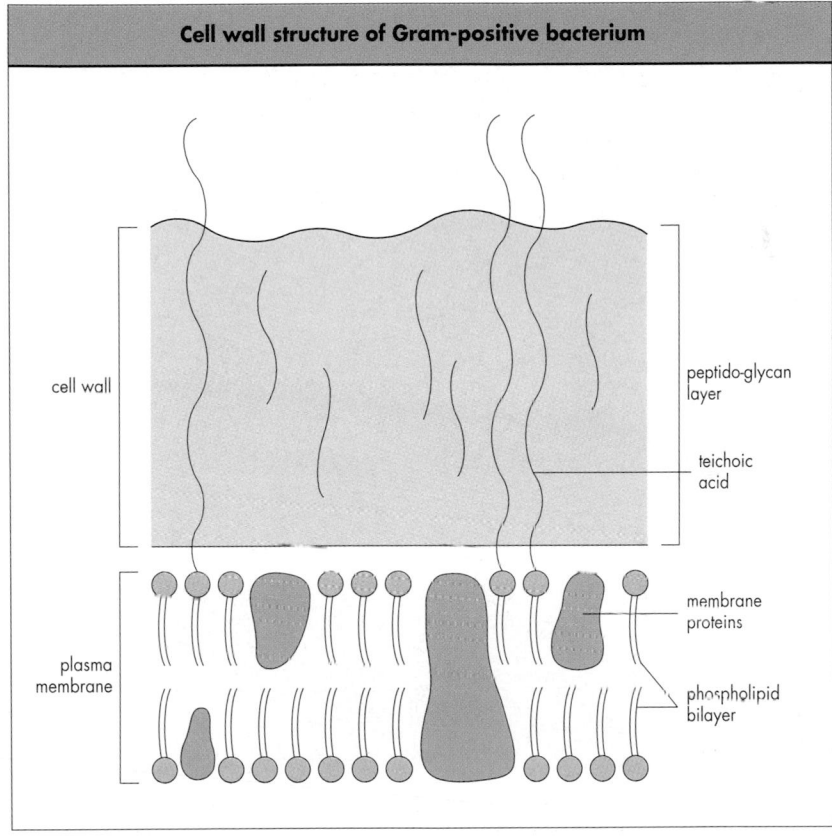

Cell wall structure of Gram-positive bacterium

cell wall

peptido-glycan layer

teichoic acid

membrane proteins

plasma membrane

phospholipid bilayer

92   Cell wall structure of Gram-positive bacterium.

lipopolysaccharides and lipoproteins (**93**). This lipopolysaccharide component of the Gram-negative cell wall constitutes the endotoxin molecules that contribute to bacterial pathogenesis.

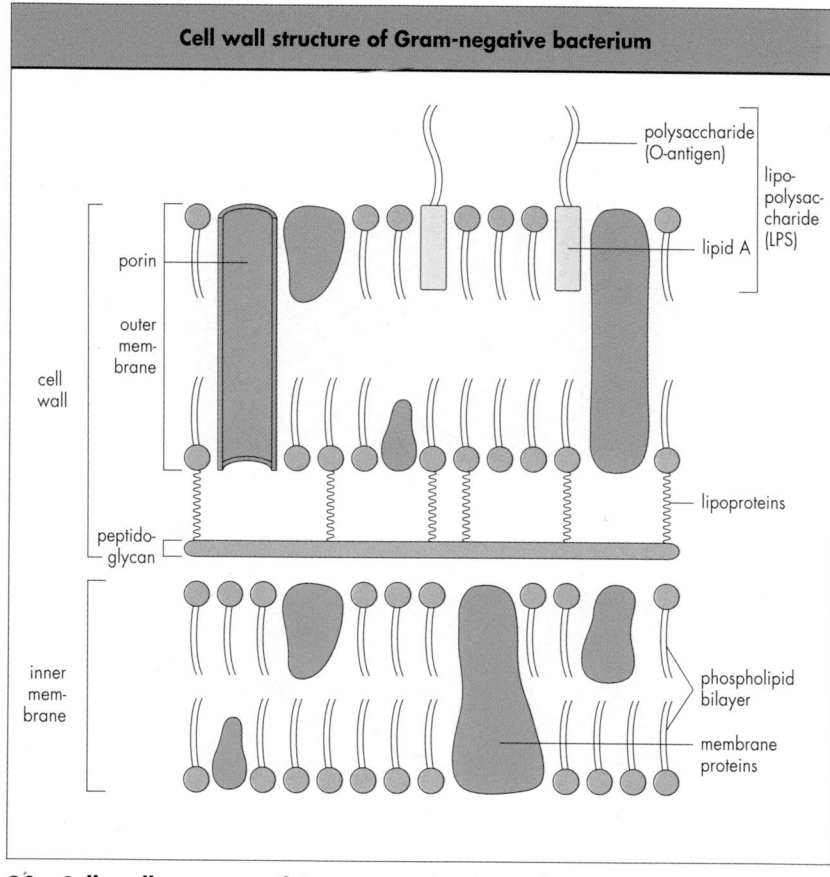

93 Cell wall structure of Gram-negative bacteria.

BACTERIAL CLASSIFICATION AND CULTURE

The shape of bacteria, and their staining properties, form the basis for classification. Bacteria may be spherical (cocci) rod-shaped (bacilli) or intermediate (cocco-bacilli). Most bacteria can be stained by the Gram reaction, Gram-positive bacteria being blue/purple and Gram-negative bacteria pink. Mycobacteria (e. g. *M. tuberculosis*) are stained by the Ziehl–Neelsen technique, the stained bacteria being pink.

94–97 show the classification of the medically important bacteria, many of which are illustrated in the following sections.

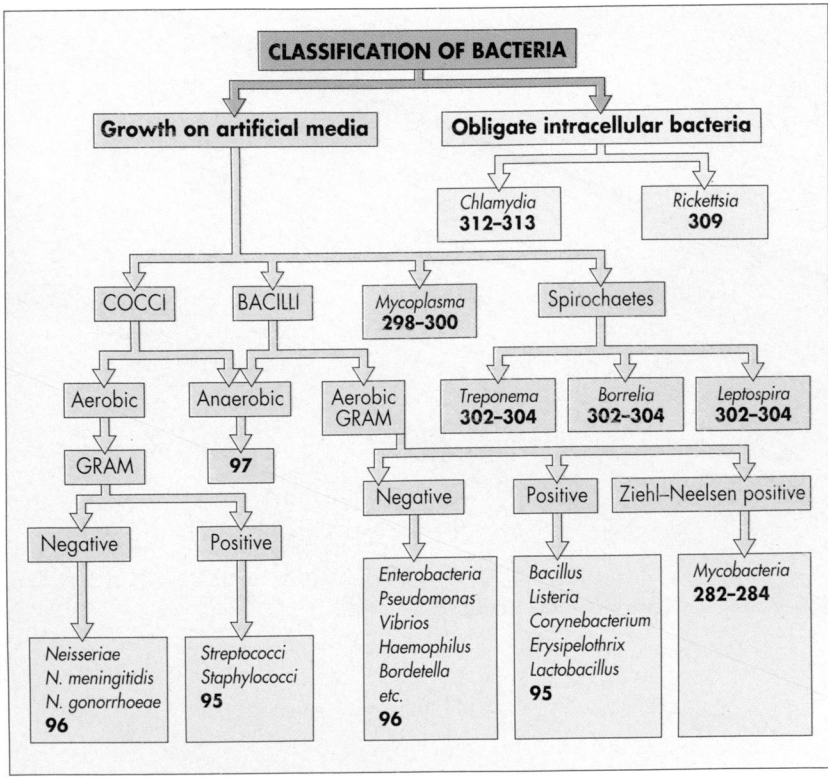

94 Classification of bacteria.

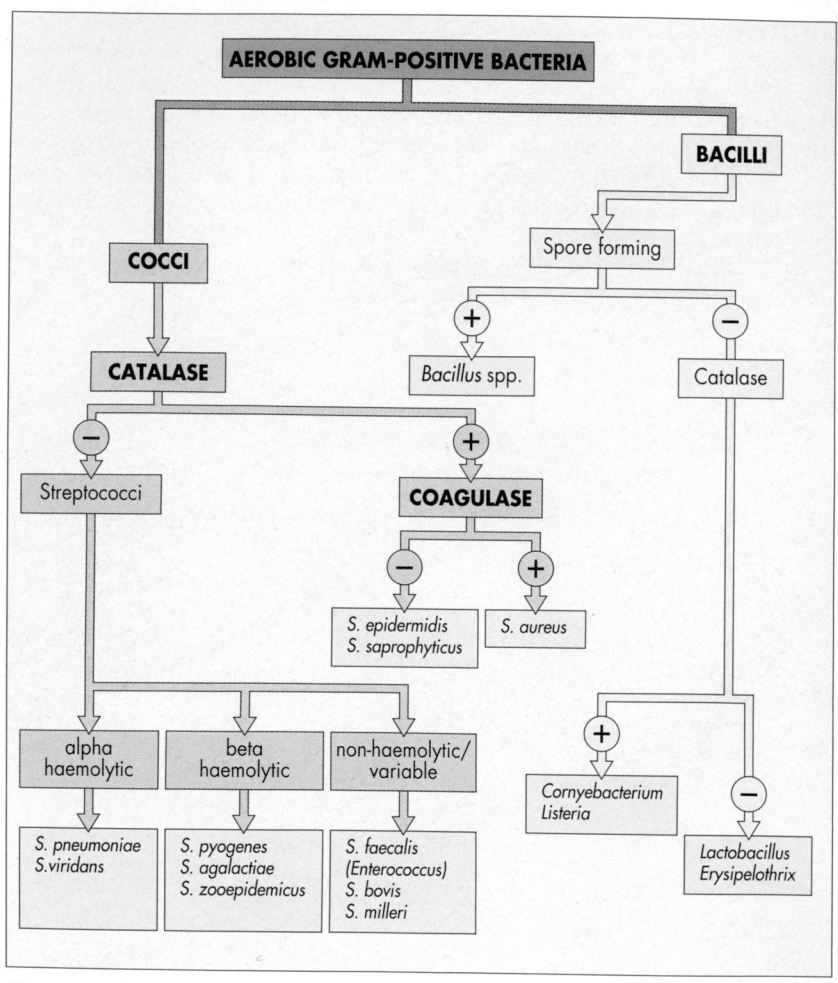

95 Aerobic Gram-positive bacteria.

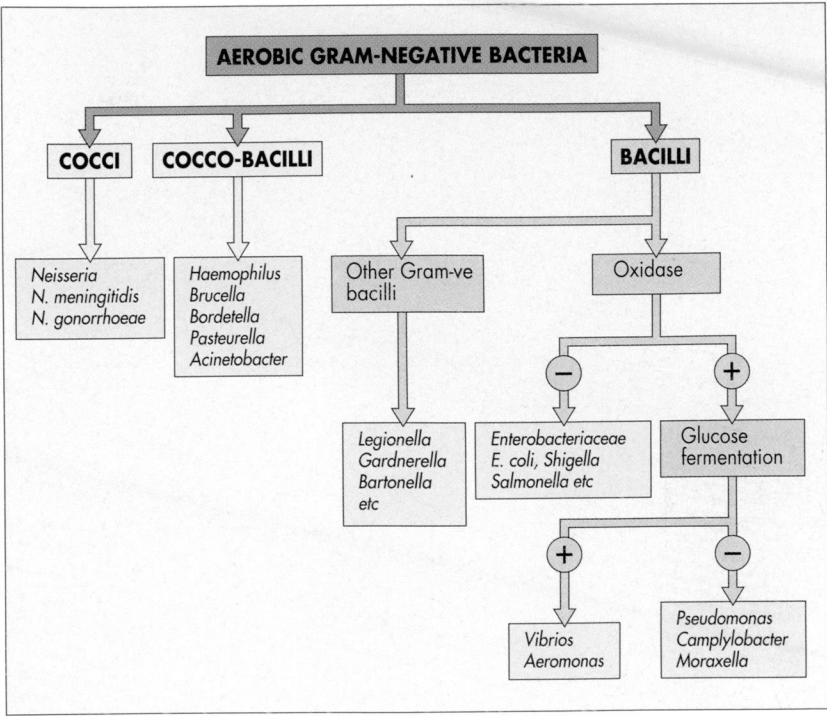

96 Aerobic Gram-negative bacteria.

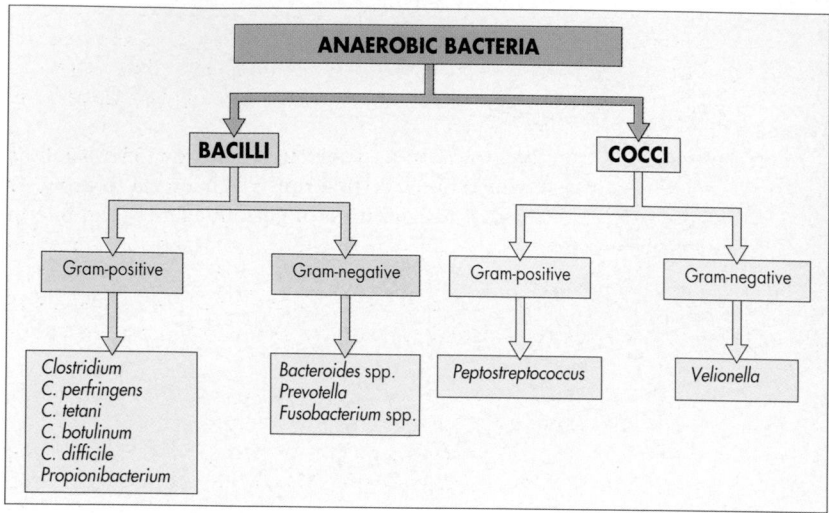

97 Anaerobic bacteria.

Most bacteria can be grown on artificial culture media, which provide the necessary nutrients for growth. Some bacteria are obligate intracellular parasites (such as the *Rickettsiae*, *Chlamydiae* and *Coxiella*) and can only be cultivated in vivo or in cell culture systems.

Cultivable bacteria may be grown on non-selective culture media, such as nutrient agar or blood agar, which allow a wide range of bacteria to grow, or selective media which, because of the addition of certain agents (e.g. bile in MacConkey media) or antibiotics (e.g. vancomycin, colistin) allow only certain bacteria to grow. Some bacteria are obligate anaerobes and will only grow in an atmosphere devoid of oxygen. In the diagnostic laboratory, different media and culture conditions are used to isolate particular bacteria from clinical specimens (**98**).

While some bacteria may be identified presumptively by characteristic microscopy and culture appearances (e.g. *Vibrio cholerae, Neisseria meningitidis*) further tests are usually necessary to confirm identification. Many of these tests are biochemical, where bacteria with similar Gram and cultural appearance can be distinguished by carbohydrate fermentation or other biochemical tests (**99**). In some bacteria (e.g. *Salmonella* spp., *N. meningitidis*) sub-types may be distinguished by antigenic differences, determined by agglutination with specific antisera (**100**).

Bacterial culture media		
Medium	Major ingredients	Uses
Blood agar	Nutrient agar + 5% horse or sheep blood	Non-selective medium for a wide range of non-fastidious Gram-negative and Gram-positive bacteria.
Buffered charcoal yeast extract (BCYE) agar	Yeast extract, charcoal, L-cysteine, HCl, α-ketoglutarate	Selective for *Legionella* spp.
Campylobacter medium	Nutrient agar base with vancomycin, trimethoprim, amphotericin	Selective medium for *Campylobacter* spp.
Cefsoludin-irgasan-novobiocin (CIN) agar	Peptone base with antibiotic supplements	Selective medium for *Yersinia* spp.
Charcoal cephalexin blood (CCBA) agar	Charcoal agar, sheep blood, cephalexin	Selective medium for *Bordetella* spp.
Chocolate (heated blood) agar	Heated blood agar. The cells are lysed and specific growth factors released	Cultivation of *Haemophilus* and *Neisseria* spp.
Cycloserine-cefoxitin-fructose-agar (CCFA)	Egg yolk base with fructose and antibiotics	Selective medium for *Clostridium difficile*
Cystine-lactose-electrolyte deficient (CLED) agar	Peptone base with lactose and L-cystine. Bromothymol blue indicator inhibits swarming of *Proteus* spp.	Isolation of bacteria in urine
Deoxycholate-citrate agar (DCA)	Peptone agar base including lactose, deoxycholate and indicator neutral red	Selective medium for *Salmonella* and *Shigella*
Kanamycin blood agar	Blood agar base with kanamycin	Selective isolation of *Bacteroides* spp.
Kligler iron agar (KIA)	Peptone agar base with lactose, glucose, phenol red and ferric citrate	A differential slope medium to distinguish *Shigella* and *Salmonella* and other Enterobacteriaceae

98 Bacterial culture media.

Bacterial culture media (cont.)

Medium	Major ingredients	Uses
Löwenstein-Jensen (LJ) medium	Egg-based medium with malachite green	Selective medium for mycobacteria
MacConkey agar	Peptone base containing bile salts, lactose and neutral red. Lactose fermenters produce acid and thus pink colonies	A low selectivity medium for enteric bacteria that distinguishes lactose fermenters and non-lactose fermenters
Mannitol salt agar	Peptone base containing mannitol, sodium chloride and phenol red	Selective and differential medium for isolating *Staphylococcus aureus*
Modified New York City (MNYC) medium	Peptone base with yeast and haemoglobin, and antibiotics including vancomycin and colistin	A selective medium to isolate *Neisseria gonorrhoeae* from urogenital specimens
Salmonella-Shigella (SS) agar	Peptone-based medium containing bile salts, lactose, neutral red and ferric citrate	A selective medium to isolate *Salmonella* and *Shigella spp.*
Sorbitol-MacConkey agar	Peptone base containing bile salts, sorbitol and neutral red	Differentiation of non-sorbitol fermenting *Escherichia coli (E. coli 0157)*
Tellurite blood agar	Blood agar with potassium tellurite	Selective medium for *Corynebacterium diphtheriae* which reduces tellurite to form black colonies
Thayer-Martin agar	Blood agar base with supplements and antibiotics including colistin and vancomycin	Selective isolation of *Neisseria* spp.
Thiosulphate citrate bile salt (TCBS) agar	Peptone base including thiosulphate, citrate, sucrose and thymol-blue.	Selective medium for *Vibrio* spp. *V. cholerae* ferments sucrose and produces yellow colonies
Xylose lysine deoxycholate (XLD) agar	Yeast extract with lysine, xylose, lactose and ferric citrate	Selective and differential medium for *Shigella* (pink colonies) and *Salmonella* (pink/black colonies)

Biochemical tests for bacterial identification

Test	Test principle	Examples of use
Bile solubility	Bile salts dissolve *Streptococcus pneumoniae*.	To distinguish *S. pneumoniae* from other alpha-haemolytic streptococci.
Catalase	Catalase breaks down H_2O_2 to produce bubbles of oxygen.	To differentiate streptococci (negative) from staphylococci (positive).
Coagulase	The enzyme coagulase clots plasma.	To differentiate coagulase positive (*S. aureus*) and negative staphylococci.
Cooked meat medium	Saccharolytic reaction causes reddening of the meat. Proteolytic reaction causes blackening.	Distinguishes *Clostridium perfringens* (saccharolytic) from other clostridia.
DNA-ase	The enzyme deoxyribonuclease hydrolyses DNA. Unhydrolysed DNA forms a precipitate with HCL.	To distinguish *S. aureus* (positive) from other staphylococci.
Dye inhibition test	Growth of different *Brucella* spp. is inhibited by the dyes basic fuchsin and thionin.	To differentiate *Brucella* spp.
Hiss' serum sugars	Detection of growth and acid production from different carbohydrate substrates.	To differentiate *Corynebacterium* spp.
Indole test	Tryptophan is broken down with the release of indole which produces a red colour with Kovac's reagent.	To distinguish *Escherichia coli* from other Enterobacteriaceae.
Koser's citrate test	Growth in citrate medium produces alkaline conditions and the indicator changes from green to blue.	To differentiate bacteria that can use citrate as a sole carbon source.
Lactose egg-yolk medium	Detects lecithinase activity, lactose fermentation, lipase hydrolysis and proteinase activity.	Differentiation of *Clostridium* spp.
Litmus milk decolorization	Enzymatic reduction and decolorization of litmus milk.	Identification of enterococci (positive) and some clostridia.

99 Biochemical tests for bacterial identification.

Biochemical tests for bacterial identification (cont.)

Test	Test principle	Examples of use
Methyl red test	Production of acid in glucose fermentation sufficient to give a red colour with the indicator methyl red.	Distinguishes *Escherichia coli* and *Enterobacter* spp.
Nagler reaction	Detects production of lecithinase and opacity in egg-yolk agar.	Distinguishes *C. perfringens* from other clostridia.
Neisseria carbohydrate fermentation tests	Detects fermentation of glucose, maltose and lactose in *Neisseria* spp.	Differentiates *N. gonorrhoeae* (glucose only) from *N. meningitidis* (glucose and maltose) from other *Neisseria*.
Nitrate reduction test	The enzyme nitrate reductase reduces nitrate to nitrite.	Differentiates nitrate positive Enterobacteriaceae from other Gram-negative bacteria.
Oxidase test	Oxidase enzymes oxidize phenylenediamine producing a blue colour.	Assists in the identification of oxidase positive bacteria, e.g. vibrios, *Neisseriae*.
Oxidation-fermentation test	Organisms are incubated in a medium containing glucose (to test for oxidation) and anaerobic (to test for fermentation) conditions	Distinguishes organisms that oxidize glucose (e.g. *Pseudomonas*) from fermenters (e.g. Enterobacteriaceae).
Peptone water sugars	A series of peptone waters containing different carbohydrates as substrates.	To distinguish different members of the Enterobacteriaceae.
Phenylalanine deaminase	Phenylalanine is broken down to produce phenylpyruvic acid which produces a green colour with ferric chloride.	Differentiates *Proteus* (positive) from other Enterobacteriaceae.
Urease test	Urease-producing bacteria hydrolyse urea producing ammonia, which changes the indicator phenol red to a red colour.	Differentiates *Proteus* (positive) from other Enterobacteriaceae.
Voges-Proskauer (VP) test	Some bacteria ferment glucose with the production of acetoin, which is detected by producing a pink colour with creatinine.	Distinguishes VP positive Enterobacteria e.g. *Klebsiella pneumoniae* from VP negative, e.g. *Escherichia coli*.
X and V test	Some bacteria will only grow in the presence of porphyrin (X) and/or NAD (V).	Differentiation of *Haemophilus* spp.

Examples of bacterial sub-typing based on antigenic properties

Bacteria	Typing system	Antigens detected
Beta haemolytic streptococci	Lancefield grouping	Group specific cell wall carbohydrates; groups A, B, C, D, G most commonly found in human infections.
Group A beta haemolytic streptococci	Griffith's typing	Cell wall M proteins differentiate Group A streptococci and determine virulence.
Streptococcus pneumoniae	Serotyping	Capsular polysaccharides distinguish over 80 serotypes.
Neisseria meningitidis	Serogroups	Capsular polysaccharides distinguish 13 serogroups, the major human pathogens being A, B, C, W135.
N. meningitidis	Sub-types	Class 2 and 3 outer membrane proteins, e.g. Serogroup B, type 15.
N. meningitidis	Serotypes (Frasch typing)	Class 1 outer membrane proteins give further differentiation particularly in Group B.
Haemophilus influenzae	Pittman types	Capsular polysaccharides distinguish 6 types, a–f. Type b responsible for most invasive infections.
Salmonella spp.	Kaufman–White scheme	Classification of salmonellae based on O (somatic) and H (flagellar) antigens.
Shigella spp.	Serogroups and serotypes	O antigens define the four major groups: A, *S. dysenteriae*; B, *S. flexneri*; C, *S. boydii*; and D, *S. sonnei*; and serotypes within groups A, B, C.
Vibrio cholerae	Serogrouping	Somatic (O) antigens. Serogroups 01 and 0139 cause cholera.
V. cholerae 01	Subtyping	01 antigens A,B,C distinguish Ogawa, Inaba and Hikojima subtypes.

100   Examples of bacterial sub-typing based on antigenic properties.

AEROBIC GRAM-POSITIVE BACTERIA

AEROBIC GRAM-POSITIVE COCCI

Characteristics of Gram-positive cocci are summarized in **101–103** and **113–115**.

Organism	Major infection	Less common infection	Vaccine Preventable	Incubation Period	Period of Infectivity
Gram-positive cocci Infections					
Staphylococci *S. epidermidis*	Bacteraemia in immunocompromised	Most commonly associated with indwelling devices	No	–	–
S. saprophyticus	Urinary tract infections		No	–	–
S. aureus	Boils, impetigo, wound infections, osteomyelitis, septicaemia	Pneumonia, endocarditis, toxic shock syndrome, food poisoning	No	–	–
Micrococcus	Occasional contaminant of clinical specimens.				
Streptococci **a) beta haemolytic**					
S. pyogenes (Group A)	tonsillitis, impetigo, cellulitis, scarlet fever (rheumatic fever, glomerulonephritis)	puerperal sepsis, erysipelas, septicaemia	No	1–3 days	–
S. agalactiae (Group B)	neonatal sepsis	puerperal sepsis osteomyelitis	No	–	–
S. zooepidemicus (Group C)	bacteraemia		No	–	–

101 Gram-positive cocci. Infections.

Gram-positive cocci
Sources and transmission of bacteria

Organism	Man	Reservoir			Transmission			Comments
		Animal	Env.	Faecal/oral	Droplet	Direct	Nosocomial	
Staphylococcus epidermidis	+	–	–	–	–	+	+	
S. saprophyticus	+	–	–	–	–	+	–	
S. aureus	+	+	±	+	+	+	+	Methicillin-resistant strains important hospital problem
Micrococci	+	–	+	–	–	+	±	
Streptococcus pyogenes	+	–	–	–	+	+	+	
S. agalactiae	+	–	–	–	+	+	–	
S. zooepidemicus	+	+		+	±	–	–	Outbreaks have occurred from unpasteurized milk

102 Gram-positive cocci. Sources and transmission of bacteria.

Gram-positive cocci
Identifying characteristics

Organism	Gram	Culture on blood agar	Biochemical	Other tests
Staphylococcus epidermidis	+ve cocci	pale colonies	catalase +ve	coagulase –ve, mannitol +ve
S. saprophyticus	+ve cocci	pale colonies	catalase +ve	coagulase –ve, mannitol +ve
S. aureus	+ve cocci	yellow colonies	catalase +ve	coagulase +ve
Micrococci	+ve cocci	yellow/orange colonies	catalase +ve	coagulase –ve, bacitracin sensitive
Streptococcus pyogenes	+ve cocci in chains	beta haemolytic	catalase –ve	bacitracin sensitive
S. agalactiae	+ve cocci	beta haemolytic	catalase –ve	CAMP +ve
S. zooepidemicus	+ve cocci	beta haemolytic	catalase –ve	Lancefield group C

103 Gram-positive cocci. Identifying characteristics.

Staphylococci

Staphylococci are a major component of the normal human flora but also include species that are important pathogens. On staining, they appear as Gram-positive cocci in clusters (**104, 105, 106**). **107** and **108** show the cultural appearances of *S. epidermidis* and *S. aureus* on blood agar.

The coagulase test is used to distinguish *S. aureus* (coagulase positive) from the other staphylococci (**109**). Staphylococci can also be distinguished by testing for DNA-ase production. *S. aureus* is DNA-ase positive (**110**).

Selective media, such as mannitol salt agar, may be used for culturing *S. aureus* when screening cases for carriage in epidemiological studies (**111**). **112** shows a culture of micrococcus on blood agar. They are Gram-positive cocci that are rarely of clinical significance.

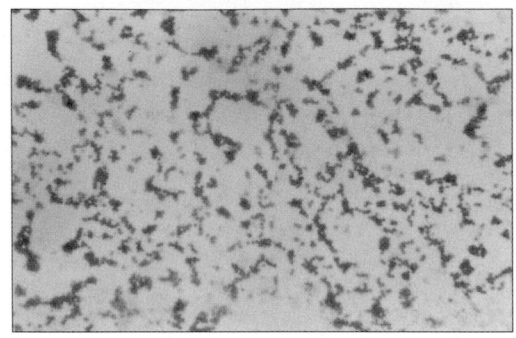

104 *Staphylococcus aureus*. Gram stain showing the typical Gram-positive cocci in clusters. *S. aureus* is an important pathogen, causing skin infections, osteomyelitis, septicaemia and pneumonia. *S. aureus* is coagulase positive. *(Gram, x1000)*

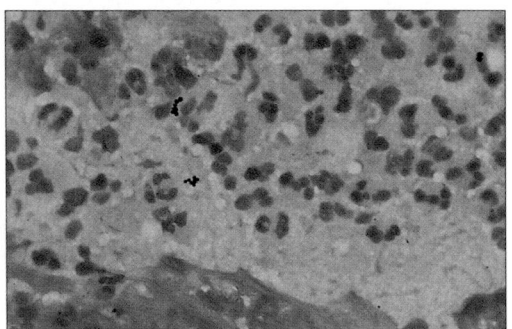

105 *Staphylococcus aureus*. Gram stain of blood culture from a patient with septicaemia caused by *S. aureus*. Staphylococcal septicaemia may result from infection of a minor injury. *(Gram, x1000)*

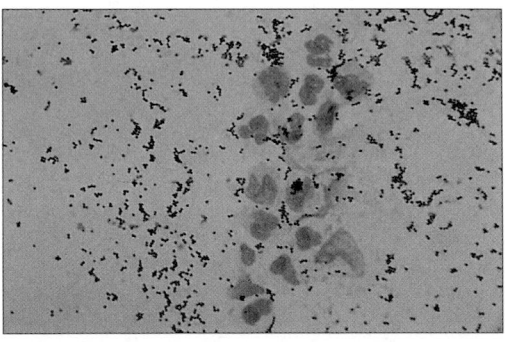

106 *Staphylococcus aureus*. Gram stain of pus from patient with a wound infected with *S. aureus*. Note the Gram-positive cocci and the pink coloured pus cells. *(Gram, x1000)*.

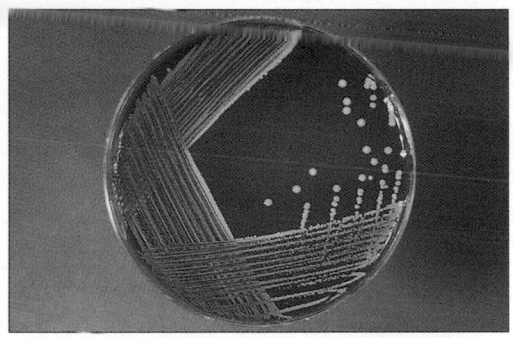

107 Staphylococcus epidermidis. Culture on blood agar, showing white colonies. *S. epidermidis* is one of the coagulase negative staphylococci. They are part of the normal skin flora, but may cause infection in neonates, the immunocompromised, and in patients with indwelling devices. *(Blood agar, 18 h at 37°C)*

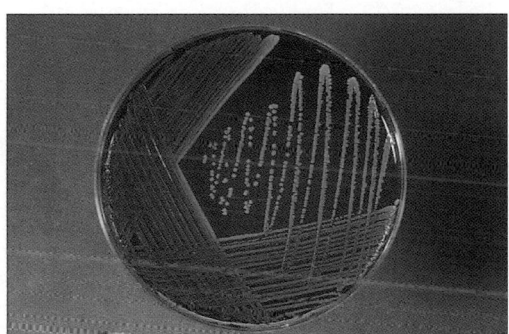

108 Staphylococcus aureus. Culture on blood agar. *S. aureus* are typically yellow or golden colonies in contrast to the pale colonies of *S. epidermidis* and other coagulase negative staphylococci. *(Blood agar, 18 h at 37°C)*

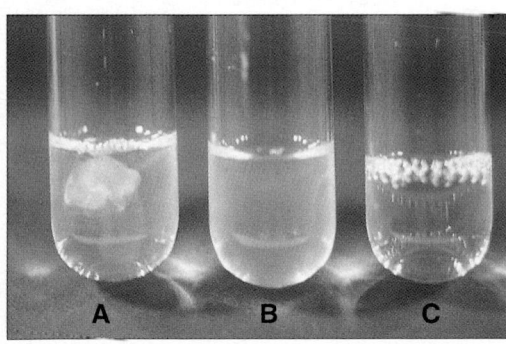

109 Tube coagulase test. *S. aureus* produces coagulase which clots plasma. A few drops of a broth culture of the test organism is added to 1:10 diluted plasma in saline and incubated for 2 h at 37°C). Coagulase positive *S. aureus* (**A**), coagulase negative *S. epidermidis* (**B**). A negative control tube is included (**C**). *(2 h at 37°C)*

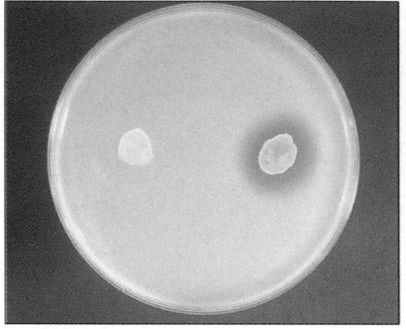

110 DNA-ase test. Coagulase positive and negative staphylococci can be distinguished by testing for DNA-ase production. After overnight incubation on a medium containing DNA, the plate is flooded with weak hydrochloric acid. The acid precipitates unhydrolysed DNA. DNA-ase producing colonies are surrounded by clear areas where DNA has been hydrolysed. *S. aureus* is DNA-ase producing. *(DNA-ase agar, 18 h at 37°C)*

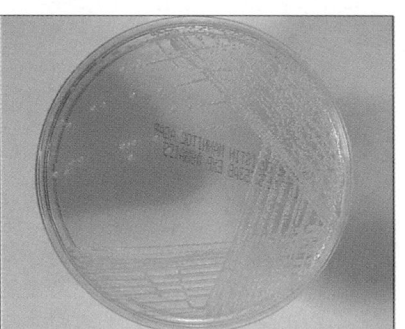

111 *Staphylococcus aureus.* Culture on mannitol salt agar, showing yellow colonies. This is a selective medium for recovering *S. aureus* when screening for carriage in infection control investigations. *(Mannitol salt agar, 18 h at 37°C)*

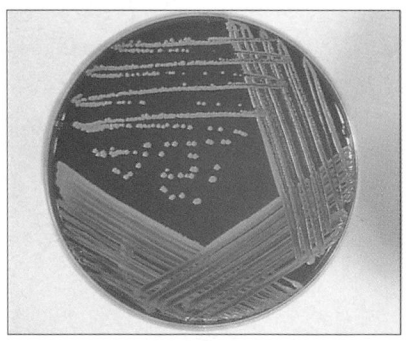

112 *Micrococcus.* Culture on blood agar, showing pale yellow colonies. Micrococci may occur as contaminants in clinical specimens. *(Blood agar, 18 h at 37°C)*

Organism	Major infection	Less common infection	Vaccine preventable	Incubation period	Period of infectivity
Gram-positive cocci Infections					
Streptococci (Cont. from **101**)					
b) alpha haemolytic					
S. pneumoniae	pneumonia, otitis media	meningitis, septicaemia	Yes (some serotypes)	—	—
S. viridans	dental caries	sub-acute bacterial endocarditis	No	—	—
c) Group D streptococci					
S. faecalis (enterococci) (*Enterococcus faecalis*)	urinary tract infections, wound infections, intra-abdominal abscess	bacteraemia endocarditis	No	—	—
S. bovis	endocarditis, bacteraemia		No	—	—
Other streptococci					
S. milleri	intra-abdominal sepsis, wound infections brain abscess	—	No	—	—

113 Gram-positive cocci. Infections (cont. from **101**).

Gram-positive cocci Sources and transmission of bacteria							
	Reservoir			Transmission			
Organism	Man	Animal	Env.	Faecal oral	Droplet	Direct	Nosocomial	Comments
S. pneumoniae	+	–	–	–	+	–	–	Penicillin resistant strains increasing
S. viridans	+	–	–	–	+/–	+	–	
E. faecalis	+	–	–	–	–	+	+	Occasional vancomycin resistant strains
S. bovis	+	+	–	–	–	+	–	
S. milleri	+	–	–	–	–	+	+	

114 Gram-positive cocci. Sources and transmission of bacteria.

Gram-positive cocci Identifying characteristics			
Organism	Gram	Culture on blood agar	Biochemical and other tests
Streptococcus pneumoniae	positive cocci in pairs	alpha haemolytic 'draughtsman colonies'	optochin sensitive, positive bile solubility
S. viridans	positive cocci	alpha haemolytic	optochin resistant, negative bile solubility
E. faecalis	positive cocci	variable haemolysis	grows on MacConkey medium, positive litmus milk test
S. bovis	positive cocci	variable haemolysis	no growth in 6.5% NaCl medium
S. milleri	positive cocci	small, beta-haemolytic colonies	Voges –Proskauer test positive

115 Gram-positive cocci. Identifying characteristics.

Streptococci

Streptococci are Gram-positive cocci that can be distinguished from staphylococci by the catalase test (**116**).

S. pyogenes, a pathogen responsible for a range of superficial and deep infections, is seen as chains of cocci in Gram stained preparations (**117**). **118** shows a Gram stain of *S. agalactiae* (Group B streptococcus) from a blood culture of a neonate with septicaemia.

Streptococci may be classified according to their haemolysis when cultured on blood agar. **119** shows beta (clear) haemolysis produced by *S. pyogenes*.

Beta haemolytic streptococci are divided into Lancefield groups, depending on cell wall polysaccharide antigens (**120**). *S. pyogenes* is Lancefield group A and *S. agalactiae* Lancefield group B.

Alpha haemolysis is a partial haemolysis producing a greenish zone around the colonies. *S. pneumoniae* (**121**) and *S. viridans* (**122**) show alpha haemolysis. These plates contain optochin discs which distinguish *S. pneumoniae* (optochin sensitive) from other alpha haemolytic streptococci. *S. pneumoniae* may also be distinguished by the bile solubility test (**123**). *S. pneumoniae* shows characteristic diplococci on Gram staining (**124** and **125**).

Streptococci that grow in the intestine are now termed enterococci. They are able to grow on MacConkey medium that contains bile (**126**). Enterococci can be distinguished from other streptococci by a positive litmus milk decolorization reaction (**127**). *S. milleri* (**128**) is a micro-aerophilic streptococcus associated with abdominal and brain abscesses.

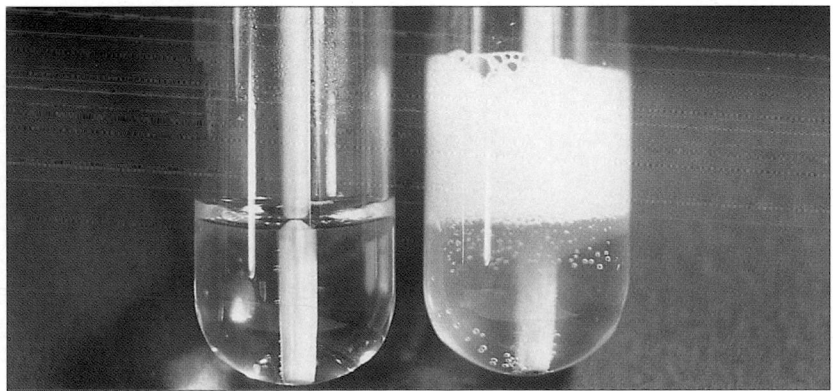

116 Catalase test. Staphylococci (catalase positive) and streptococci (catalase negative) can be distinguished by the catalase test. Catalase positive organisms break down hydrogen peroxide to oxygen and water. A small inoculum of the bacteria is added to a tube containing 2–3 ml H_2O_2. Active bubbling occurs with catalase positive organisms. Left, catalase negative; right, catalase positive *(1 min after mixing with H_2O_2).*

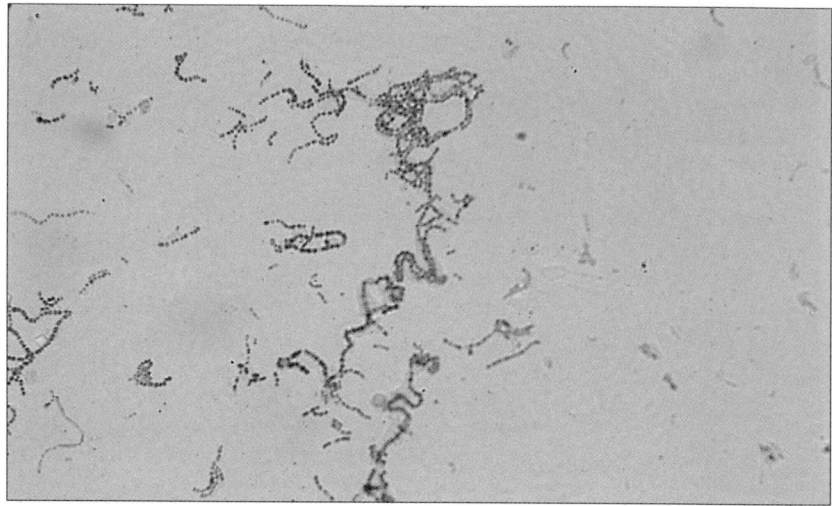

117   *Streptococcus pyogenes.* Gram stain showing typical Gram-positive cocci in chains. Streptococci of different Lancefield groups have a similar Gram appearance. *(Gram, x1000)*

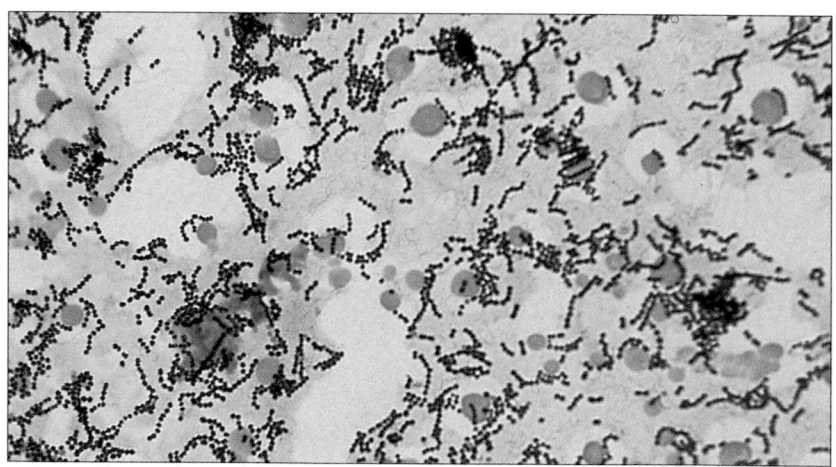

118   *Streptococcus agalactiae* (Lancefield group B). Gram stain showing Gram-positive cocci in a blood culture from a neonate. Group B streptococci are an important cause of neonatal sepsis and meningitis. *(Gram, x1000)*

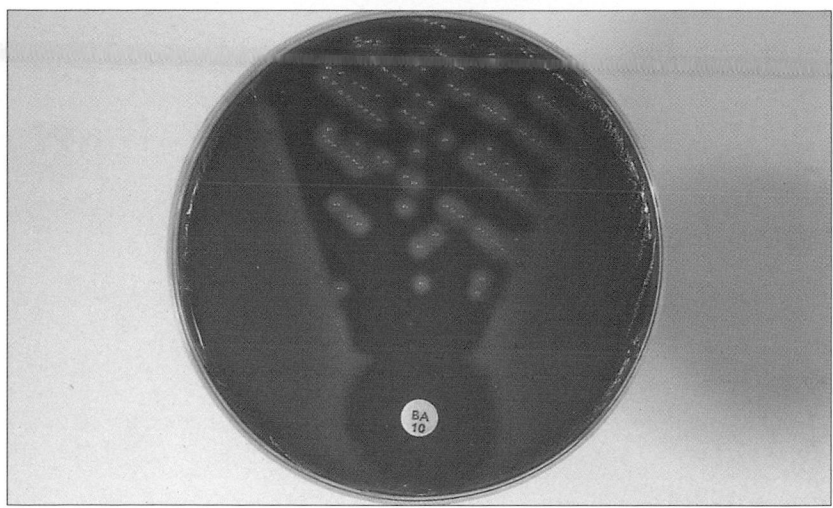

119 *Streptococcus pyogenes* culture. Cultured on blood agar, showing beta (clear) zones of haemolysis around the colonies. The plate also contains a bacitracin disk to which *S. pyogenes* (unlike most other beta haemolytic streptococci) is sensitive. *(Blood agar, 18 h at 37°C)*

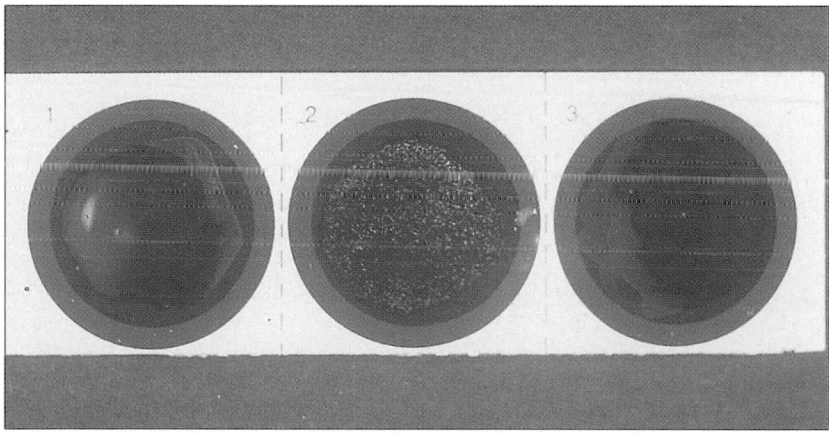

120 Lancefield grouping. Beta haemolytic streptococci are classified into Lancefield groups according to surface carbohydrate antigens. A slide agglutination test can be used with antisera to the different Lancefield groups. Positive agglutination with the appropriate antisera will determine the group. Positive agglutination in centre circle.
(Agglutination after 2 min at room temperature)

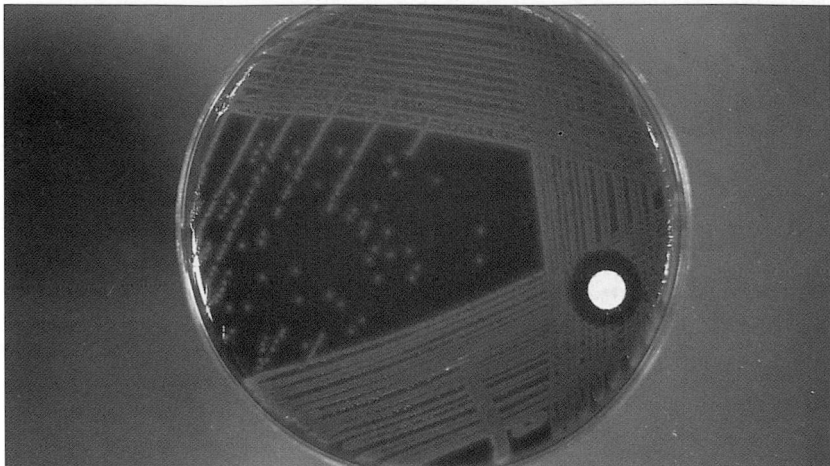

121 *Streptococcus pneumoniae.* Cultured on blood agar. Note the alpha (green) haemolysis and the 'draughtsman' shape of colonies. The plate contains an optochin disk, to which *S. pneumoniae* is sensitive, in contrast to other alpha haemolytic streptococci. *(Blood agar, 18 h at 37°C)*

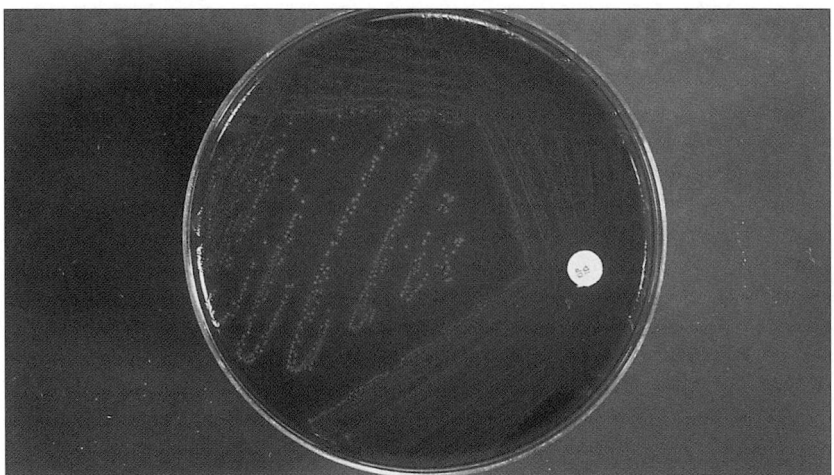

122 *Streptococcus viridans.* Culture on blood agar, showing alpha haemolysis and optochin resistance. Viridans streptococci are normal oral flora, but are an important cause of bacterial endocarditis in patients with congenital or acquired abnormalities of heart valves. *(Blood agar, 18 h at 37°C)*

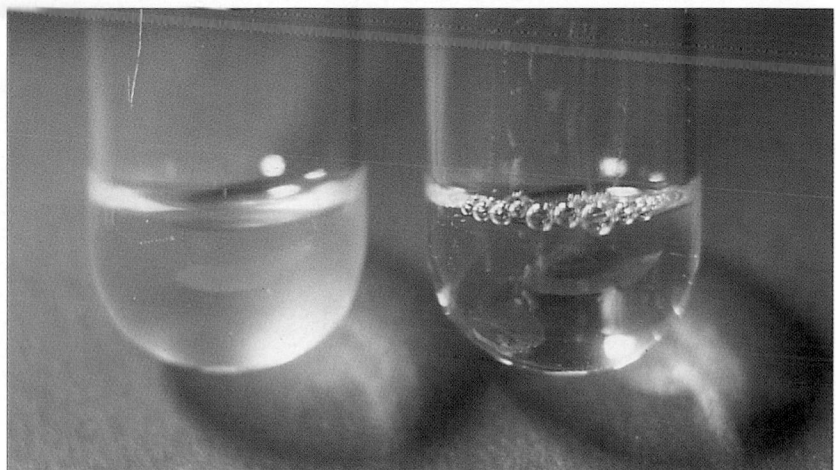

123 Bile solubility test. This is a further test for distinguishing pneumococci from other alpha haemolytic streptococci. A heavy inoculum of the test organism is emulsified in saline and the bile salt, sodium deoxycholate, added. The bile salt dissolves *S. pneumoniae* and clears the turbidity. Left, *S. viridans*; right, *S. pneumoniae*. *(Solubility demonstrated 3 min after the addition of bile salt)*

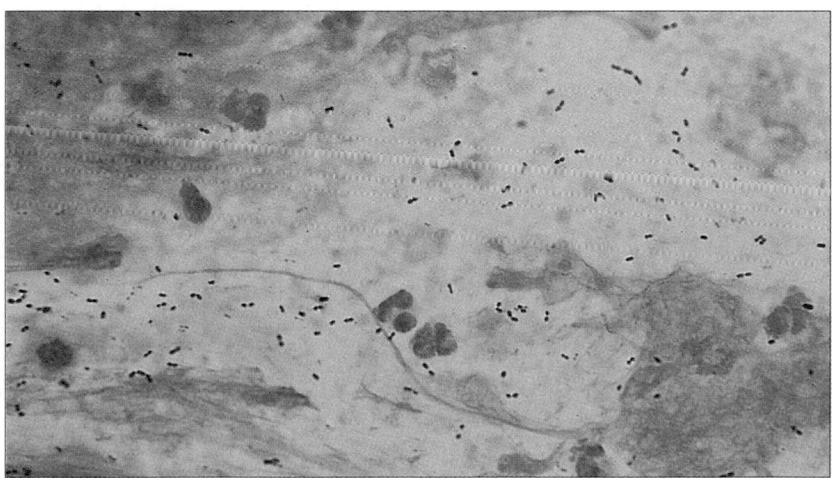

124 *Streptococcus pneumoniae.* Gram stain showing Gram-positive diplococci with a lanceolate shape typical of *Streptococcus pneumoniae* (pneumococcus). This is a Gram stain of sputum from a patient with pneumococcal pneumonia. *(Gram, x1000)*

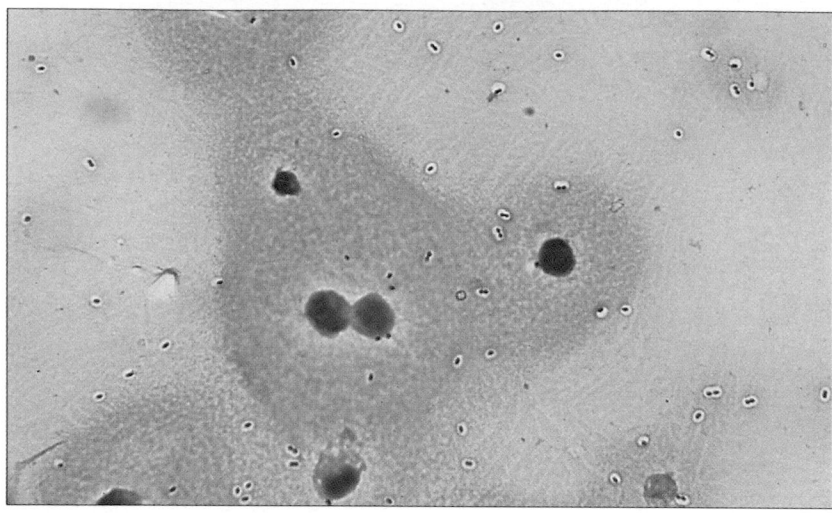

125 *Streptococcus pneumoniae.* Gram stain of the cerebro-spinal fluid of a patient with pneumococcal meningitis. The clear areas surrounding the diplococci are formed by the capsules. *(Gram, x1000)*

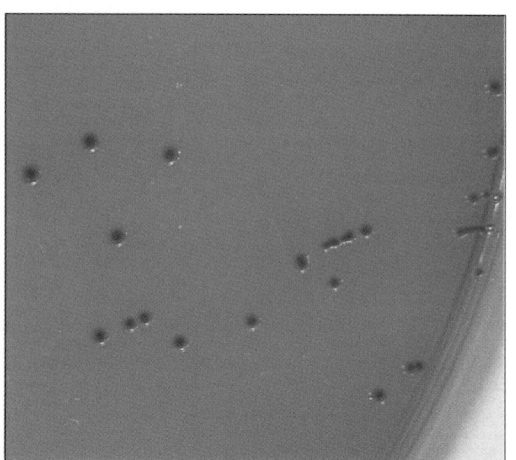

126 *Enterococcus faecalis.* Growth on MacConkey agar showing red dot colonies. Enterococci are a group of streptococci found in the human intestine. They will grow on MacConkey medium, unlike other streptococci. Enterococci are implicated in urinary tract infections, wound infections and bacterial endocarditis. *(MacConkey agar, 18 h at 37°C)*

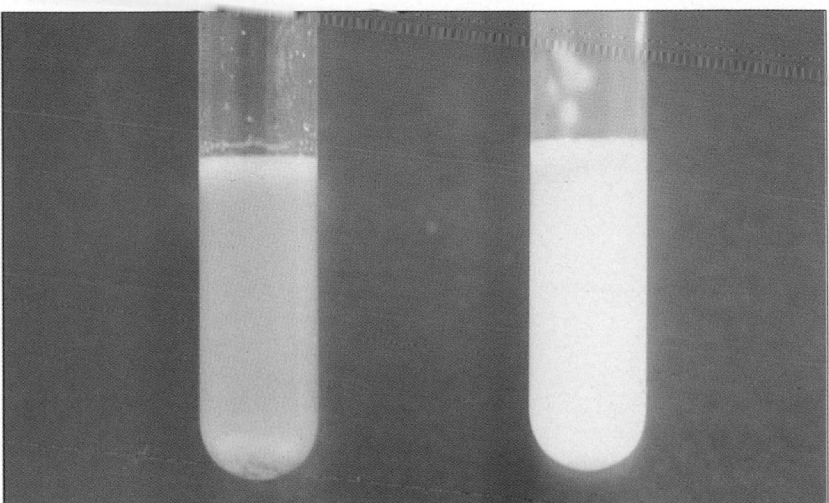

127 *Enterococcus faecalis.* Litmus milk decolorization test. The test organism is incubated for 4 h at 37 °C in the litmus milk reagent. Enterococci (right) decolorize the litmus. The negative control is *S. viridans.* *(4 h at 37°C)*

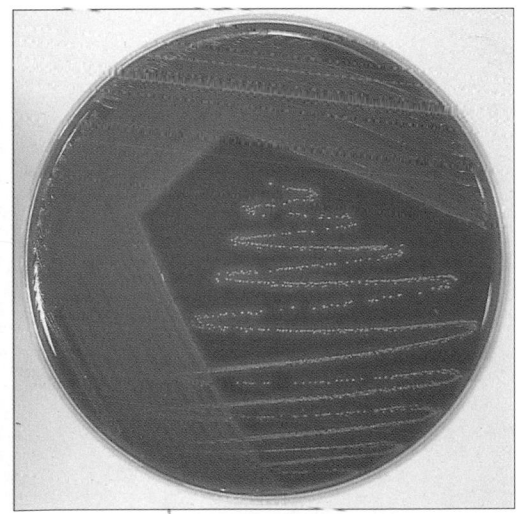

128 *Streptococcus milleri.* *S. milleri* is a commensal in the alimentary tract and is associated with intra abdominal abscesses. It produces small colonies on blood agar. *(Blood agar, 18 h at 37°C)*

AEROBIC GRAM-POSITIVE BACILLI

Characteristics of Gram-positive bacilli are summarized in **129–131**.

Bacillus spp.

Bacillus species are spore-forming Gram-positive bacilli. Many are non-pathogenic but *B. anthracis* is the cause of the disease anthrax. **132** shows anthrax bacilli stained by the McFadyean reaction and **133** shows *B. anthracis* cultured on blood agar. *B. cereus* is a cause of food poisoning (**134**). It can be cultured on the selective medium—mannitol, egg yolk, phenol red, polymyxin agar (MYPA) (**135**).

Listeria spp.

Listeria monocytogenes is a cause of infection in neonates and the immuno-compromised. It is a small Gram-positive bacillus (**136**) and produces pale colonies on blood agar (**137**).

Aerobic Gram-positive bacilli Infections					
Organism	Major infection	Less common infection	Vaccine preventable	Incubation period	Period of infectivity
a) Spore forming **Bacillus**					
B. anthracis	Anthrax		(Yes)	2–5 days	—
B. cereus	Food poisoning	Wound infections, endocarditis	No		
b) Non spore forming **Listeria**					
L. monocytogenes	Neonatal sepsis, meningitis	Septicaemia in immunocompromised	No	3 days – 3 weeks	
Corynebacterium					
C. diphtheriae	Diphtheria	Skin infections	Yes	2–5 days	Up to 4 weeks
C. urealyticum	Cystitis				
C. jeikeium	Infection associated with prosthetic devices and intravenous or csf catheters		No		
Erysipelothrix					
E. rhusiopathiae	Erysipeloid	Bacteraemia, endocarditis	No	—	—
Lactobacillus spp.	—	Rarely associated with endocarditis, abscesses	No	—	—

129 **Aerobic Gram-positive bacilli.** Infections.

Corynebacterium spp.

C. diphtheriae is the cause of diphtheria. Neisser staining shows the meta-chromatic volutin granules in diphtheria bacilli (**138**). Gram staining of *Corynebacteria* shows small Gram-positive rods, often arranged as 'Chinese lettering'(**139**). *C. diphtheria* is divided into three biotopes: gravis, intermedius and mitis. All produce black colonies on tellurite medium (**140**). There is some variation in the colonial appearance of the different biotopes (**141–143**). Only toxigenic strains of *C. diphtheriae* cause diphtheria. The Elek test (**144**) is used to demonstrate toxin production.

Several corynebacteria are non-pathogenic, and these can be differentiated from *C. diphtheriae* by biochemical tests, using Hiss's serum sugars (**145–147**). Some 'diphtheroids', now designated *C. jeikeium*, are a cause of bacteraemia associated with intravenous catheters.

Lactobacillus spp.

Lactobacilli (**148** and **149**) are part of the normal flora of the alimentary tract and vagina and are rarely associated with disease.

	Gram-positive bacilli Sources and transmission of bacteria							
	Reservoir			Transmission				
Organism	Man	Animal	Env.	Faecal/oral	Droplet	Direct	Nosocomial	Comments
Bacillus anthracis	–	+	+	–	+	+	–	Category III pathogen
B. cereus	–	–	+	+	–	+	–	
Listeria monocytogenes	+	+	+	+	–	+ (neonatal)	–	
Corynebacterium diphtheriae	+	–	–	–	+	+	–	Toxin production demonstrated by Elek test
C. urealyticum	+	–	–	–	–	+	–	
C. jeikeium	+	–	–	–	–	+	+	
Erysipelothrix rhusiopathiae	–	+	+	–	–	+	–	Infections mostly in farm/veterinary workers
Lactobacillus spp.	+	–	–	–	–	±	–	

130 Gram-positive bacilli. Sources and transmission of bacteria.

Gram-positive bacilli
Identifying characteristics

Organism	Gram	Culture	Biochemical and other tests				
Bacillus anthracis	large positive bacilli	grey/white on blood agar, non-haemolytic	red-mauve bacilli on staining with Loeffler's methylene blue, positive gelatin liquefaction				
B. cereus	large positive bacilli	beta haemolytic on blood agar	Grey colonies on mannitol egg yolk polymyxin agar				
Listeria monocytogenes	small positive bacilli	beta haemolytic on blood agar	'tumbling motility', grows well at 4°C				
			Biochemical differentiation by Hiss' sugars				
			Glu	Mal	Suc	Starch	Urea
C. diphtheriae	pleomorphic positive bacilli volutin granules demonstrated by Albert's stain.	black colonies on tellurite medium	+	+	–	+	–
C. hofmannii	positive bacilli	"	–	–	–	–	+
C. urealyticum	"	"	–	–	–	–	+
C. jeikeium	"	"	+	±	–	±	–
Erysipelothrix rhusiopathiae	small positive bacilli	alpha haemolysis on blood agar	non-motile: produces H$_2$S in triple sugar agar				
Lactobacillus spp.	large positive bacilli	variable colony appearance and size	catalase –ve				

131 Gram-positive bacilli. Identifying characteristics.

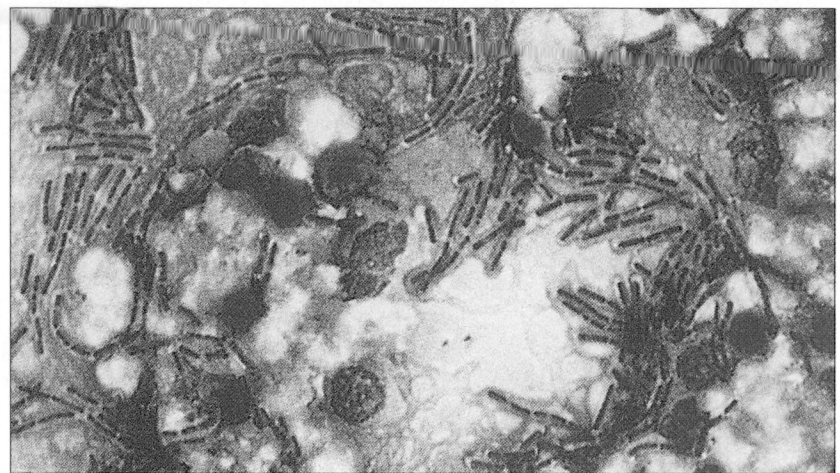

132   *Bacillus anthracis.* Stained with Loeffler's polychrome methylene blue (McFadyean's reaction). The capsule of *B. anthracis* stains red-mauve. *(Polychrome methylene blue, x1000)*

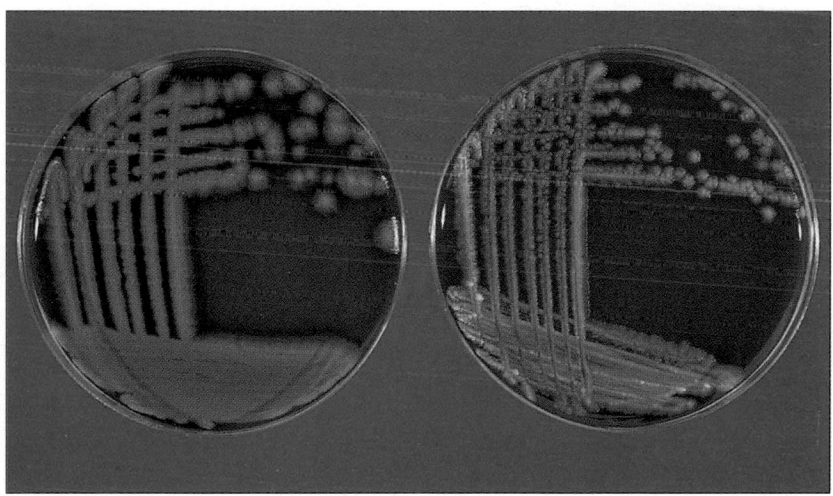

133   *Bacillus anthracis/B. cereus.* Culture on blood agar, showing large, grey-white colonies with wavy edges. Saprophytic Bacillus species are usually haemolytic. Anthrax is highly infectious and great care must be taken if specimens are processed in the laboratory. *(Blood agar, 18 h at 37°C)*

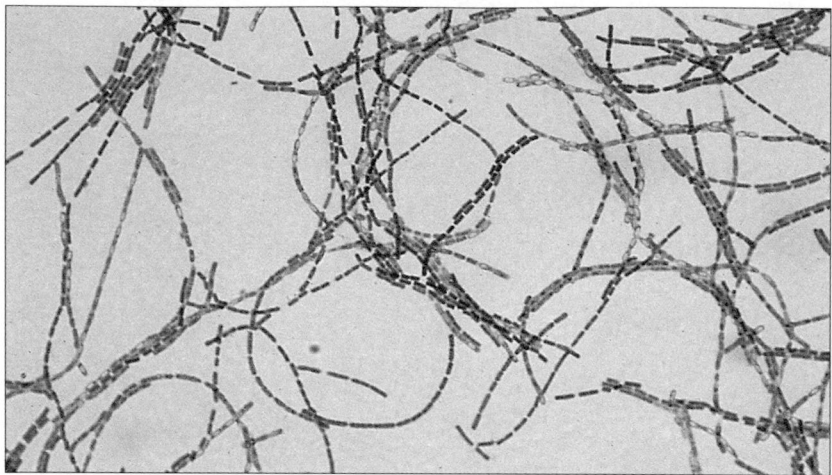

134   Bacillus cereus. Gram stain showing the large, Gram-positive bacilli, often arranged in chains. *B. cereus* is a cause of food poisoning and a selective medium—mannitol, egg yolk, phenol red, polymyxin agar (MYPA) is used to isolate it from faeces or food. *(Gram, x1000)*

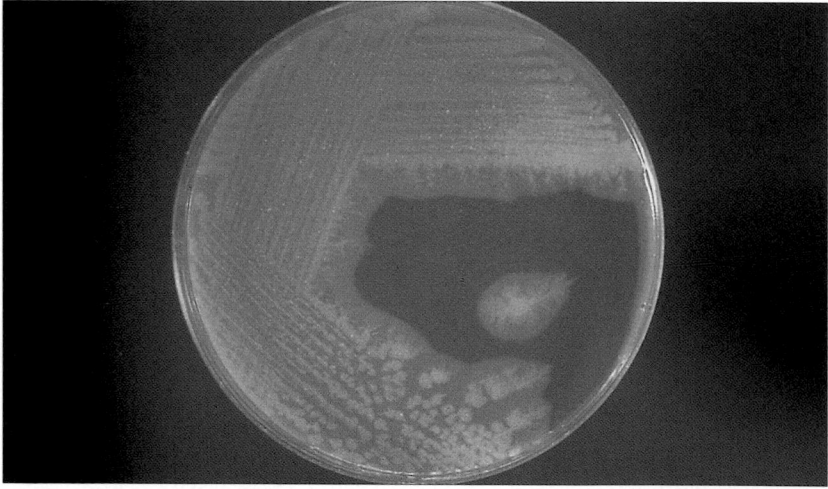

135   Bacillus cereus, culture on MYPA. *B. cereus* produces large, grey-white colonies, surrounded by an area of white precipitate. MYPA may be used as a selective medium in the investigation of food poisoning to isolate *B. cereus* from faeces or food. *(Mannitol, egg yolk, phenol red, polymyxin agar, 18 h at 37°C)*

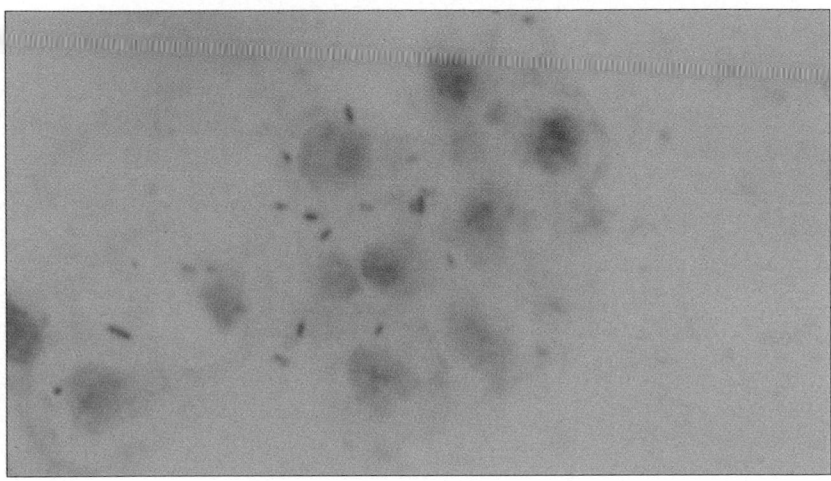

136 *Listeria monocytogenes.* Gram stain of csf from a neonate with meningitis due to *L. monocytogenes* showing small, Gram-positive bacilli. *(Gram, x1000)*

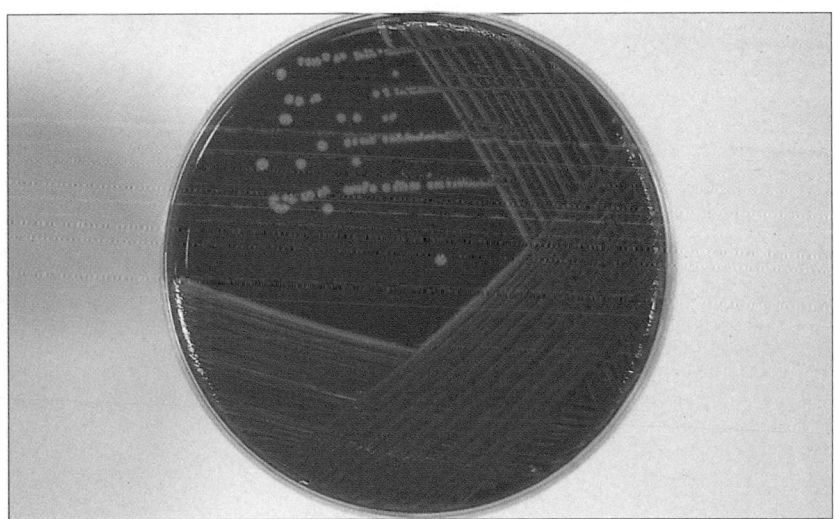

137 *Listeria monocytogenes.* Culture on blood agar, showing small, pale colonies with a zone of beta haemolysis. *L. monocytogenes* can grow at 4°C. *(Blood agar, 18 h at 37°C)*

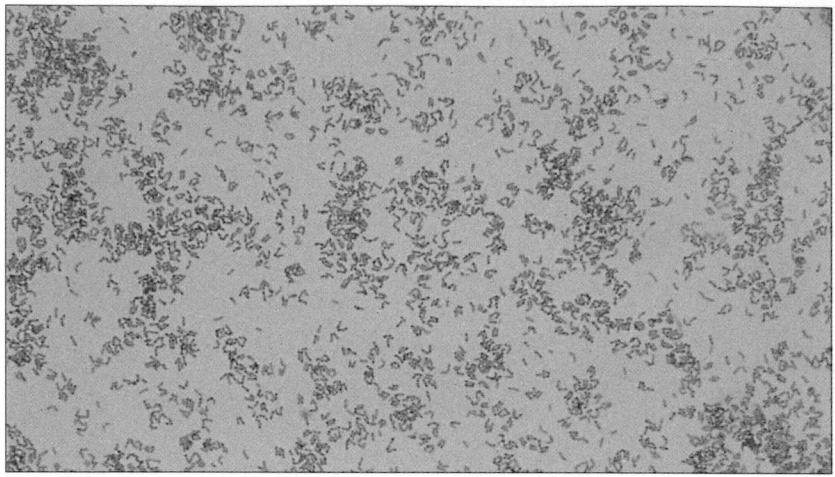

138 *Corynebacterium diphtheriae*, Neisser stain. The stain shows the volutin granules within the bacilli which are characteristic of *C. diphtheriae*. *(Neisser stain, x1000)*

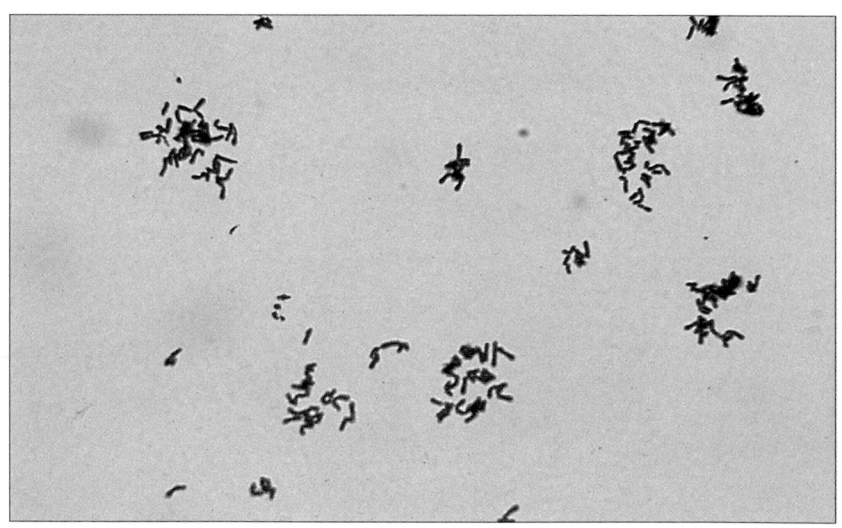

139 Gram stain of diphtheroids. The term diphtheroids includes various *Corynebacterium* species that are skin commensals. The Gram stain shows a typical 'Chinese lettering' arrangement of the bacilli. *(Gram, x1000)*

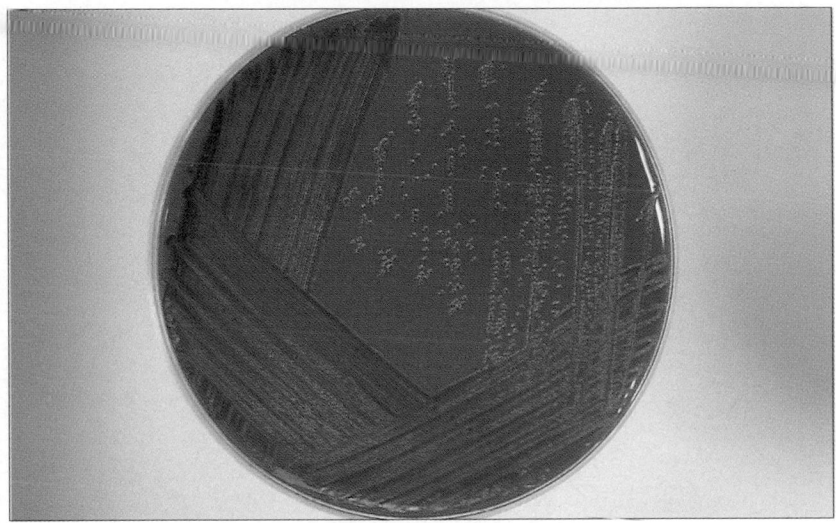

140 *Corynebacterium diphtheriae,* **tellurite blood medium.** *C. diphtheriae* reduces tellurite and produces grey-black colonies. Commensal diphtheroids are grey. *(Tellurite blood agar, 48 h at 37°C)*

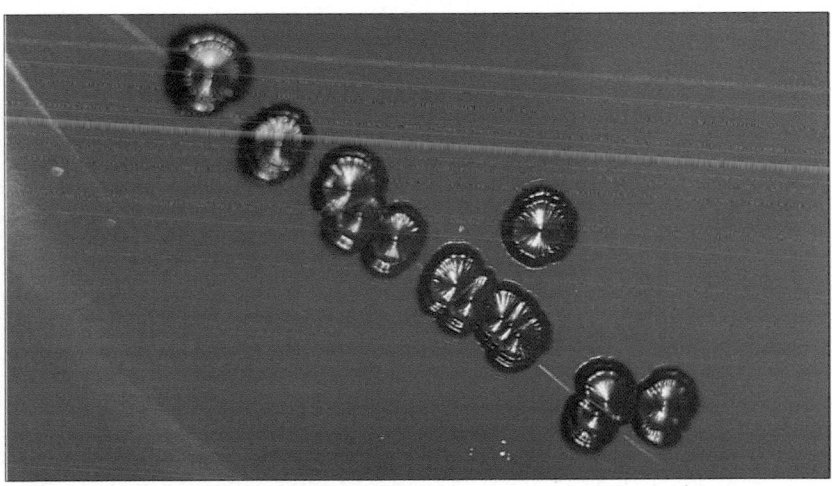

141 *Corynebacterium diphtheriae,* **gravis type.** Close-up of colonies showing striated margins (daisy head appearance). *(Tellurite blood agar, 48 h at 37°C)*

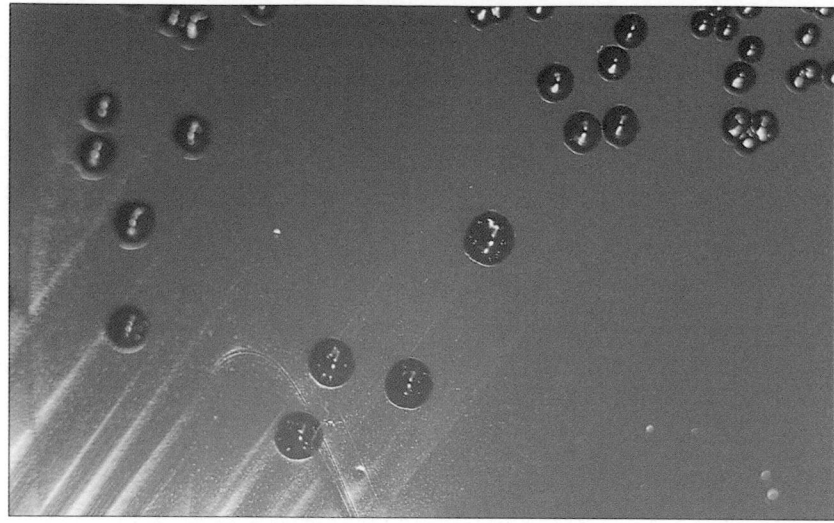

142 *Corynebacterium diphtheriae, mitis type.* Close-up showing small colonies with black centres. *(Tellurite blood agar, 48 h at 37°C)*

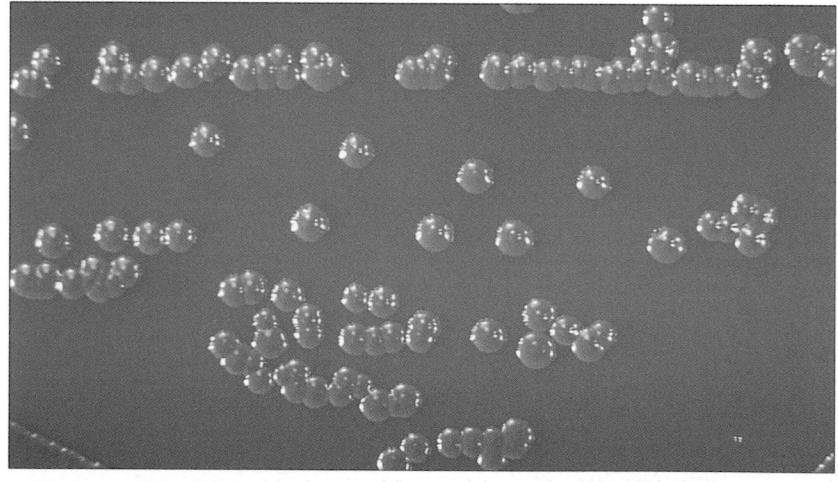

143 *Corynebacterium hofmannii.* Close-up of colonies showing raised, cone-shaped appearance. *(Tellurite blood agar, 24 h at 37°C)*

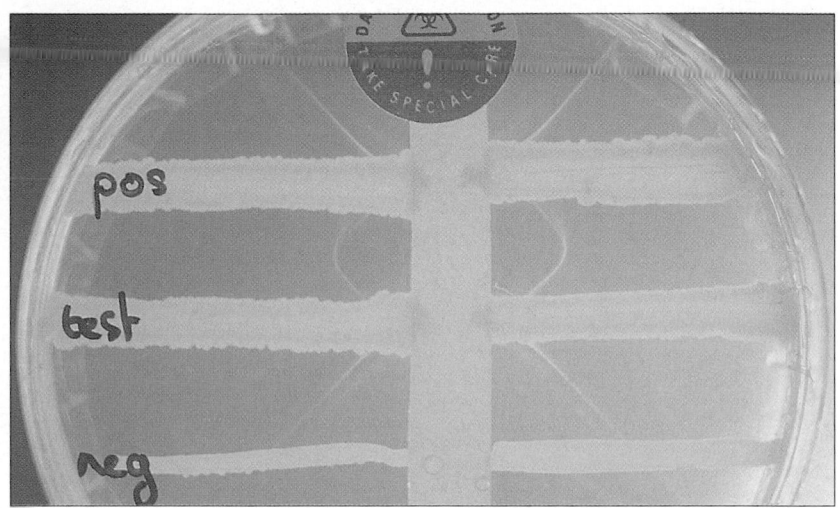

144 Elek plate to demonstrate toxigenicity of *Corynebacterium diphtheriae*. The filter paper strip contains diphtheria antitoxin and is placed in the Petri dish and the medium poured. The test strain, and toxigenic and non-toxigenic strains are inoculated at right angles to the strip. A toxigenic strain produces a V-shaped line of precipitation between the toxin and the anti-toxin. *(Elek's medium, 48 h at 37°C)*

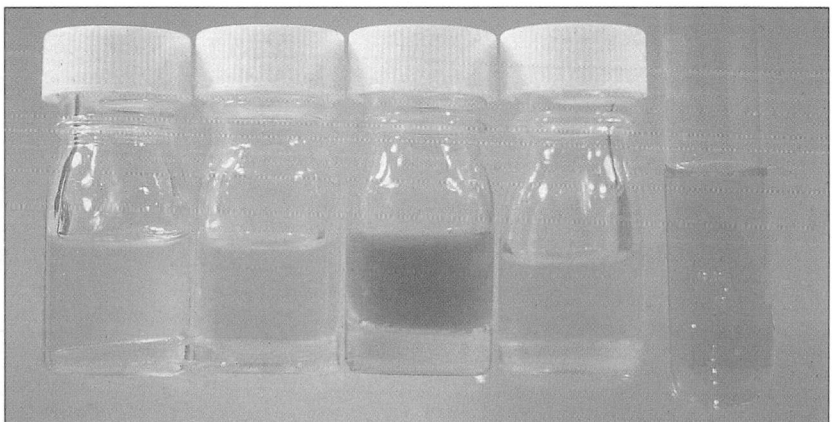

145 Biochemical differentiation of *Corynebacteria* by Hiss' serum sugars. The tubes contain glucose, maltose, sucrose, starch and urea, respectively. *C. diphtheriae gravis* produces acid from glucose, maltose and starch. *(Hiss' serum water sugars with phenol red indicator, 24 h at 37°C)*

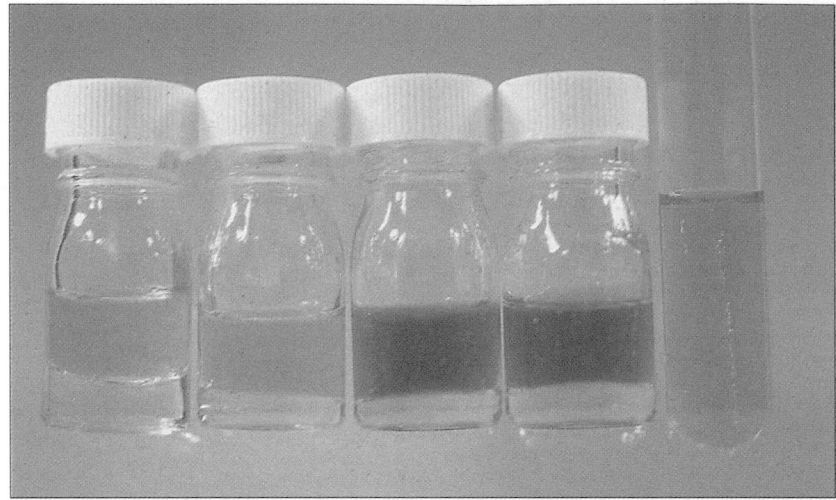

146 Biochemical differentiation of *Corynebacteria* by Hiss' serum sugars.
C. diphtheriae mitis is positive for glucose and maltose.

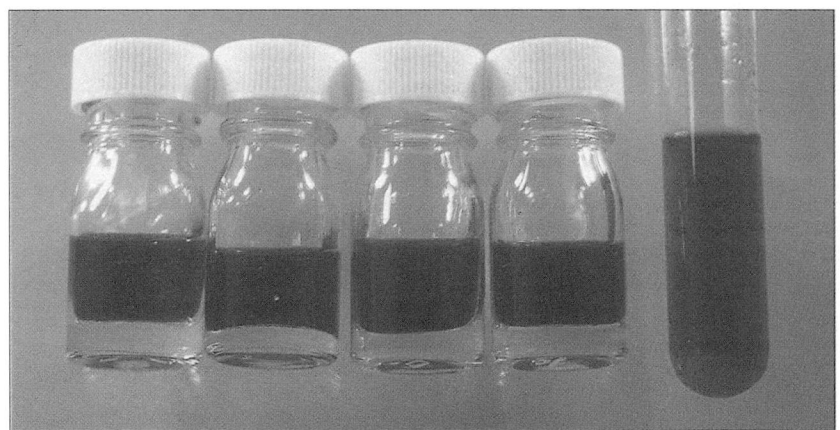

147 Biochemical differentiation of *Corynebacteria* by Hiss' serum sugars. *C. hofmannii*, a throat commensal, does not ferment the sugars, but is urease positive.

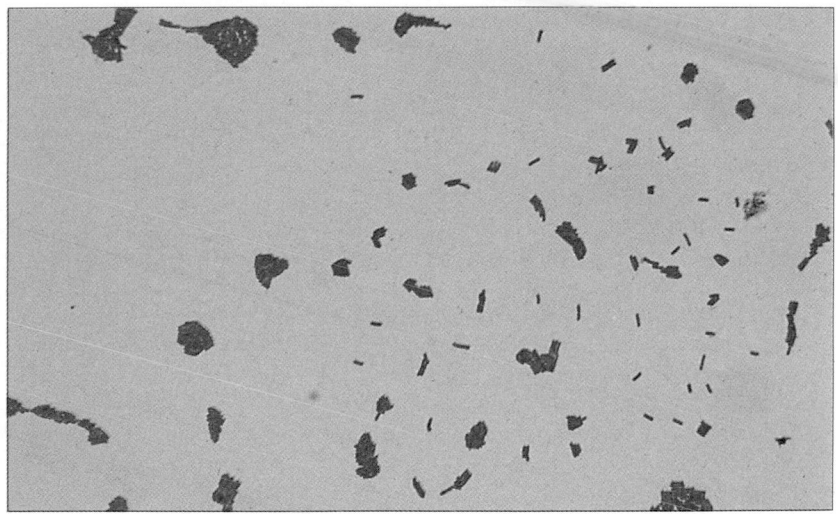

148 Gram stain of Lactobacilli. Lactobacilli are large, Gram-positive rods, that occur singly and in chains. They are part of the normal vaginal flora. *(Gram, x1000)*

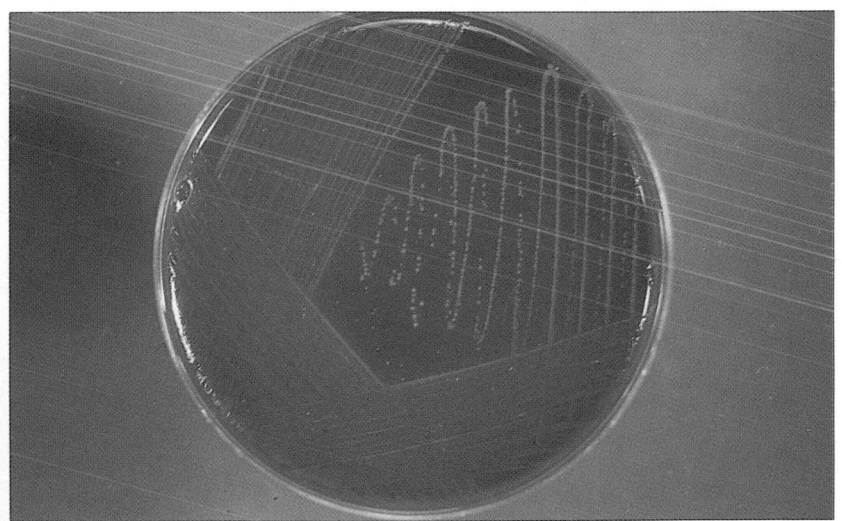

149 Culture of Lactobacillus on blood agar. Lactobacilli grow best in a 5% CO_2 atmosphere, producing small, pale colonies. *(Blood agar, 18 h at 37°C)*

AEROBIC GRAM-NEGATIVE BACTERIA

AEROBIC GRAM-NEGATIVE BACILLI

Enterobacteriaceae

Characteristics of this family are summarized in **150–154**. The Enterobacteriaceae comprise a wide range of species including intestinal commensal bacteria and important pathogens such as *Shigella* and *Salmonella*. Gram staining cannot differentiate between the different Enterobacteriaceae. **155** shows the typical appearance; in this case it is *Escherichia coli*. Enterobacteria (coliforms) will all grow on MacConkey medium, which can distinguish lactose fermenting (pink) from non-lactose fermenting (pale) species. **156** shows the lactose fermenting *E. coli* cultured on MacConkey medium and **157** the pale, non-lactose fermenting colonies of *Proteus mirabilis*. **158** shows the mucoid lactose fermenting colonies of *Klebsiella pneumoniae*. **159** shows the differentiation between coliform bacteria (larger green/blue colonies) and staphylococci (smaller, white colonies) from a urine sample grown on cystine–lactose electrolyte-deficient (CLED) medium. MacConkey medium containing sorbitol in place of lactose can be used to distinguish the *E. coli* serotype 0157, which causes haemorrhagic colitis, from other *E. coli*. *E. coli* 0157 does not ferment sorbitol and forms pale colonies on sorbitol MacConkey (**160** and **161**). *Proteus* spp. have the characteristic of 'swarming' when cultured on blood agar (**162**). **163** shows lactose fermenting *E. coli* and non-lactose fermenting *Shigella sonnei* cultured on MacConkey medium. More selective media such as xylose lysine deoxycholate (XLD) may be used to isolate *Shigella* or *Salmonella* from faecal specimens (**164** and **165**). Other selective media for these species include Salmonella–Shigella (SS) agar and deoxycholate citrate agar (DCA) (**166** and **167**).

A wide range of sugar fermentation and other biochemical tests may be used to differentiate between the different Enterobacteriaceae. **168–172** show examples of sugar fermentation reactions using peptone water sugars. **173** shows the tube indole test that can distinguish between *E. coli* and *K. pneumoniae*. **174–178** show other biochemical tests commonly used in the differentiation of Enterobacteriaceae. Combinations of these tests are now available in a variety of commercial systems; examples are shown in **179** and **180**.

Where resources are limited, particularly in developing countries, biochemical differentiation can be done by using inexpensive composite media. **181–183** show Kligler's-iron-agar composite medium, and **184–186** motility-indole urea medium, used to distinguish the pathogens *Shigella* and *Salmonella* from other enterobacteria. *Salmonella* spp. include the causes of typhoid and paratyphoid fevers, and a large number of serotypes responsible for less severe gastrointestinal disease. The serotypes are distinguished by their O (somatic) and H (flagella) antigens (the Kauffman–White typing scheme). **187** shows a slide agglutination test to determine the salmonella O serotypes, using specific O antisera.

Typhoid and paratyphoid fevers may also be diagnosed by identifying specific O and H antibodies in the patient's serum using the Widal test (**188** and **189**). Dilutions of the serum are incubated with standard H and O suspensions of *S. typhi* or *S. paratyphi* and the highest titres (reciprocal dilutions) read for H-flocculation and O-agglutination determined. The Enterobacteriaceae also contain the genus *Yersinia*, which includes the cause of plague, *Y. pestis* (**190**), and *Y. enterocolitica*, causing mesenteric adenitis and entero-colitis (**191**).

	Enterobacteriaceae Infections					
Organism	Major infection	Less common infection	Vaccine preventable	Incubation period	Period of infectivity
Escherichia					
E. coli	Urinary tract, wound infection, septicaemia, neonatal meningitis	gastroenteritis by some serotypes	–	–	–
Klebsiella					
K. oxytoca	urinary tract	septicaemia	–	–	–
K. pneumoniae	urinary tract, chest infections				
Enterobacter					
E. cloacae	wound, urinary tract	septicaemia	–	–	–
E. aerogenes				–	–
Shigella					
S. dysenteriae	bacillary dysentery	–	–	3–4 days	
S. flexneri	bacillary dysentery	–	–	"	} 1–4 weeks
S. boydii	bacillary dysentery	–	–	"	
S. sonnei	bacillary dysentery	–	–	"	
Salmonella					
S. typhi	typhoid fever	osteomyelitis	+	7–21 days	Variable
S. paratyphi A	paratyphoid fever		±	7–21 days	5–21 days
S. paratyphi B	paratyphoid fever	septicaemia	±	7–21 days	some long-
S. typhimurium *	gastroenteritis	osteomyelitis	–	1–3 days	term excreters

* S. typhimurium is given as the example of a large number of non-typhi salmonella serotypes.

150 Enterobacteriaceae. Infections.

Enterobacteriaceae Infections					
Organism	Major infection	Less common infection	Vaccine preventable	Incubation period	Period of infectivity
Citrobacter					
C. freundii	urinary tract, wound infections	septicaemia	–	–	–
Edwardsiella					
E. tarda	wound infection		–	–	–
Serratia					
S. marcescens	wound infection	septicaemia	–	–	–
Hafnia		rarely UTI,			
H. alvei	–	septicaemia	–	–	–
Proteus					
P. mirabilis	urinary tract, wound infection	septicaemia	–	–	–
P. vulgaris	" "		–	–	–
Providencia					
P. stuartii	urinary tract, burns infections		–	–	–
Morganella					
M. morganii	urinary tract	septicaemia	–	–	–
Yersinia					
Y. enterocolitica	gastroenteritis		–	–	–
Y. pseudotuberculosis	mesenteric adenitis	septicaemia	–	–	–
Y. pestis	bubonic plague (rat plague)	pneumonia	killed vaccine available	1–6 days	see **153**

151   Enterobacteriaceae. Infections.

Enterobacteriaceae Sources and transmission of bacteria							
	Reservoir			Transmission				
Organism	Man	Animal	Env.	Faecal/oral	Droplet	Direct	Nosocomial	Comments
Escherichia coli	+	+	+	+	−	+	+	
Klebsiella oxytoca	+	−	+	−	−	+	+	
K. pneumoniae	+	−	+	−	+	+	+	
Enterobacter cloacae	+	−	+	−	−	+	+	
E. aerogenes	+	−	+	−	−	+	+	Large epidemics
Shigella dysenteriae	+	−	−	+	−	−	−	of multiple
S. flexneri	+	−	−	+	−	−	−	antimicrobial
S. boydii	+	−	−	+	−	−	−	resistant strains
S. sonnei	+	−	−	+	−	−	−	may occur
Salmonella typhi	+	−	−	+	−	−	−	
S. paratyphi A	+	−	−	+	−	−	−	
S. paratyphi B	+	+	−	+	−	−	−	
S. typhimurium	+	+	−	+	−	−	−	

152 Enterobacteriaceae. Sources and transmission of bacteria.

Enterobacteriaceae
Sources and transmission of bacteria

Organism	Reservoir			Transmission					Comments
	Man	Animal	Env.	Insect	Faecal /oral	Droplet	Direct	Nosocomial	
Citrobacter freundii	+	−	+	−	−	−	+	+	
Edwardsiella tarda	+	−	+	−	−	−	+	+	
Serratia marcescens	+	−	+	−	−	−	+	+	
Hania alvei	+	−	+	−	−	−	+	+	
Proteus mirabilis	+	−	+	−	−	−	+	+	
P. vulgaris	+	−	+	−	−	−	+	+	
Providencia stuartii	+	−	+	−	−	−	+	+	
Morganella morganii	+	−	+	−	−	−	+	+	
Yersinia enterocolitica	+	+	−	−	+	−	−	−	
Y. pseudotuberculosis	+	+	−	−	+	−	−	−	
Y. pestis	−	+	−	+	−	+	−	−	Pneumonic form directly transmissible

153 Enterobacteriaceae. Sources and transmission of bacteria.

Enterobacteriaceae
Biochemical characterization

	Lac	Gluc [a]	Man	Suc	Cit	Dulc	Ind	U'rea	Motile	H₂S	MR [b]	VP [c]	PD [d]	NO₃
Escherichia coli	+	+g	+	±	-	±	+	-	+	-	+	-	-	+
Klebsiella oxytoca	+	+g	+	+	+	±	+	+	-	-	-	+	-	+
K. pneumoniae	+	+g	+	+	+	±	-	+	-	-	-	+	-	+
Enterobacter cloacae	+	+g	+	+	+	-	-	±	+	-	-	+	-	+
Enterobacter aerogenes	+	+g	±	+	+	-	-	-	+	-	-	+	-	+
Shigella dysenteriae	-	+	+	-	-	-	±	-	-	-	+	-	-	+
Shigella sonnei	±	+	+	-	-	-	-	-	-	-	+	-	-	+
Salmonella typhi	-	+	+	-	-	-	-	-	+	+	+	-	-	+
Salmonella paratyphi A	-	+g	+	-	-	+	-	-	+	-	+	-	-	+
Salmonella paratyphi B	-	?	+	-	-	+	-	-	+	-	+	-	-	+
Salmonella typhimurium	-	+g	+	-	+	+	-	-	+	+	+	-	-	+
Citrobacter freundii	-	+g	+	±	+	±	-	±	+	+	+	-	-	+
Edwardsiella tarda	-	+g	-	-	-	-	+	-	+	+	+	-	-	+
Serratia marcescens	-	±/g	+	+	+	-	-	-	+	-	-	+	-	+
Hafnia alvei	-	+g	+	-	-	-	-	-	+	-	±	+	-	+
Proteus mirabilis	-	+g	-	±	±	-	-	+	+	+	+	±	+	+
Proteus vulgaris	-	+g	-	+	±	-	+	+	+	+	+	-	+	+
Providencia stuartii	-	+g	-	±	+	-	+	±	+	-	+	-	+	+
Morganella morganii	-	+g	-	-	-	-	+	+	+	-	+	-	+	+
Yersinia enterocolitica	-	+	+	+	-	-	±	±	-	-	+	-	-	+
Yersinia pseudotuberculosis	-	+	+	+	-	-	-	+	-	-	+	-	-	+
Y. pestis	-	+	+	-	-	-	-	-	-	-	+	-	-	+

(a) Gas production. (b) Methyl Red. (c) Voges–Proskauer. (d) Phenylalanine deaminase.

154 Enterobacteriaceae. Biochemical characterization.

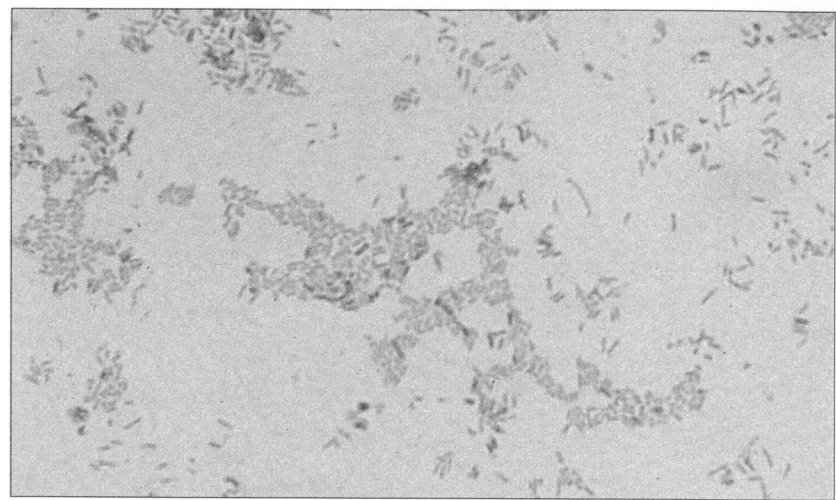

155 *Escherichia coli*, **Gram stain.** The stain shows the Gram-negative bacilli typical of the Enterobacteriaceae. Most have a similar morphology and cannot be distinguished by Gram staining. *(Gram, x1000)*

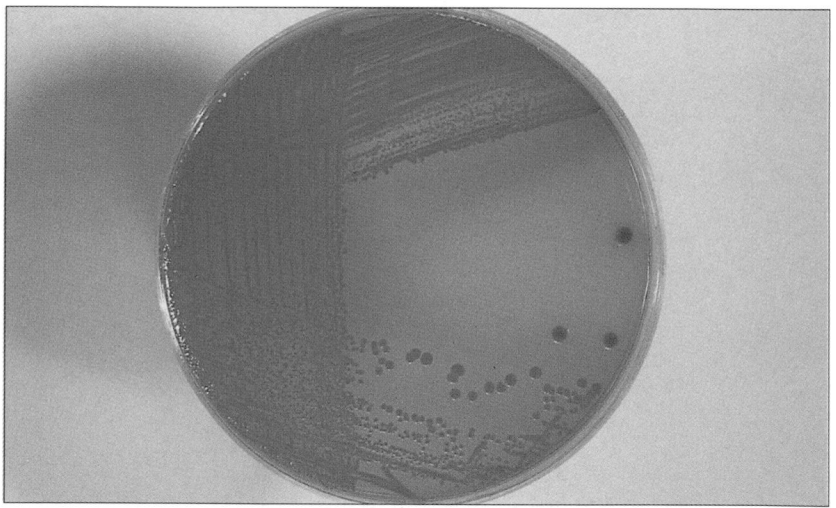

156 *Escherichia coli* **cultured on MacConkey medium.** *E. coli* produces pink, lactose-fermenting colonies. MacConkey medium is a selective medium for enteric bacteria, containing bile salts, lactose and the pH indicator, neutral red. Lactose-fermenting colonies produce acid and turn the indicator red. *(MacConkey agar, 18 h at 37°C)*

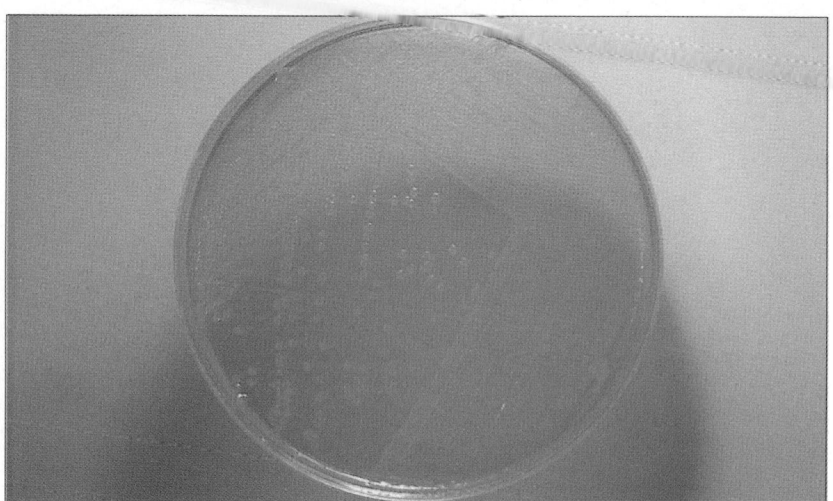

157 *Proteus mirabilis* **on MacConkey medium.** *P. mirabilis* is a non-lactose fermenter and produces pale colonies on MacConkey medium. *(MacConkey agar, 18 h at 37°C)*

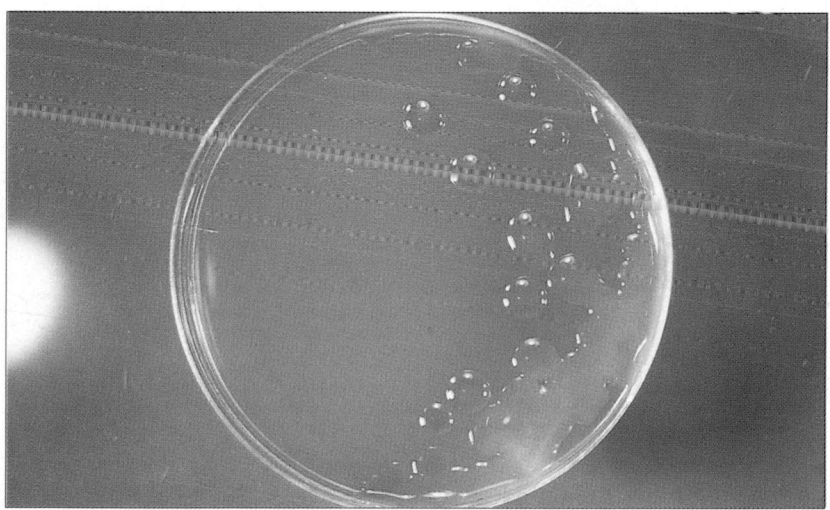

158 *Klebsiella pneumoniae* **on MacConkey medium.** *K. pneumoniae* is a lactose-fermenter and produces pink, mucoid colonies. *(MacConkey agar, 18 h at 37°C)*

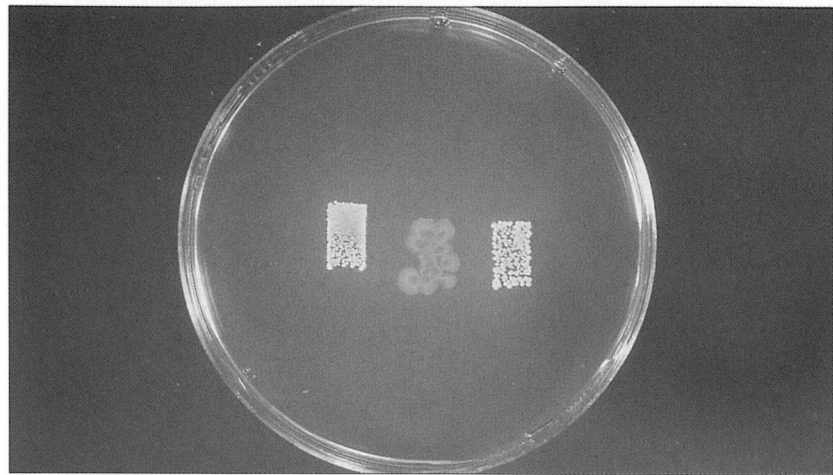

159 *Escherichia coli* **and** *Staphylococcus epidermidis* **on CLED medium.**
Cystine lactose electrolyte deficient (CLED) agar is used as a selective medium for urine samples. *E. coli* produces large colonies with a bluish colour; *S. epidermidis* produces small, white colonies. *(Cystine-lactose electrolyte deficient agar, 18 h at 37°C)*

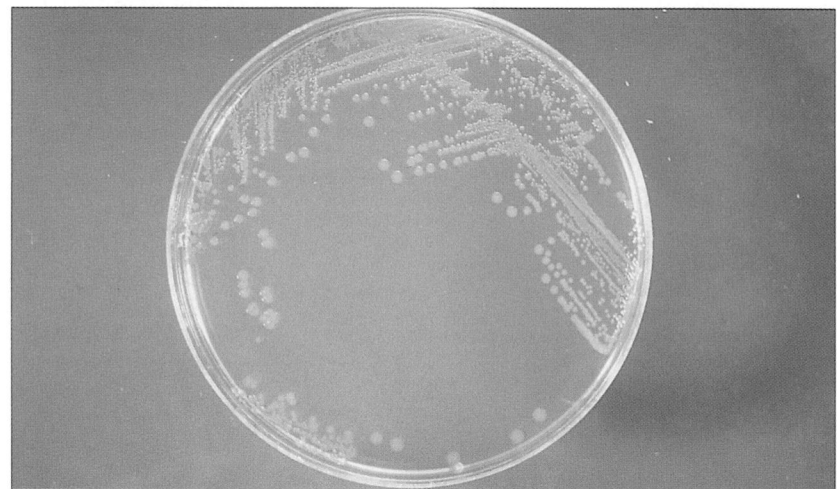

160 *Escherichia coli* **0157 on sorbitol-MacConkey medium.** *E. coli* serogroup 0157 is an important pathogen causing haemorrhagic colitis and the haemolytic uraemic syndrome. It does not ferment sorbitol and produces pale colonies on MacConkey medium in which lactose is replaced by sorbitol. *(Sorbitol MacConkey agar, 18 h at 37°C)*

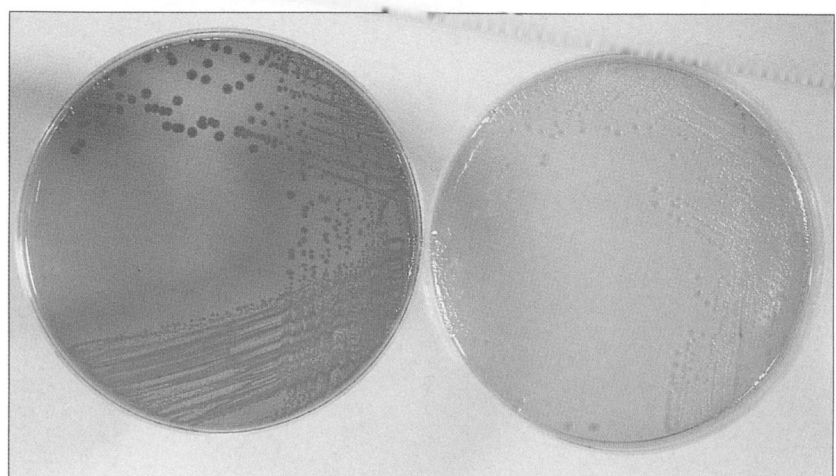

161   *E. coli* 0157 on MacConkey and sorbitol MacConkey. *E. coli* 0157 is a
lactose-fermenter and produces pink colonies on standard MacConkey (left), compared
to the non-sorbitol-fermenters on the selective medium(right). *(MacConkey and sorbitol
MacConkey agar, 18 h at 37°C)*

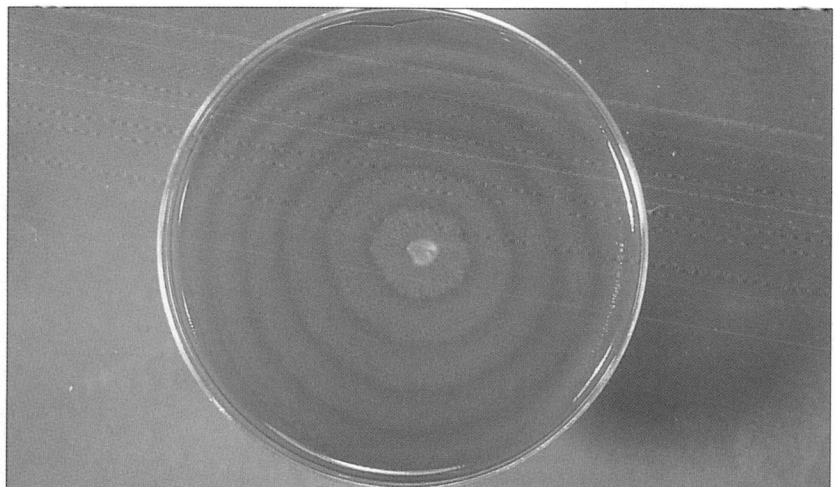

162   *Proteus mirabilis* cultured on blood agar. *P. mirabilis* produces swarming
growth on blood agar which may often conceal other bacteria in a mixed growth.
(Blood agar, 18 h at 37°C)

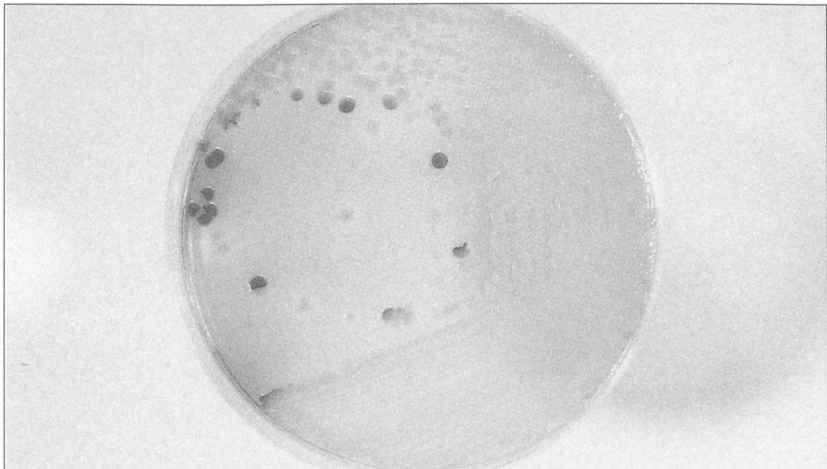

163 *Escherichia coli* and *Shigella sonnei* on MacConkey medium. *Shigella* colonies are pale, non-lactose-fermenting and often have a characteristic wavy edge. *E. coli* show the typical pink, lactose-fermenting colonies. *(MacConkey agar, 18 h at 37°C)*

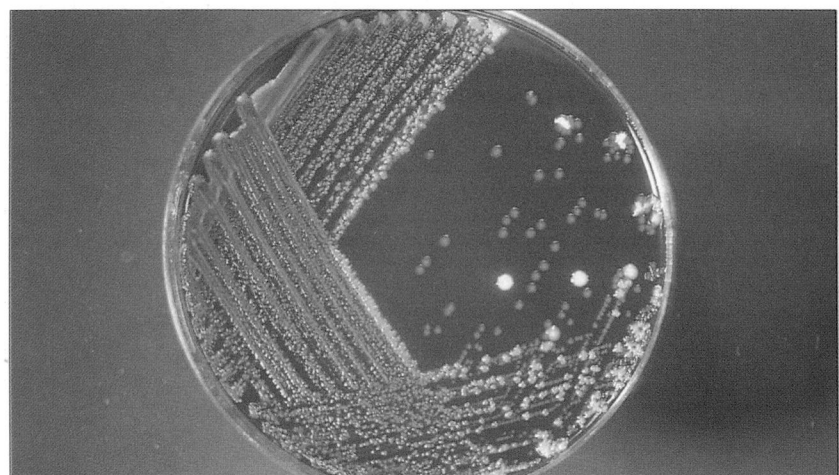

164 *Shigella sonnei* and *Escherichia coli* on xylose–lysine–deoxycholate (XLD) medium. XLD is a selective medium for the isolation of *Shigella* and *Salmonella* from faecal specimens. XLD contains the indicator phenol red which is red at alkaline pH and yellow at acid pH. *Shigella* form red colonies as they do not ferment xylose; *E. coli* produce pale yellow colonies. *(Xylose–lysine–deoxycholate agar, 18 h at 37°C)*

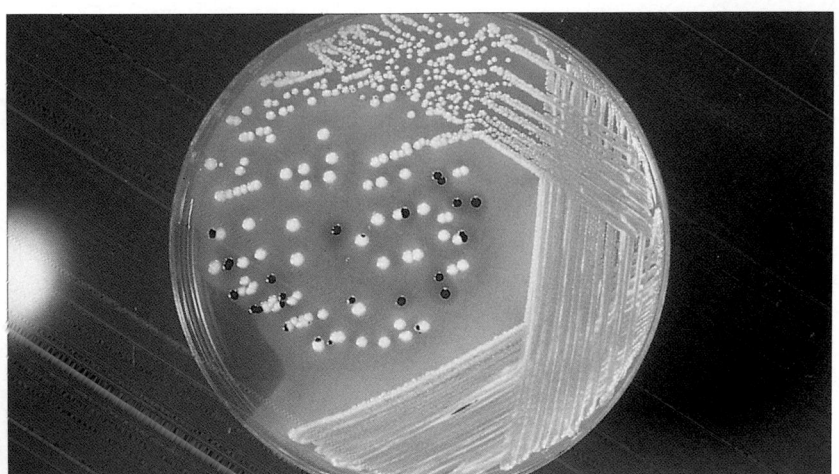

165 *Salmonella enteritidis* and *Escherichia coli* on XLD medium.
Salmonella produce red colonies with black centres due to H$_2$S production. *E. coli* are
yellow colonies.*(XLD medium, 18 h at 37°C)*

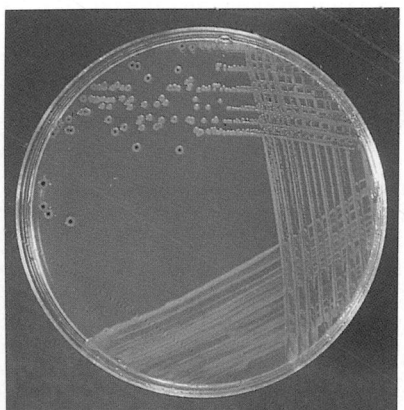 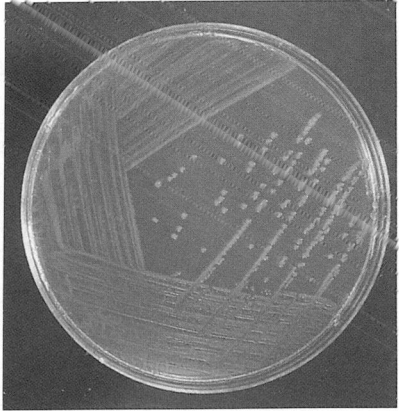

166,167 *Salmonella enteritidis* on SS agar (166) and DCA agar (167).
SS (*Salmonella/Shigella*) agar and DCA (deoxycholate-citrate agar) are also selective
media for isolation of these pathogens from faecal specimens. On both, *Salmonella*
produce pale, non-lactose-fermenting colonies. *(SS and DCA agar, 18 h at 37°C)*

168–172 Peptone-water sugar reactions of Enterobacteriaceae. A series of peptone-water sugars; glucose, mannite, lactose, sucrose, dulcite, and urea can be used for the biochemical differentiation of Enterobacteriaceae. Acid production changes the indicator to red and gas production is shown by bubbles in the inverted tube. *(Peptone-water sugars, Andrade's indicator, 24 h at 37°C)*

169   *Escherichia coli.*
170   *Shigella sonnei.*
171   *Salmonella typhimurium.*
172   *Proteus mirabilis.*

Reactions in peptone-water sugars						
Code:	glucose green	mannite purple	lactose red	sucrose blue	dulcite pink	urea black
Escherichia coli	A G	A G	A G	– –	– –	–
Shigella sonnei	A –	A –	– –	– –	– –	–
Salmonella typhimurium	A G	A G	– –	– –	A G	–
Proteus mirabilis	A G	– –	– –	– –	– –	+

A = acid production (pink)   G = gas production (bubbles in tube)

168

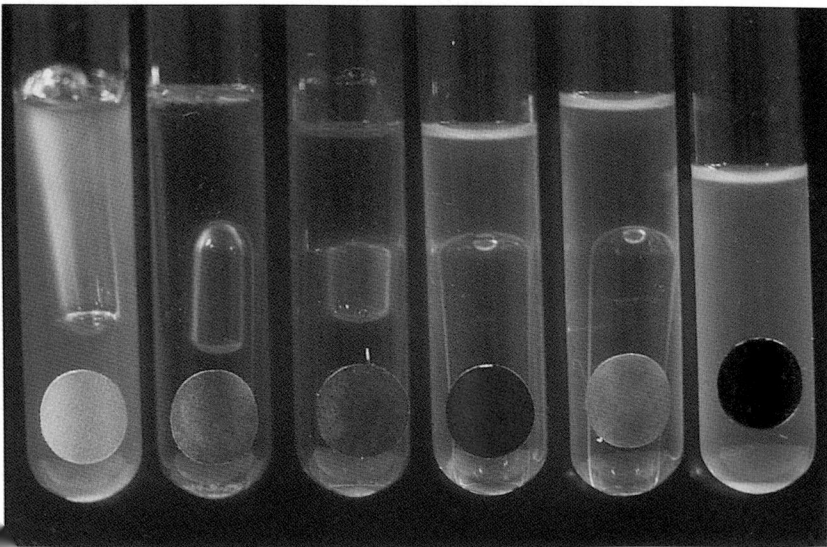

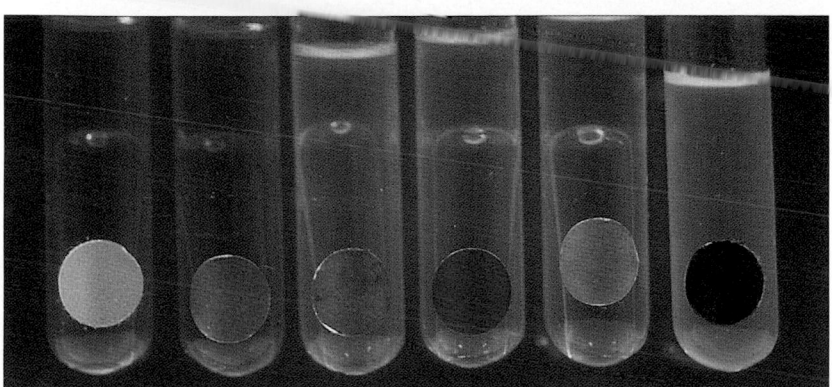

170

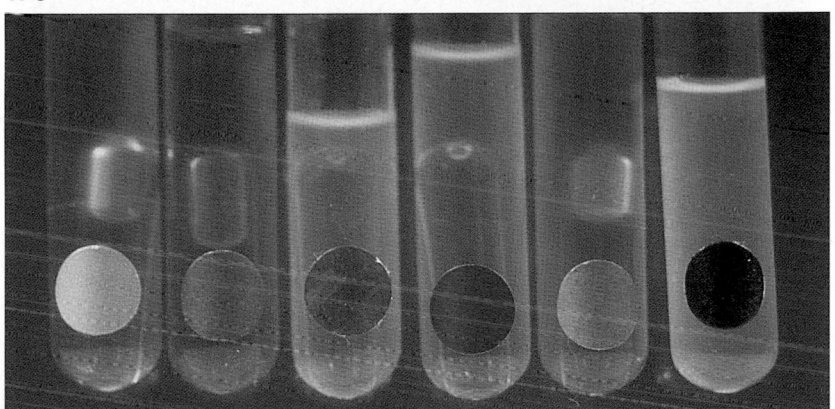

171

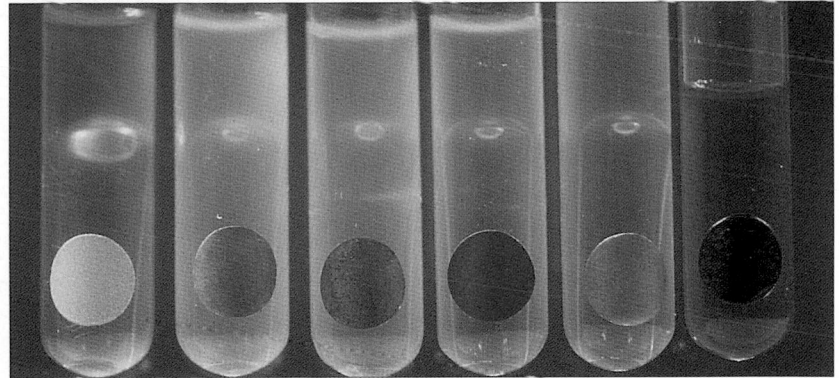

172

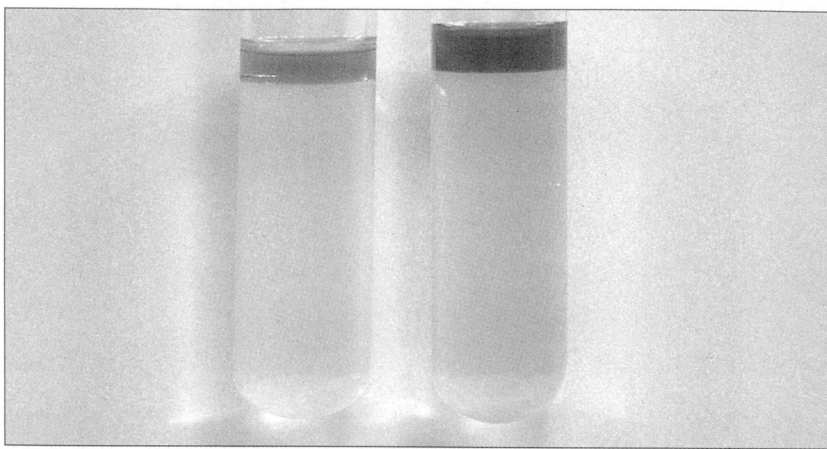

173 Tube indole test. Indole positive bacteria break down the amino acid tryptophan to indole, which reacts with Kovac's reagent to produce a red colour. *E. coli* is indole positive (right); *K. pneumoniae* is indole negative (left). *(Peptone water, 24 h at 37°C)*

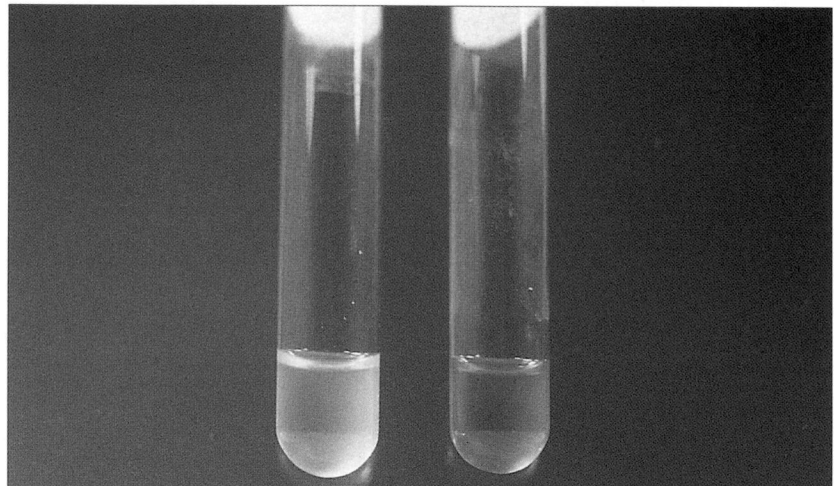

174 Methyl red test. Enterobacteriaceae differ in the extent to which pH is lowered in glucose fermentation. With methyl red indicator, only those that reduce pH to approximately 5 will change the indicator to a red colour. *E. coli*: methyl red positive (right), *Enterobacter aerogenes*: methyl red negative (left). *(Glucose phosphate/peptone water, 24 h at 37°C)*

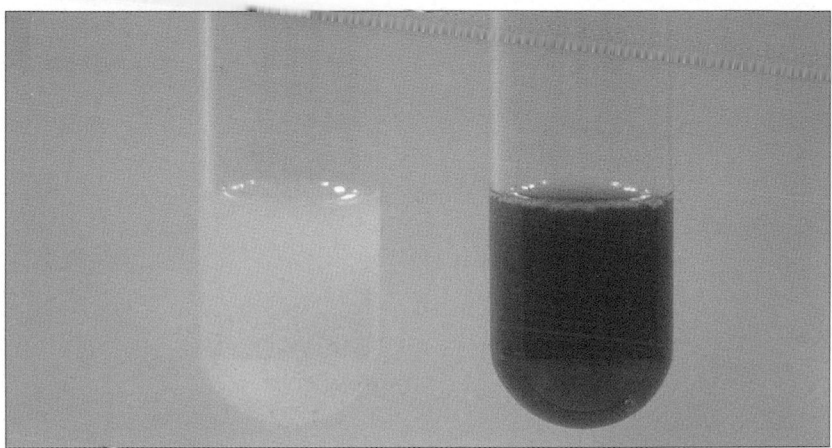

175 Voges–Proskauer (V-P) test. Some Enterobacteriaceae ferment glucose with the production of acetyl methylcarbinol, which is oxidized and reacts with alpha-naphthol to produce a red colour. *Enterobacter aerogenes*, V-P positive (right); *E. coli*, V-P negative (left). *(Glucose phosphate/peptone water, 48 h at 37°C, alpha-naphthol and KOH added and viewed after 5 min)*

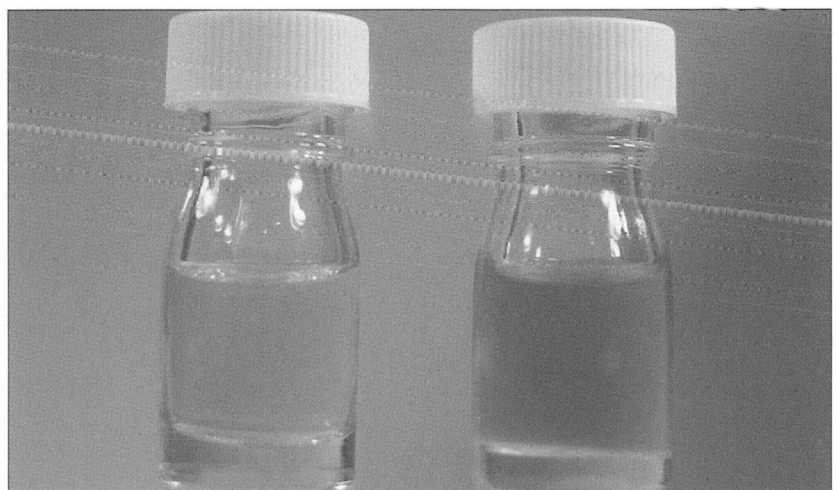

176 Koser's citrate medium. This test distinguishes Enterobacteriaceae that can utilize citrate as the sole source of carbon. The indicator bromo-thymol blue turns from green to blue due to the alkaline reaction. *Citrobacter freundii*, positive (right); *E. coli*, negative (left). *(Koser's citrate medium, 18 h at 37°C)*

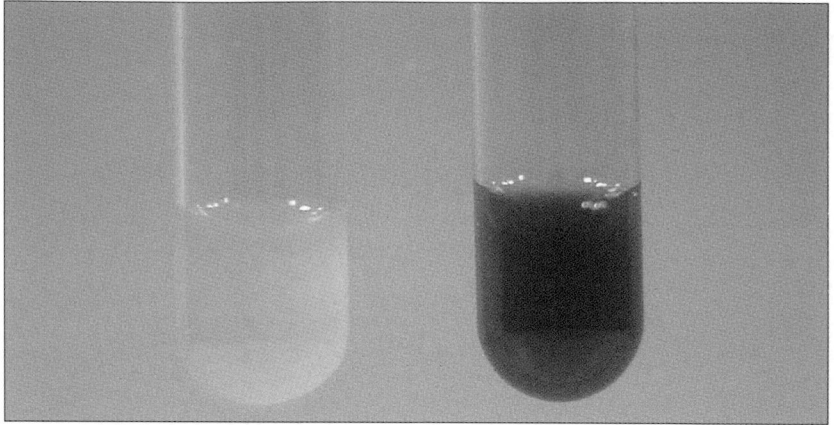

177 Nitrate reduction test. The test organism is incubated in a broth containing nitrate. After 4 h, the broth is tested for the reduction of nitrate to nitrite, which reacts to form a red colour with sulphanilic acid and alpha-naphthylamine. Positive nitrate reduction, *E. coli* (right); negative *Ps. aeruginosa* (left). *(Nitrate broth, 4 h at 37°C)*

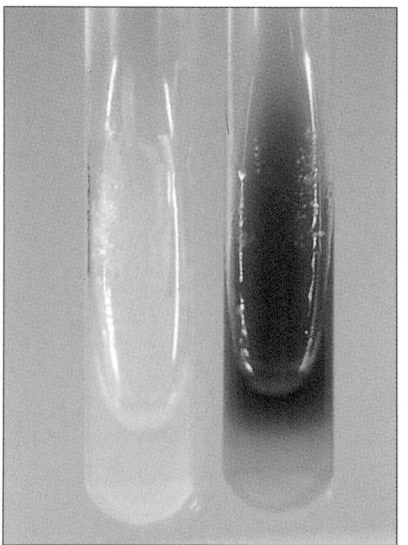

178 Phenylalanine deaminase test. Certain Enterobacteriaceae (*Proteus, Providencia*) will break down phenylalanine to produce phenylpyruvic acid, which gives a green/brown colour with ferric chloride. Phenylalanine positive, *Proteus mirabilis* (right); negative, *E. coli* (left). *(Phenylalanine agar, 18 h at 37°C; then four drops 10% w/v ferric chloride added; observe after 5 min)*

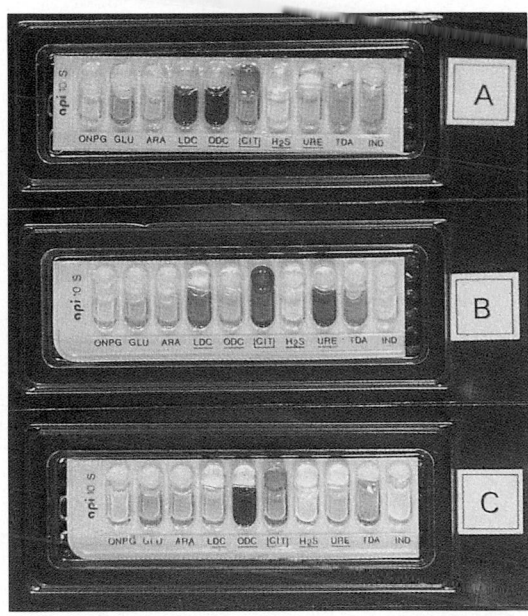

179 API-10S kit for Enterobacteriaceae.

These kits use dried reagents in cupules to which a suspension of the test organisms is added. The strips are incubated overnight and the reactions determined. This allows the rapid processing of large numbers of isolates.

Tests in strips from left to right: ONPG, GLU, ARA, LDC, ODC, CIT, H_2S, UREA, TDA, INDOLE, NO_2.

A *Escherichia coli*
B *Klebsiella pneumoniae*
C *Shigella sonnei*
(API-10S kits, 18 h at 37°C)

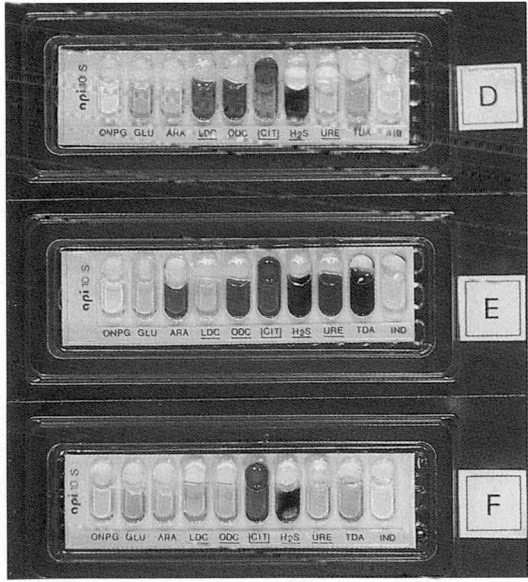

180 API-10S diagnostic strips (*cont.*).

D *Salmonella typhimurium*
E *Proteus mirabilis*
F *Citrobacter freundi*
(API-10S kits, 18 h at 37°C)

Reactions in Kligler's iron agar (KIA)			
	base (glucose fermentation) if yellow	slope (lactose fermentation) if yellow	gas production	H$_2$S production
Before culture	pink	pink	–	–
Escherichia coli	yellow	yellow	+	–
Shigella sonnei	yellow	pink	–	–
Salmonella enteritidis	yellow/black	pink/black	+/–	+
Proteus mirabilis	yellow/black	pink/black	+	+

181   Reactions in Kligler's iron agar (KIA).

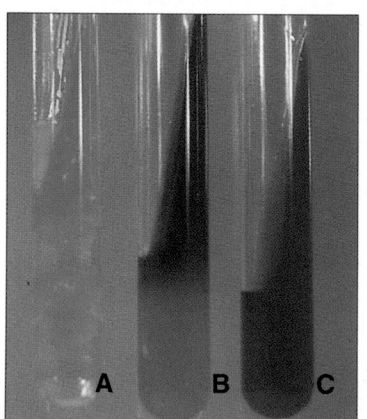

182   Enterobacteriaceae reactions in Kligler iron agar (KIA). KIA is a composite medium containing glucose, lactose, phenol red, and ferric citrate. A yellow base indicates glucose fermentation, a yellow base and slope indicates both glucose and lactose fermentation. Bubbles in the medium indicate gas production from glucose. Blackening of the medium indicates H$_2$S production. **A,** E. coli; **B,** Sh. sonnei; **C,** uninoculated. (Kligler iron agar, 18 h at 37°C)

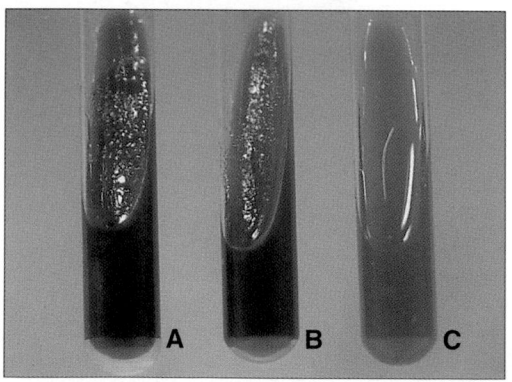

183   Kligler iron agar.
A, S. enteritidis; **B,** Proteus mirabilis; **C,** uninoculated. (Kligler iron agar, 18 h at 37°C)

Reactions in motility-indole-urea (MIU) medium

	motility	indole	urea
Escherichia coli	+	+	–
Shigella sonnei	–	–/+	–
Salmonella enteritidis	+	–	–
Proteus mirabilis	+	–	+

184   Reactions in motility-indole-urea (MIU) medium .

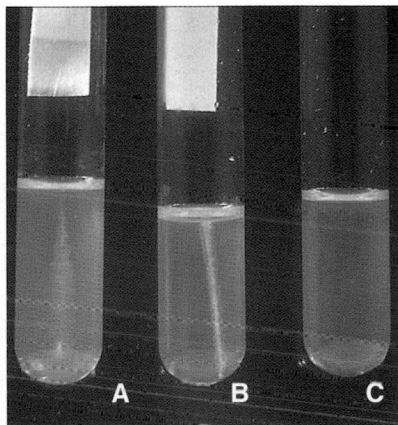

185   Enterobacteriaceae reactions in motility-indole-urea (MIU). MIU is a composite medium containing tryptone, phenol red and urea and a paper strip moistened in Kovac's reagent. It is inoculated by a straight wire through the centre of the medium. Non-motile organisms (e.g. *Shigella*) grow only in the line of the inoculum, but motile organisms (most *Salmonellae*) grow throughout the medium, which becomes turbid. Urease positive organisms (e.g. *Proteus* spp.) turn the medium red. Indole positive organisms (e.g. *E. coli*) turn the Kovac's strip red. **A,** *E. coli;* **B,** *Sh. sonnei;* **C,** uninoculated. *(Motility-indole-urea agar, 18 h at 37°C.)*

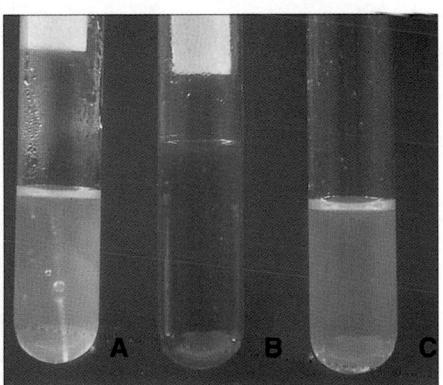

186   Enterobacteriaceae reactions in MIU.
A, *S. enteritidis;* **B,** *Proteus mirabilis;* **C,** uninoculated. *(Motility-indole-urea agar, 18 h at 37°C)*

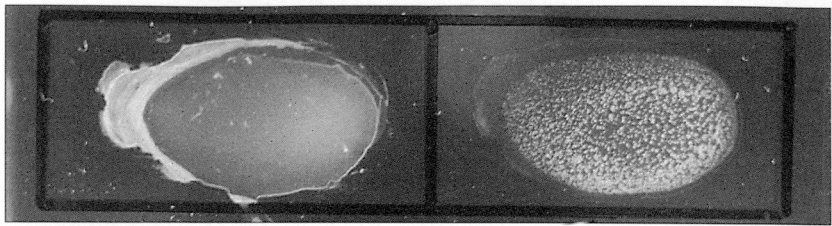

187 *Salmonella* identification by O serotyping. A presumptive *Salmonella* isolate (from culture and biochemical testing) is tested for its O and H antigen type. For O agglutination, an emulsion of the isolate is prepared in saline on a slide and a drop of specific O antiserum added. After 30 sec, the mixture is observed for visible clumping. *(Agglutination after 30 sec)*

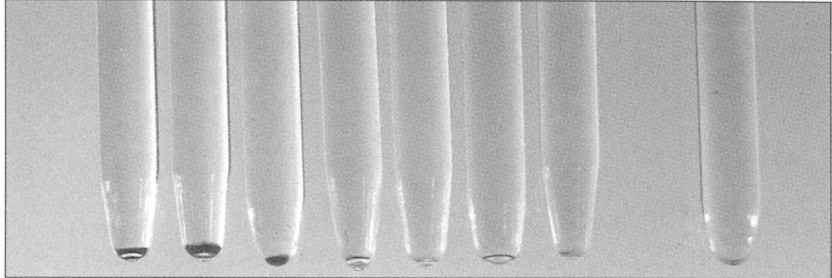

188 Widal test for serological diagnosis of typhoid fever. The Widal test measures the patient's antibodies against *Salmonella typhi* O and H antigen preparations. Serial dilutions of the patient's serum are added to the antigens in tubes and the highest dilution giving granular agglutination with the O antigen and floccular agglutination with the H antigen is reported. Dilutions 1:20–1:1280 and negative control. O titre, 1:80. *(Incubated 2 h at 37°C)*

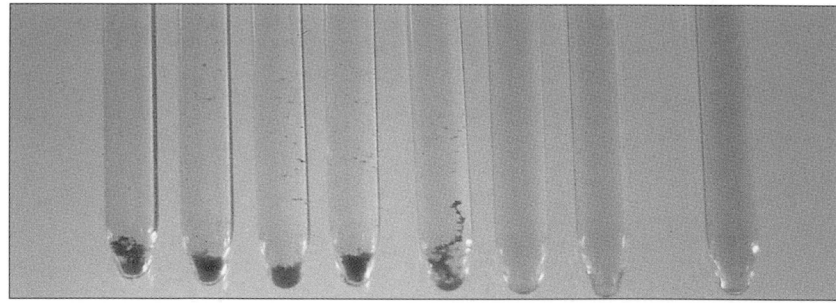

189 Widal test, H agglutination.
H titre, 1:320. *(Incubated 3 h at 37°C)*

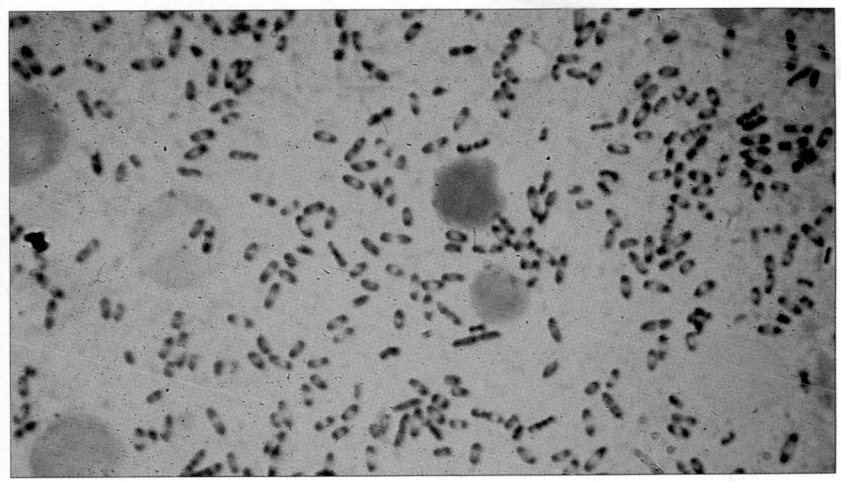

190 *Yersinia pestis* (the plague bacillus), Wayson's stain. Wayson's staining shows cocco-bacilli with bipolar staining. *(Wayson's stain, x1000)*

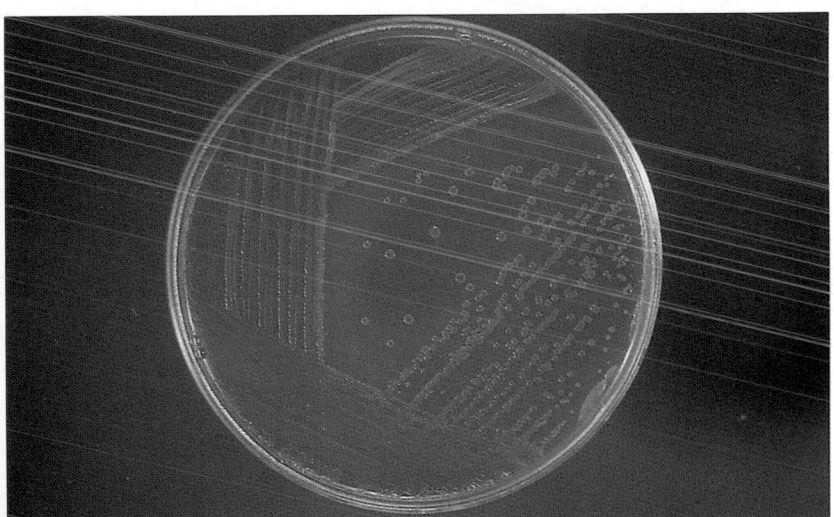

191 *Yersinia enterocolitica*, culture on CIN medium. CIN medium (cefsoludin–irgasan–novobiocin medium) is a selective medium for isolating Y. enterocolitica from faeces. After 48 h incubation, Y. enterocolitica appears as pink colonies with a red centre. *(CIN agar, 48 h at 37°C)*

GRAM-NEGATIVE COCCI AND COCCO-BACILLI

Major characteristics and effects of this group are summarized in **192–200**

Neisseria spp.

Neisseria spp.includes the two important pathogens *N. meningitidis* and *N. gonorrhoeae*, as well as commensal organisms such as *N. lactamica*. **201** is a Gram stain of the cerebrospinal fluid from a patient with meningococcal meningitis, showing the paired Gram-negative cocci of *N. meningitidis*. **202** shows colonies of *N. meningitidis* cultured on heated blood ('chocolate') agar. Gram stain and culture of *N. gonorrhoeae* are shown in **203** and **204**. Selective media, such as Modified New York City (MNYC) media are necessary to isolate *N. gonorrhoeae* from clinical specimens. *Neisseria* spp. are oxidase positive (**205**), and can be distinguished from each other by carbohydrate utilization tests (**206–208**). *Moraxella catarrhalis* (formerly *N. catarrhalis*) is a cause of respiratory infections (**209**). *M. lacunata* (**210**) is a cause of conjunctivitis.

Bordetella spp.

Bordetella pertussis, the cause of whooping cough, occurs as Gram-negative cocco-bacilli (**211**). Clinical specimens are cultured on a selective medium such as charcoal-cephalexin blood agar (CCBA) and need to be incubated for 2–3 days. The colonies have a metallic or mercury-like appearance (**212**).

Haemophilus spp.

Haemophilus spp. include a number pathogenic to humans. *H. influenzae* has both capsulated and non-encapsulated strains. Capsulated strain serotype b is a cause of meningitis and epiglottitis. **213**, **214**, and **215** show the Gram appearance of *H. influenzae*. Culture of *Haemophilus* spp. requires the growth factors haemin (X) and/or nicotinamide-adenine diphosphate (V). *H. influenzae* requires both, which are provided by heated blood agar (**216**). Differentiation of *Haemophilus* spp. by X and V factor-dependence is shown in **217** and **218**. **219** demonstrates increased growth of *H. influenzae* on blood agar close to a streak of *S. aureus* (satellitism) which provides additional V factor.

Pasteurella spp.

Pasteurella multocida is part of the oral flora of dogs and cats and may cause infection in bite wounds (**220** and **221**).

Brucella spp.

Brucellosis in humans may be caused by *Brucella abortus* (from cattle), *B. melitensis* (from sheep and goats) or *B. suis* (from pigs). **222** is a Gram stain of *B. abortus*, showing the small, Gram-negative, cocco-bacilli.

The different *Brucella* spp. may be distinguished by growth inhibition by the dyes thionine and fuchsin (**223**). Contamination of milk by brucella may be demonstrated by the milk ring test (**224**). The Rose–Bengal test is a serological screening test for brucellosis in cattle (**225**).

	Gram-negative cocci and cocco-bacilli Infections				
Organism	Major infection	Less common infection	Vaccine preventable	Incubation period	Period of infectivity
Neisseria					
N. meningitidis (13 serogroups)	Meningitis, septicaemia	Arthritis	Yes (serogroups A/C)	2–10 days	Until 24 h after rifampicin prophylaxis
N. gonorrhoeae	Gonorrhoea, pelvic inflammatory disease	Arthritis, conjunctivitis	No	2–7 days	Months if untreated
Moraxella					
M. catarrhalis	Pneumonia	Conjunctivitis, otitis media	No	–	–
M. lacunata	Conjunctivitis	–	No	–	–
Francisella					
F. tularensis	Tularaemia	–	Yes	2–10 days	Not directly transmitted

192 Gram-negative cocci and cocco-bacilli. Infections.

Gram-negative cocci and cocco-bacilli Sources and transmission of bacteria								
	Reservoir			Transmission				
Organism	Man	Animal	Env.	Insect	Faecal/ oral	Droplet	Direct	Nosocomial	Comments
Neisseria meningitidis	+	–	–	–	–	+	–	–	Epidemics of serogroup A occur in Africa
N. gonnorrhoeae	+	–	–	–	–	–	+	–	Penicillin resistant strains increasing
Moraxella catarrhalis	+	–	–	–	–	+	–	–	
Moraxella lacunata	+	–	–	–	–	–	+	–	
Francisella tularensis	–	+	+	+	+	+	+	–	Category III pathogen

193 Gram-negative cocci and cocco-bacilli. Sources and transmission of bacteria.

Gram-negative cocci and cocco-bacilli Identifying characteristics				
Organism	Gram stain	Culture on blood agar	Oxidase	Biochemical tests
Neisseria meningitidis	–ve diplococci	grey colonies	+	ferment glucose and maltose
N. gonnorrhoeae	–ve diplococci	no growth	+	ferment maltose
Moraxella catarrhalis	–ve diplococci	white colonies	+	DNA-ase +ve
Moraxella lacunata	–ve cocco-bacilli	poor growth: culture on Dorset egg medium	+	do not ferment glucose
Francisella tularensis	–ve cocco-bacillus	no growth	–	identification by agglutination

194 Gram-negative cocci and cocco-bacilli. Identifying characteristics.

Gram-negative cocco-bacilli Infections					
Organism	Major infection	Less common infection	Vaccine preventable	Incubation period	Period of infectivity
Acinetobacter					
A. calcaoaceticus	Wound infections, bacteraemia	Pneumonia	No	–	–
Bordetella					
B. pertussis	Pertussis (whooping cough)	–	Yes	7–21 days	21 days
B. parapertussis	Parapertussis		No	–	–
Haemophilus					
H. influenzae (type b)	Meningitis, epiglottitis, pneumonia, otitis media	Arthritis, osteomyelitis	Yes	2–4 days	In acute stage
H. influenzae (non capsulated)	Bronchitis, otitis media		No	–	–
H. parainfluenzae	Acute respiratory infections		No	–	–
H. aegyptius	Conjunctivitis, Brazilian haemorrhagic fever		No	–	–
H. ducreyi	Chancroid (venereal infection)		No	3–14 days	1–3 weeks

195 Gram-negative cocco-bacilli. Infections.

Gram-negative cocco-bacilli Sources and transmission of bacteria								
	Reservoir			**Transmission**				
Organism	Man	Animal	Env.	Faecal oral	Droplet	Direct	Nosocomial	Comments
Acinetobacter calcaoaceticus	+	–	+	–	+	+	+	
Bordetella pertussis	+	–	–	–	+	–	–	
B. parapertussis	+	–	–	–	+	–	–	
Haemophilus influenzae (b)	+	–	–	–	+	–	–	
H. influenzae	+	–	–	–	+	–	–	
H. parainfluenzae	+	–	–	–	+	–	–	
H. aegyptius	+	–	–	–	–	+	–	
H. ducreyi	+	–	–	–	–	+	–	

196 Gram-negative cocco-bacilli. Sources and transmission of bacteria.

Gram-negative cocco-bacilli
Identifying characteristics

Organism	Gram stain	Culture	Biochemical and other tests
Acinetobacter calcaoaceticus	–ve cocco-bacilli	grows on blood agar and MacConkey	Oxidase negative, nitrate negative
Bordetella pertussis	–ve cocco-bacilli	no growth on blood agar	Mercury-like colonies on CCBA[a] medium, oxidase positive, urea –ve
B. parapertussis	–ve cocco-bacilli	grows on blood agar	oxidase positive, urea +ve

Organism	Gram stain	Culture	Culture dependent on X[b] and V[c] factors	
			X	V
Haemophilus influenzae	–ve cocco-bacilli	} culture on		
H. parainfluenzae	"	} heated	+	+
H. aegyptius	"	} blood agar	–	+
H. ducreyi	"	difficult to culture from clinical specimens	+	+
			+	–

(a) Charcoal cephalexin blood agar (b) X = haematin (c) V = NADP

197 Gram-negative cocco-bacilli. Identifying characteristics.

Gram-negative cocco-bacilli
Infections

Organism	Major infection	Less common infection	Vaccine preventable	Incubation period	Period of infectivity
Pasteurella					
P. multocida	Wound infection following animal bites	Septicaemia	No	–	–
Brucella					
B. abortus	Brucellosis	–	–		
B. melitensis	Brucellosis	–	–	5–30 days	not person-to-person
B. suis	Brucellosis	–	–		

198 Gram-negative cocco-bacilli. Infections.

Gram-negative cocco-bacilli Sources and transmission of bacteria							
	Reservoir			**Transmission**			
Organism	Man	Animal	Env.	Faecal/oral	Droplet	Direct	Nosocomial	Comments
Pasteurella multocida	–	+	–	–	–	+	–	
Brucella abortus	–	+	–	+	+	+	–	Cattle
B. melitensis	–	+	–	+	+	+	–	Sheep, goats
B. suis	–	+	–	+	+	+	–	Pigs

199 Gram-negative cocco-bacilli. Sources and transmission of bacteria.

Gram-negative cocco-bacilli Identifying characteristics				
Organism	Gram stain	Culture	Biochemical and other tests	
Pasteurella multocida	–ve cocco-bacilli	Small, non-haemolytic colonies on blood agar	Oxidase +ve, urease –ve	
Brucella abortus	–ve cocco-bacilli	Small, smooth colonies after 48 h on blood agar Clinical specimen may take up to 4 weeks to grow	Differentiation by dye inhibition tests	
			thionine	fuchsin
			+	–
B. melitensis	"	"	–	–
B. suis	"	"	–	+
+ = Inhibition				

200 Gram-negative cocco-bacilli. Identifying characteristics.

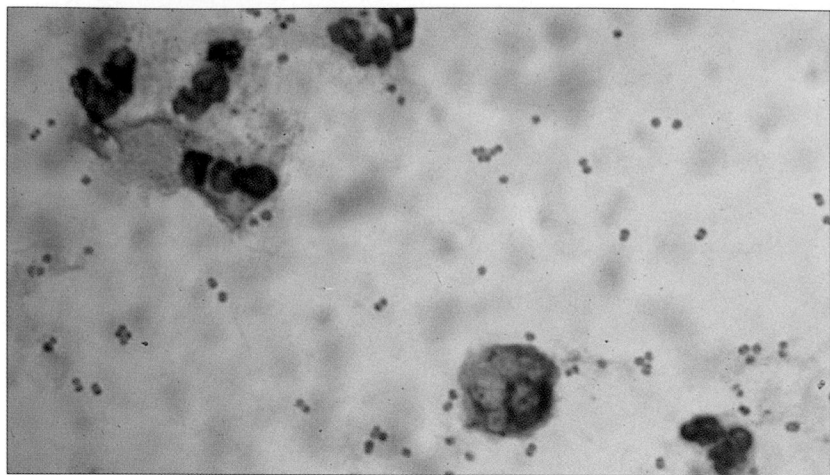

201 Gram stain of csf from a patient with meningococcal meningitis. The stain shows the Gram-negative diplococci of *Neisseria meningitidis* arranged in pairs and the pink-stained leucocytes. *(Gram, x1000)*

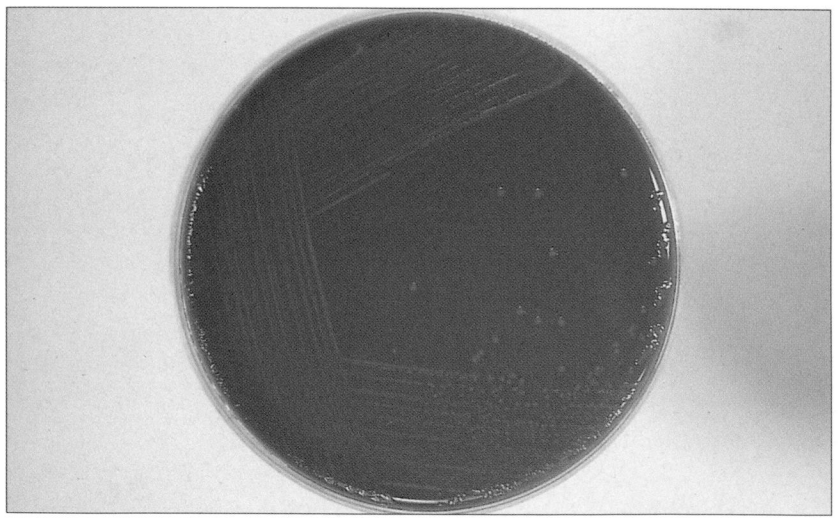

202 *Neisseria meningitidis*, chocolate agar. Cultured on heated blood ('chocolate') agar, showing pale grey colonies, which are oxidase positive. *(Heated blood agar, 18 h at 37°C)*

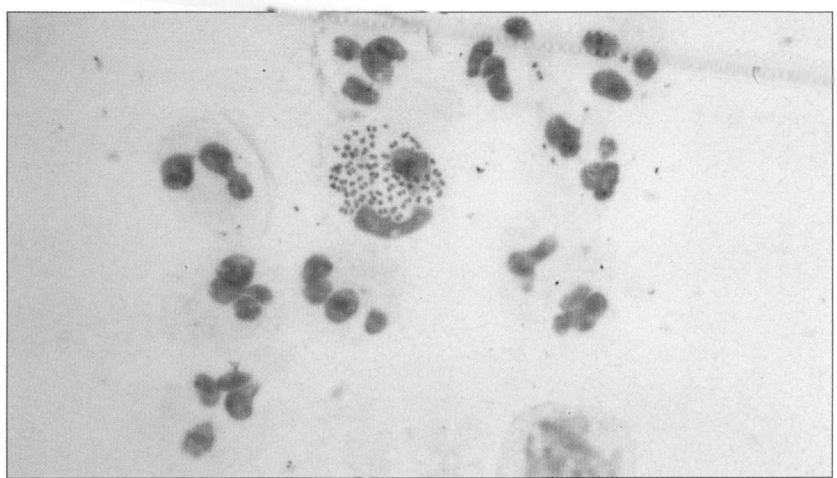

203 *Neisseria gonorrhoeae,* **Gram stain.** Gram stain of urethral pus from a patient with gonorrhoea. Note that the diplococci occur mostly intracellularly. *(Gram, x1000)*

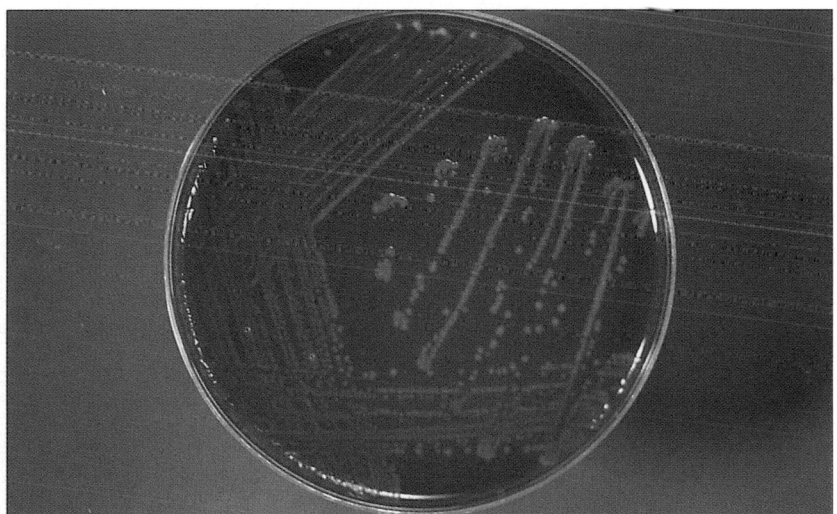

204 Culture of *Neisseria gonorrhoeae,* Modified New York City (MNYC) medium. MNYC is a selective medium for isolation of *N. gonorrhoeae* from urogenital specimens. *(MNYC agar, 18 h in CO_2 at 37° C)*

205   *Neisseria gonorrhoeae* oxidase test. *Neisseria* spp. are oxidase positive. The isolate is scraped onto a filter paper moistened with oxidase reagent containing phenylene diamine, which is oxidized to purple indophenol. *(Oxidase reagent soaked paper, read after 30 sec)*

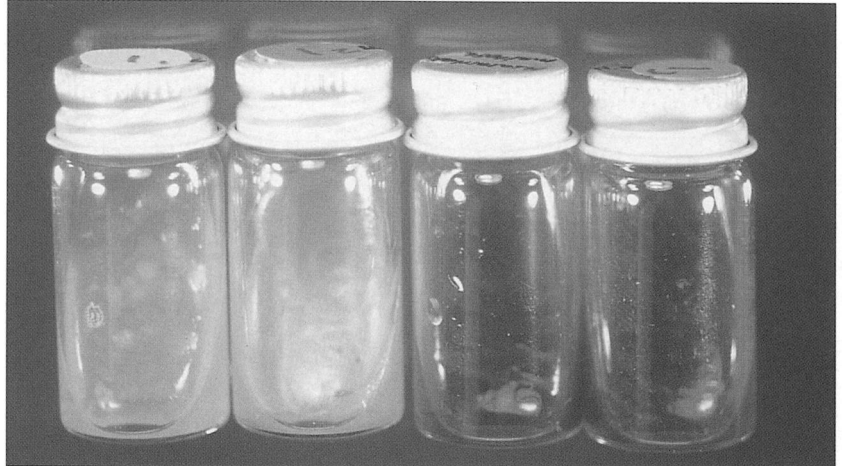

206   Carbohydrate utilization test for *Neisseria*. *Neisseria* spp. (in this case *Neisseria meningitidis*) can be distinguished by carbohydrate utilization reactions using glucose, maltose, lactose, sucrose. Acid production is indicated by a yellow colour. *(*Neisseria *sugar medium with phenol red indicator, 18 h at 37°C)*

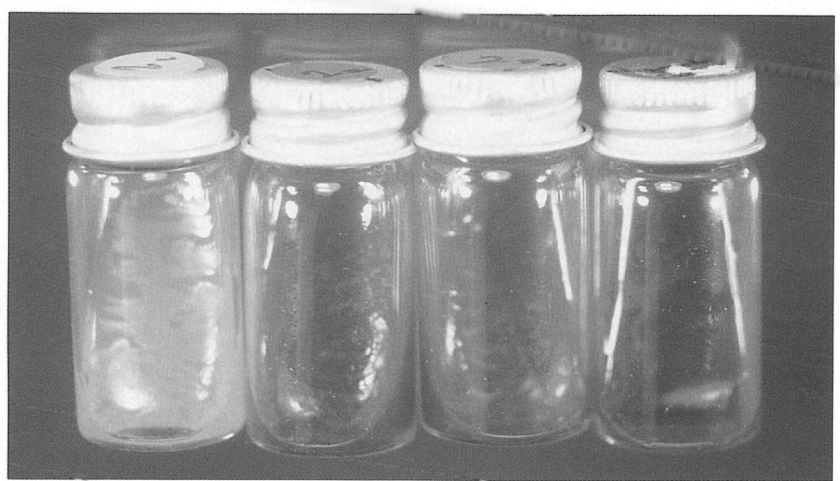

207 Carbohydrate utilization test for *Neisseria*. *N. gonorrhoeae* ferments glucose only. *(Neisseria sugar medium with phenol red indicator, 18 h at 37°C)*

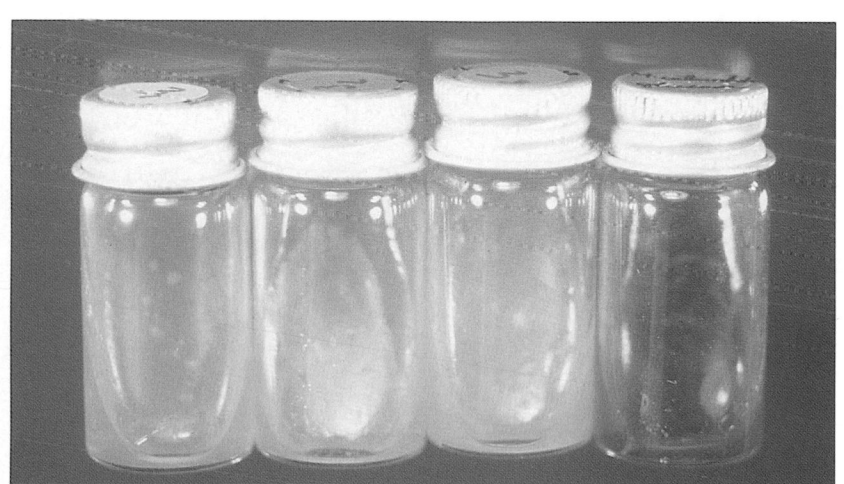

208 Carbohydrate utilization test for *Neisseria*. *N. lactamica* ferments glucose, maltose and lactose. *(Neisseria sugar medium with phenol red indicator, 18 h at 37°C)*

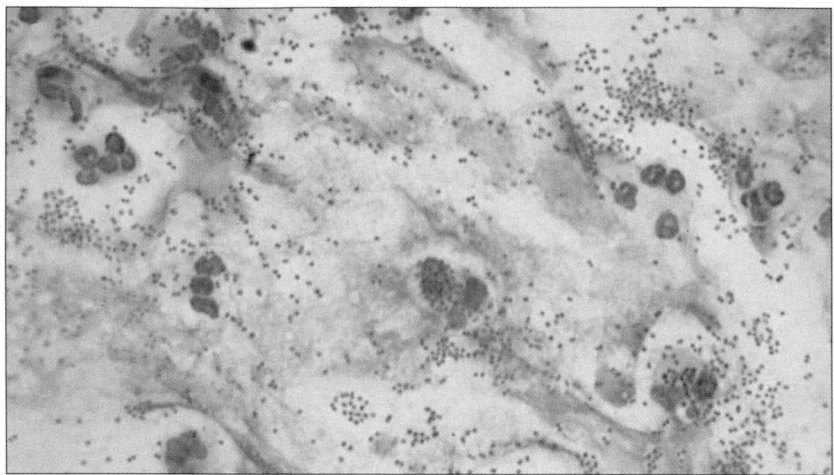

209   Moraxella catarrhalis. Gram stain of sputum showing large Gram-negative cocci. *M. catarrhalis* is a commensal of the upper respiratory tract, but may also cause upper respiratory and other infections. *(Gram, x1000)*

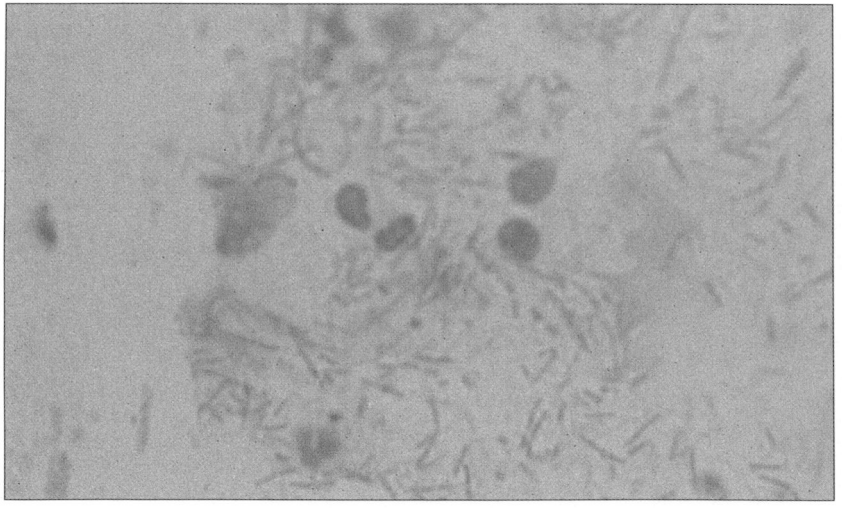

210   Moraxella lacunata. Gram stain of eye discharge from patient with conjunctivitis, showing Gram-negative cocco-bacilli, often appearing brick shaped and joined end to end. *(Gram, x1000)*

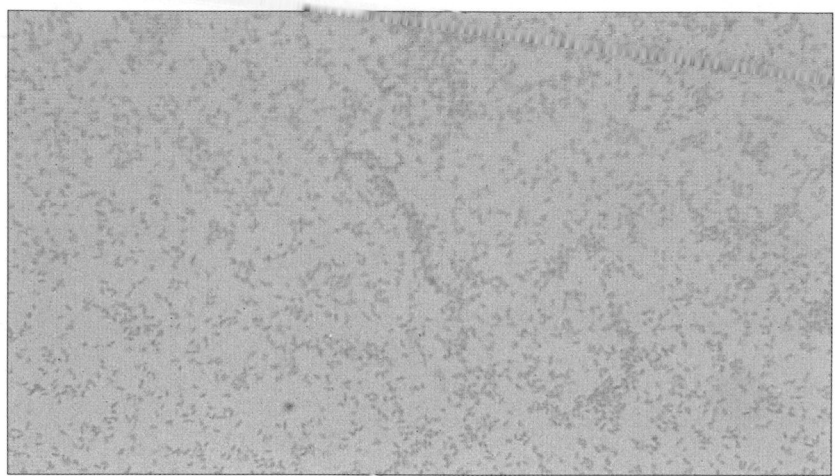

211 ***Bordetella pertussis.*** The Gram-negative cocco-bacilli occur singly or in pairs. Pertussis (whooping cough) continues to be an important infection of children. Specimens are collected by a per-nasal swab and plated on a selective medium such as charcoal cephalexin blood agar (CCBA). *(Gram, x1000)*

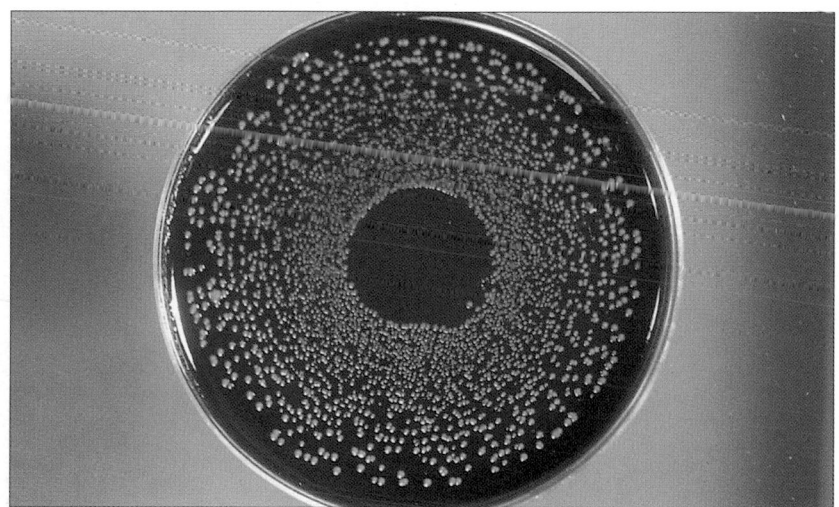

212 ***Bordetella pertussis,* culture from a per-nasal swab.** Culture on CCBA. After 2–5 days culture in a moist aerobic atmosphere, *B. pertussis* produces small, shiny, mercury-like colonies. *(CCBA medium, 5 days at 37°C)*

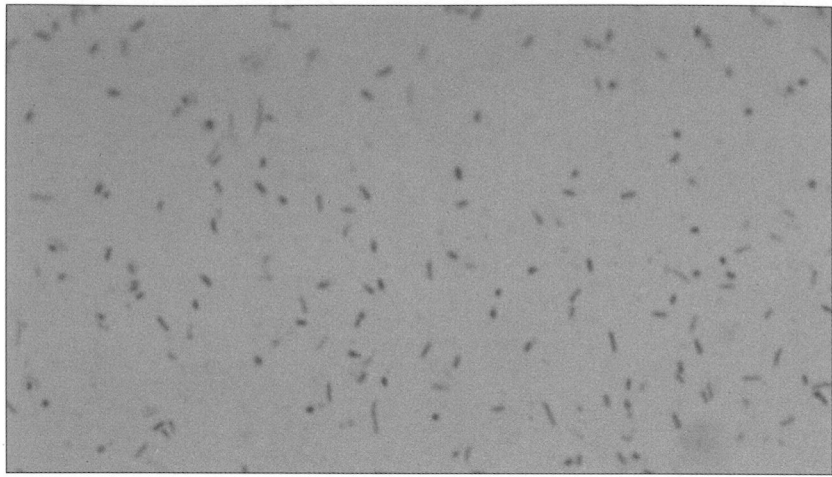

213 *Haemophilus influenzae.* This is a Gram stain from a culture showing the Gram-negative cocco-bacilli. *(Gram, x1000)*

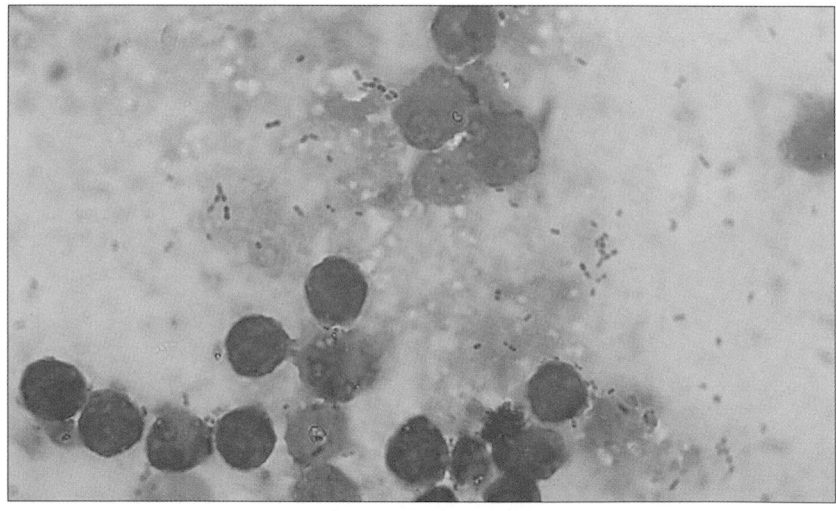

214 *Haemophilus influenzae* **meningitis.** Gram stain of csf from a patient with meningitis due to *H. influenzae.* The Gram-negative cocco-bacilli are sometimes difficult to see among the pink stained polymorphs. *(Gram, x1000)*

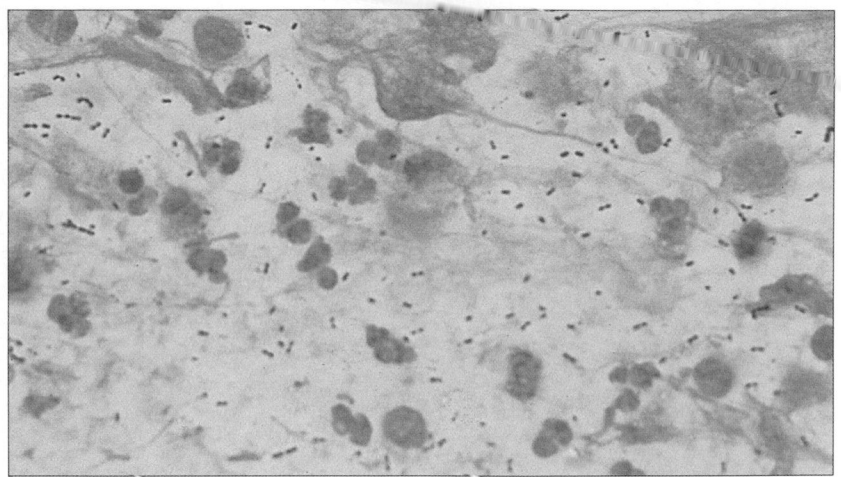

215   *Haemophilus influenzae.* Gram stain of sputum showing *H. influenzae* (Gram-negative cocco-bacilli) and *S. pneumoniae* (Gram-positive diplococci). *(Gram, x1000)*

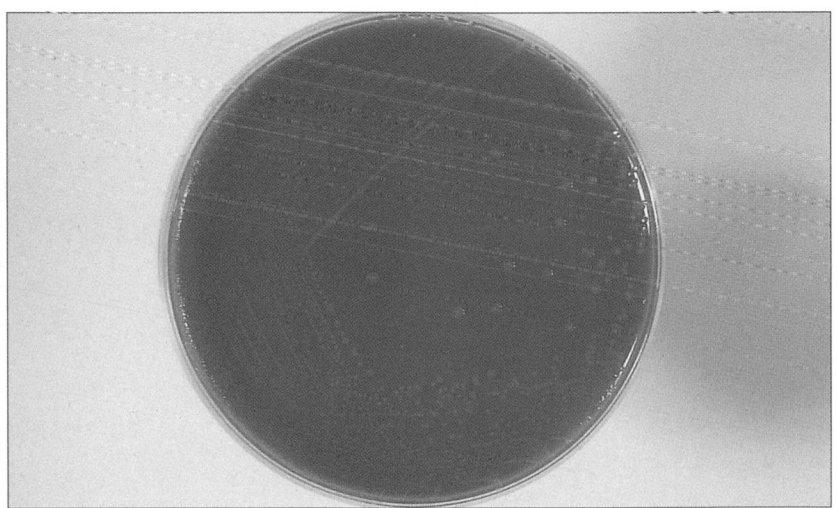

216   *Haemophilus influenzae* cultured on 'chocolate' agar. *H. influenzae* requires the growth factor haemin (X factor) and nicotinamide adenine dinucleotide, NAD (V factor). V factor is released when blood is heated. The colonies are grey with a mucoid appearance. *(Heated blood agar, 18 h at 37°C)*

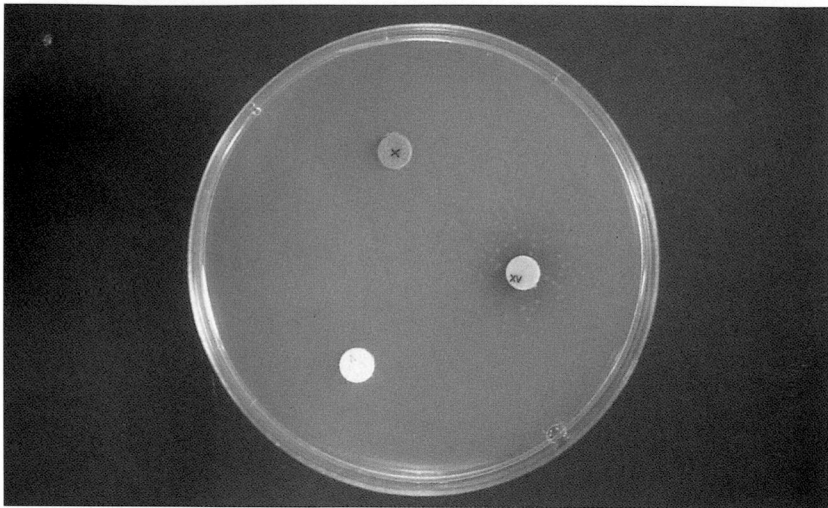

217   X and V dependence of *Haemophilus influenzae.* Growth on nutrient agar with X, V, and X+V disks. *H. influenzae* requires both X and V factors and grows only around the disk containing X and V. *(Nutrient agar, 18 h at 37°C)*

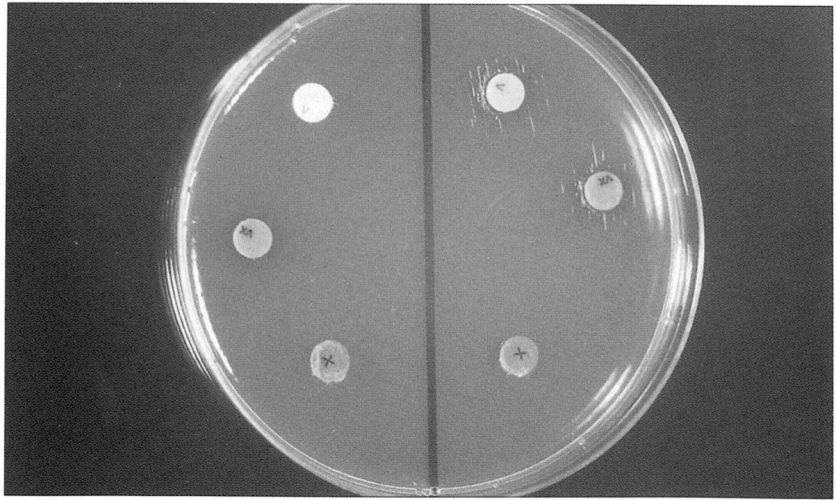

218   *Haemophilus influenzae* and *H. parainfluenzae.* The two halves of the plate are inoculated with *H. influenzae* and *H. parainfluenzae*. *H. parainfluenzae* requires only V factor, and grows round the V and the X+V disks. *(Nutrient agar, 18 h at 37°C)*

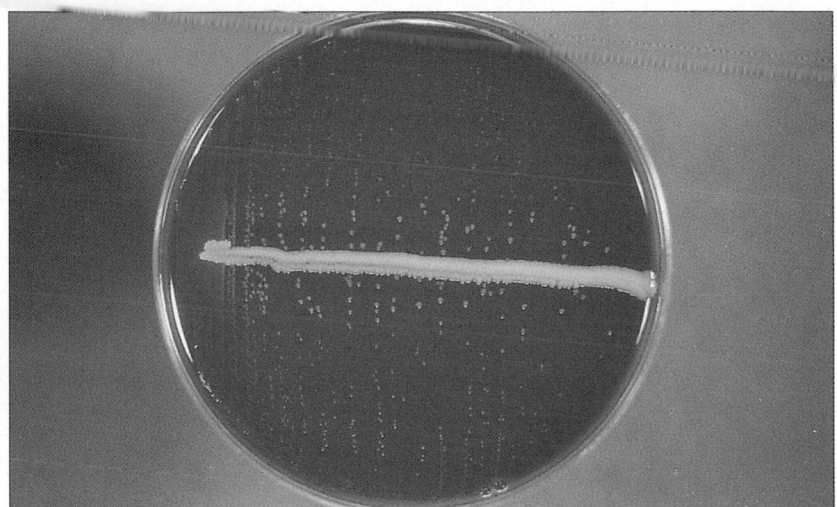

219 Effect of *Staphylococcus aureus* on growth of *H. influenzae.* Growth on blood agar showing satellitism adjacent to a streak of *S. aureus*. *S. aureus* produces surplus V factor, increasing the growth of adjacent *H. influenzae*. *(Blood agar, 18 h at 37°C)*

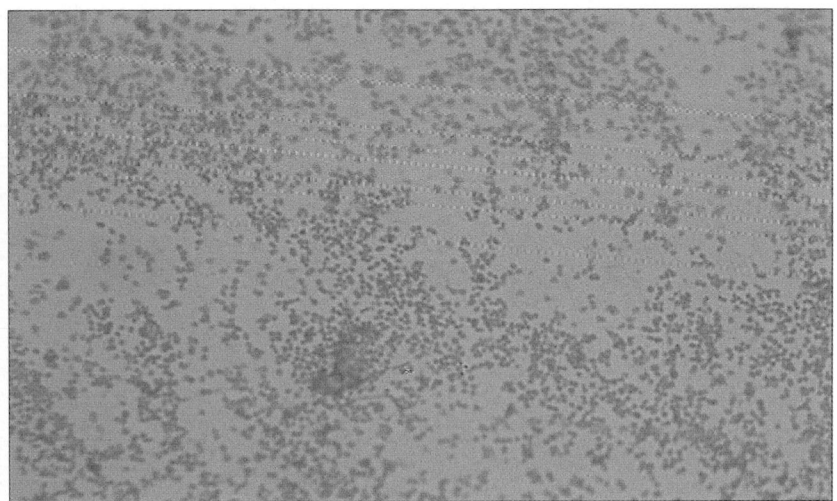

220 *Pasteurella multocida,* Gram stain. *Pasteurella multocida* appears as Gram-negative cocco-bacilli. *P. multocida* is part of the oral flora of dogs, and may be a cause of infection in bite wounds. *(Gram, x1000)*

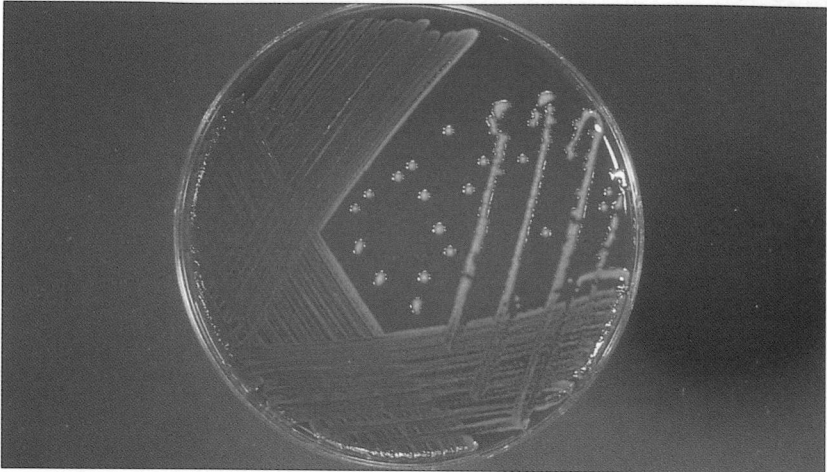

221 Culture of *Pasteurella multocida*. Culture on blood agar showing small, translucent, non-haemolytic colonies, with a blue coloration. *P. multocida* is oxidase positive and does not grow on MacConkey medium. *(Blood agar, 18 h at 37°C)*

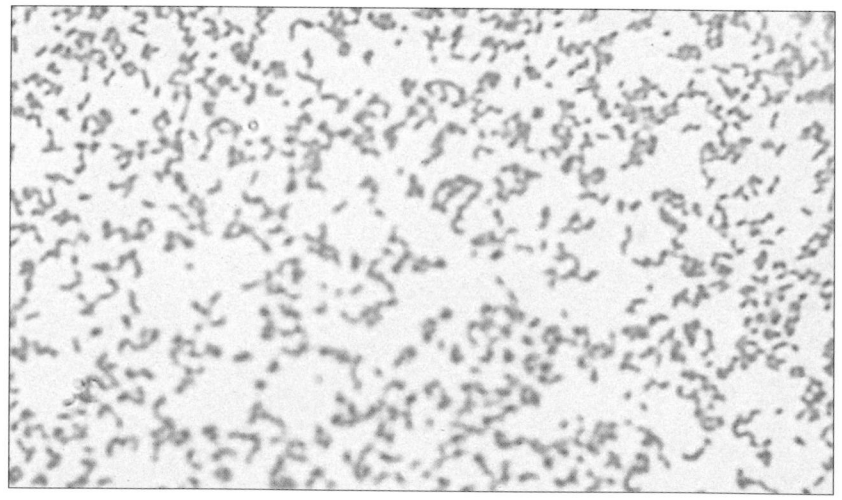

222 *Brucella abortus*. Gram stain, showing Gram-negative cocco-bacilli. The organisms may show bipolar staining and are rarely found in direct smears from uncultured specimens. *(Gram, x1000)*

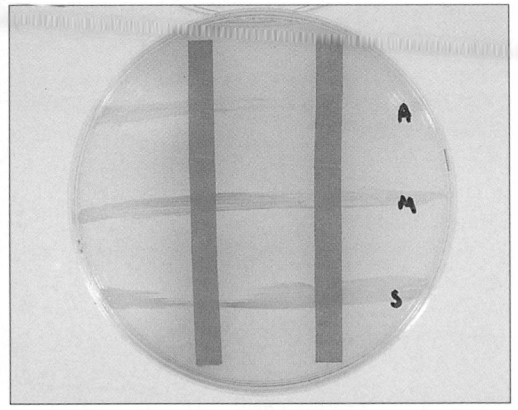

223 Dye inhibition tests for the identification of *Brucella* species. *Brucella* spp. may be distinguished by their susceptibility to the dyes, basic fuchsin and thionine. Filter papers soaked in the dyes are incorporated in the media and the isolates streaked across them. Fuchsin/thionine:
A = *B. abortus* +/−
M = *B. melitensis* +/+
S = *B. suis* −/+
(Blood agar, 4 days in CO_2 at 37°C; + = growth)

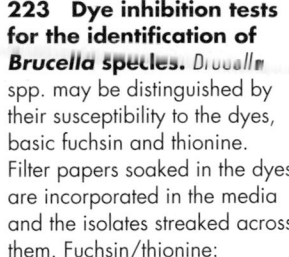

224 *Brucella* milk-ring test. Milk from animals infected with brucellosis may contain brucella agglutinins. Haematoxylin stained, killed *Brucellae* are added to a sample of the milk. A positive test is shown by agglutination and the formation of a blue ring in the sample. (Incubation for 1 h at 37°C)

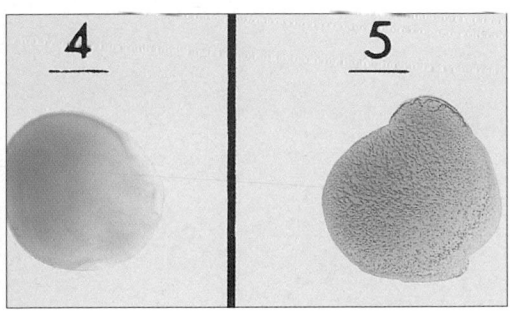

225 Rose bengal test for *Brucella*. The rose bengal test is a serological screening test for *Brucella* antibodies in animals. (Card agglutination read after 3 min; 5 = positive)

VIBRIO, CAMPYLOBACTER, LEGIONELLA AND GARDNERELLA

Characteristics of these bacteria are summarized in **226–228**.
Cholera is caused by the vibrios *V. cholerae* 01 and *V. cholerae* 0139. *V. cholerae* is a comma shaped, Gram-negative bacillus (**229**). Vibrios can be seen in unstained faecal specimens by dark-field microscopy and grow readily in alkaline peptone water (**230**). The selective medium thiosulphate/citrate/bile-salt/sucrose agar (TCBS) is used to isolate *V. cholerae* from faeces, giving yellow, oxidase-positive colonies (**231**). Different *V. cholerae* serotypes will grow on TCBS and confirmation of 01 or 0139 serotype is done by slide agglutination (**232**).

There are two biotypes of *V. cholerae* 01, Classical and El-Tor. They may be distinguished by determining sensitivity (Classical) or resistance (El-Tor) to

Vibrios and related species, *Legionella*, *Gardnerella* Infections					
Organism	Major infection	Less common infection	Vaccine preventable	Incubation period	Period of infectivity
Vibrio					
V. cholerae	cholera	—	Yes	2–3 days	may be prolonged
V. parahaemolyticus	food poisoning		No	12–36 h	asymptomatic carriage
Aeromonas					
A. hydrophila	gastroenteritis	bacteraemia in immunocompromised	No	—	—
Plesiomonas					
P. shigelloides	gastroenteritis	septicaemia	No	—	—
Campylobacter					
C. jejuni	diarrhoea, enterocolitis	bacteraemia	No	1–10 days	several weeks
Helicobacter					
H. pylori	gastritis, peptic ulcer	—	No	—	—
Legionella					
L. pneumophila	'Legionnaires' disease, fever, cough, myalgia	Pontiac fever	No	2–10 days	not directly transmitted
Gardnerella					
G. vaginalis	bacterial vaginosis	—	No		

226 Vibrios and related species, *Legionella*, *Gardnerella*. Infections.

polymyxin (**233**). *V. parahaemolyticus* is a cause of food-poisoning. It produces green colonies on TCBS (**234**).

Aeromonas hydrophila is a curved, Gram-negative bacillus that is a cause of diarrhoea and, occasionally, septicaemia. It grows on blood agar containing ampicillin, producing small haemolytic colonies (**235**). **236** and **237** show *Campylobacter jejuni*, a frequent cause of gastroenteritis. The Gram stain shows delicate 'seagull-shaped' Gram-negative bacilli. *C. jejuni* is cultured on a selective medium containing vancomycin and colistin and grows best in micro-aerophilic conditions at 42°C.

Helicobacter pylori is associated with gastritis and peptic ulcer. It may be demonstrated by Giemsa staining of gastric biopsies (**238**) or cultured on blood agar (**239**) from a biopsy of gastric mucosa. *Legionella pneumophila*, the cause of Legionnaires' disease, requires culture for up to five days on a selective medium such as buffered charcoal yeast extract agar (BCYE) (**240**). Specimens may also be investigated directly for *L. pneumophila* by immunofluorescence (**241**).

Gardnerella vaginalis is associated with bacterial vaginosis. Gram stain of discharge shows epithelial cells surrounded by the pleomorphic Gram-negative bacilli (**242**). **243** shows *G. vaginalis* cultured on a *Gardnerella*-selective agar.

Vibrios, *Legionella, Gardnerella* Sources and transmission of bacteria							
	Reservoir			Transmission			
Organism	Man	Animal	Env.	Faecul/oral	Droplet	Direct	Nosocomial	Comments
Vibrio cholerae	+	−	+	+	−	−	−	Cholera caused by Serotypes 01 and 0139
V. parahaemolyticus	−	+	±	+	−	−	+	
Aeromonas hydrophila	+	±	+	+	−	−	−	
Plesiomonas shigelloides	−	+	+	+	−	−	−	
Campylobacter jejuni	−	+	−	+	−	−		
Helicobacter pylori	+				+		+	
Legionella pneumophila	−	−	+	−	−	−	−	
Gardnerella vaginalis	+	−	−	−	−	+		

227 Vibrios, *Legionella, Gardnerella*. Sources and transmission of bacteria.

Vibrios, Legionella, Gardnerella
Identifying characteristics

Organism	Gram stain	Culture	Biochemical and other tests
Vibrio cholerae	−ve comma-shaped bacilli	yellow colonies on TCBS [a]	Oxidase +ve. Classical and El-Tor biotypes: distinguished by colistin sensitivity and VP test.
V. parahaemolyticus	−ve comma-shaped bacilli	green colonies on TCBS	Oxidase +ve
Aeromonas hydrophila	−ve bacilli	beta haemolytic on blood agar	Oxidase +ve, VP+ve
Plesiomonas shigelloides	−ve bacilli	non-haemolytic on blood agar	Oxidase +ve, VP−ve
Campylobacter jejuni	−ve, thin, S-shaped bacilli	growth preferred at 43°C, micro-aerophilic up to 7 days for growth on chocolate agar	Inositol fermenter, oxidase +ve
Helicobacter pylori	curved −ve bacilli	grey colonies on BCYE [b] agar after 3–4 days	Oxidase +ve
Legionella pneumophila	−ve bacilli	grey colonies on selective media in CO_2	Diagnosis by immunofluorescent test
Gardnerella vaginalis	−ve cocco-bacilli		'clue cells' on microscopy

(a) thiosulphate, citrate, bile salt and sucrose (b) buffered charcoal - yeast extract agar

228 Vibrios, Legionella, Gardnerella. Identifying characteristics.

229 *Vibrio cholerae.*
Gram stain from alkaline peptone-water culture, showing Gram-negative, comma-shaped bacilli of *V. cholerae*. Their characteristic appearance can help in the presumptive diagnosis of cholera. *(Gram, x1000)*

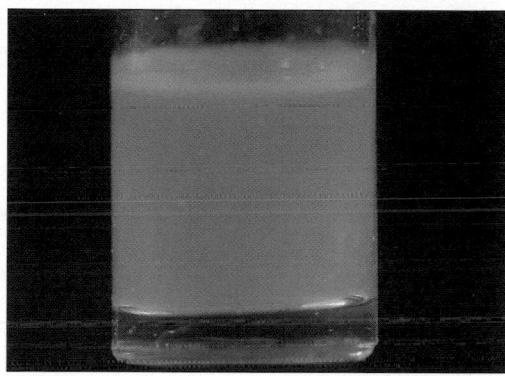

230 Culture of *Vibrio cholerae* in alkaline peptone-water. After 6 h at room temperature, visible growth can be seen at the air-liquid interface. Alkaline peptone-water is a useful transport medium for faeces or rectal swabs from suspected cholera cases. *(Alkaline peptone-water, 6 h at room temperature)*

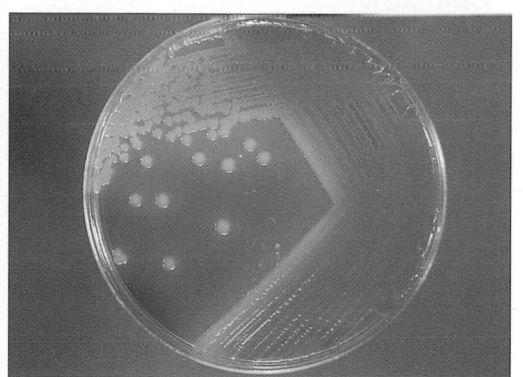

231 *Vibrio cholerae.*
Culture on thiosulphate, citrate, bile-salt, sucrose (TCBS) agar. *V. cholerae* ferments sucrose and produces yellow colonies. *V. cholerae* is oxidase positive. *(TCBS agar, 18 h at 37° C)*

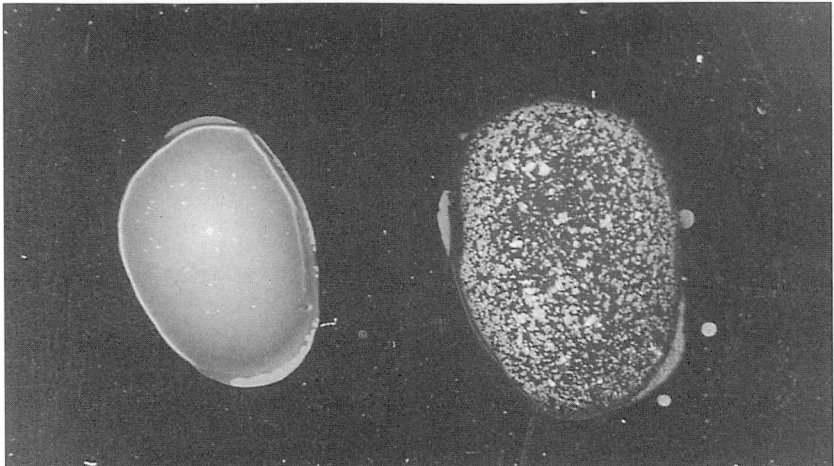

232 *Vibrio cholerae* **agglutination.** Agglutination of *V. cholerae* serogroup 01 with 01 antiserum by slide agglutination. A dilute suspension of *V. cholerae* from a nutrient agar culture is mixed with a drop of 01 antiserum on the slide and inspected after 30 sec. *(Slide agglutination, read after 30 sec)*

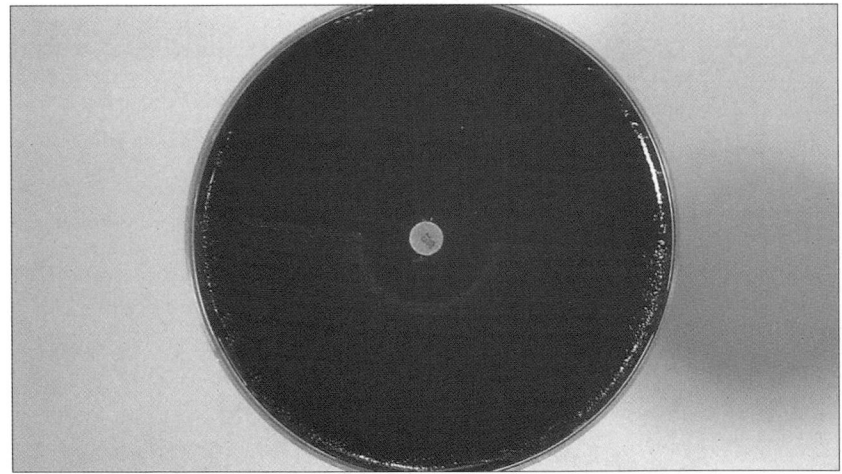

233 *Vibrio cholerae* **biotypes.** *V. cholerae* 01 is divided into two biotypes, classical and El-Tor. Most cases of cholera are now due to the El-Tor biotype. Culture on sensitivity test agar containing a 50 IU polymyxin disk can differentiate El-Tor (resistant) from classical (sensitive). *(Sensitivity test agar, 18 h at 37°C)*

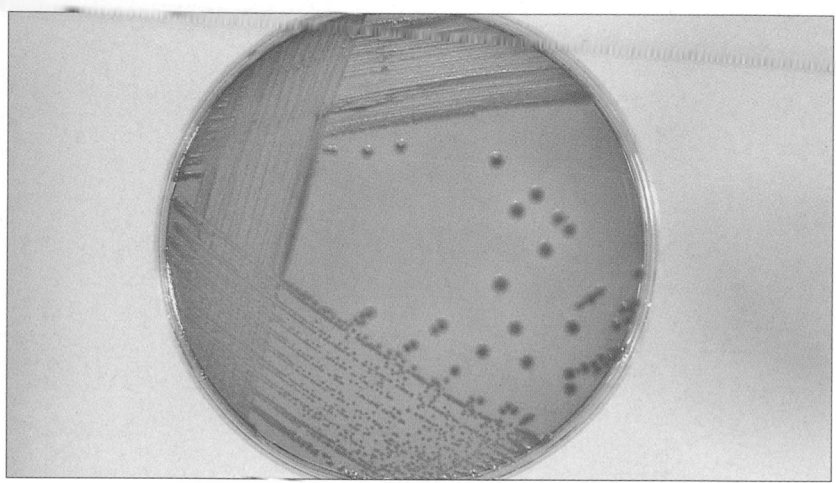

234 Culture of *Vibrio parahaemolyticus*. *V. parahaemolyticus* culture on TCBS showing green (non sucrose-fermenting) colonies. *V. parahaemolyticus* is a cause of food poisoning associated with shellfish and other seafood. *(TCBS agar, 18 h at 37°C)*

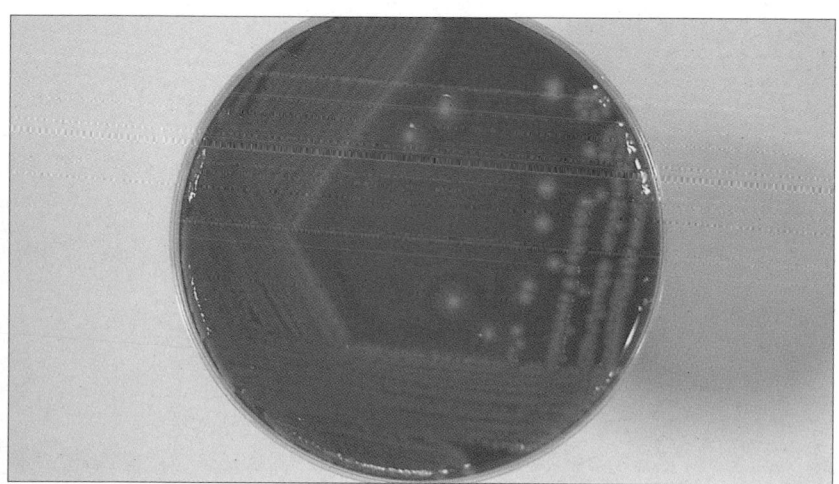

235 *Aeromonas hydrophila*. Culture on blood agar containing 10 µg/ml ampicillin. The small, beta haemolytic colonies are oxidase positive. *(Blood agar, 18 h at 37°C)*

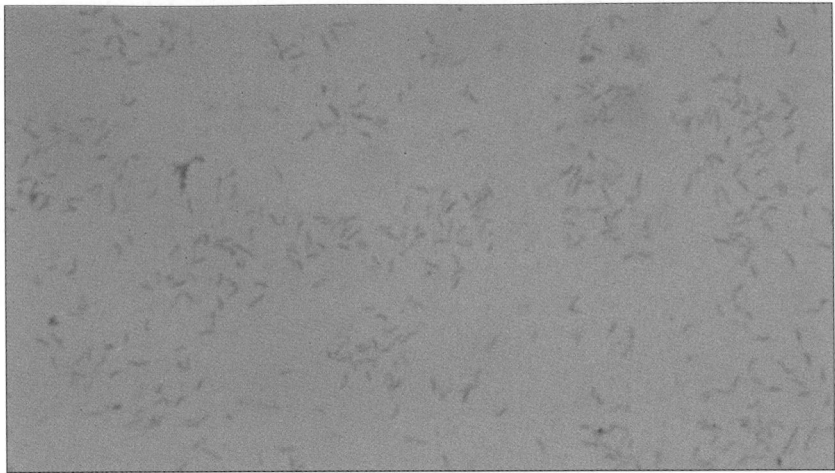

236 *Campylobacter jejuni*, Gram. The Gram stain shows characteristic Gram-negative, spirally curved bacilli, often described as 'gull wings'. *(Gram, x1000)*

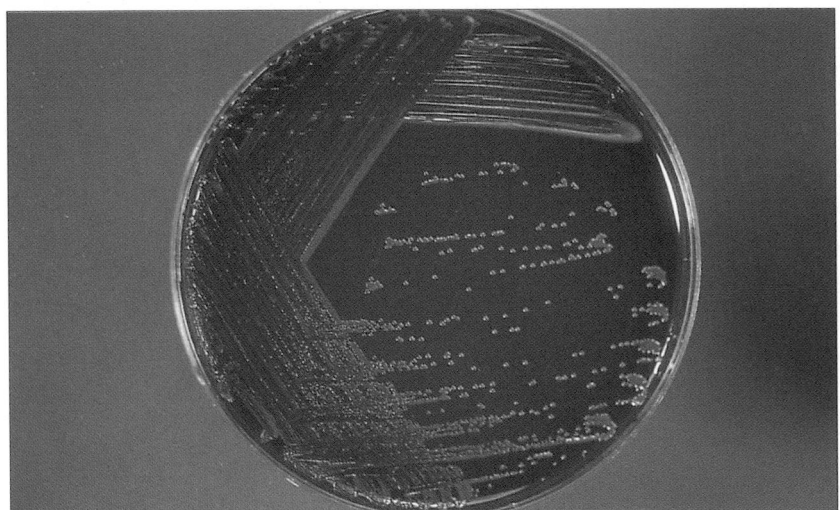

237 Culture of *Campylobacter jejuni*. *C. jejuni* are micro-aerophilic and grow best at 42°C. On *Campylobacter* selective medium, containing antibiotics including vancomycin and polymixin, the colonies are small, grey and droplet-like. *(Campylobacter selective medium, 48 h, 10% O₂ at 43°C)*

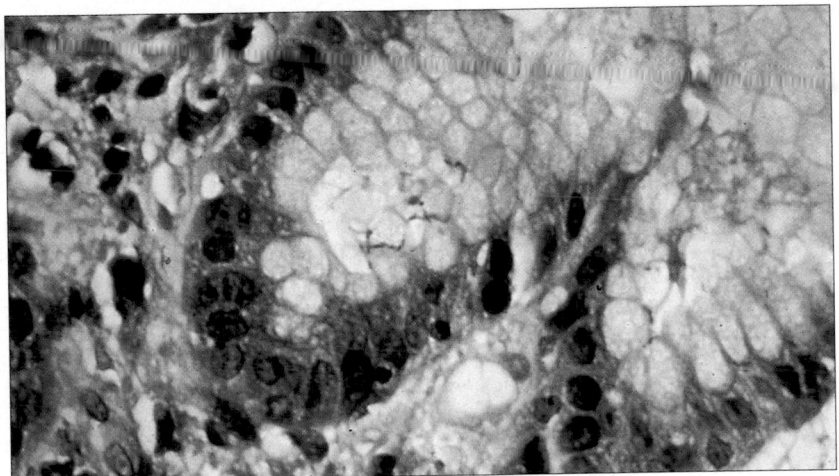

238 *Helicobacter pylori,* **Giemsa.** Giemsa stain from biopsy of gastric mucosa showing *H. pylori* on mucosal cells. *(Giemsa, x1000)*

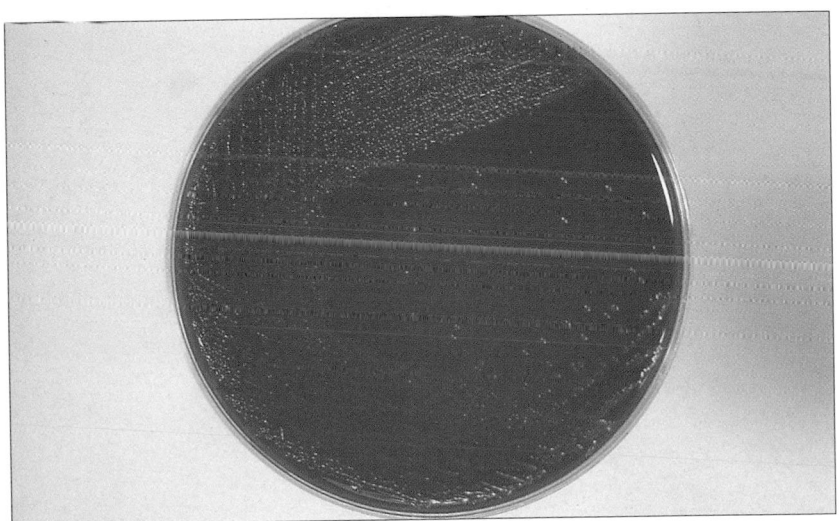

239 *Helicobacter pylori,* **blood agar.** The culture shows pale colonies, which may be grown from gastric biopsy specimens. *(Blood agar, 18 h at 37°C)*

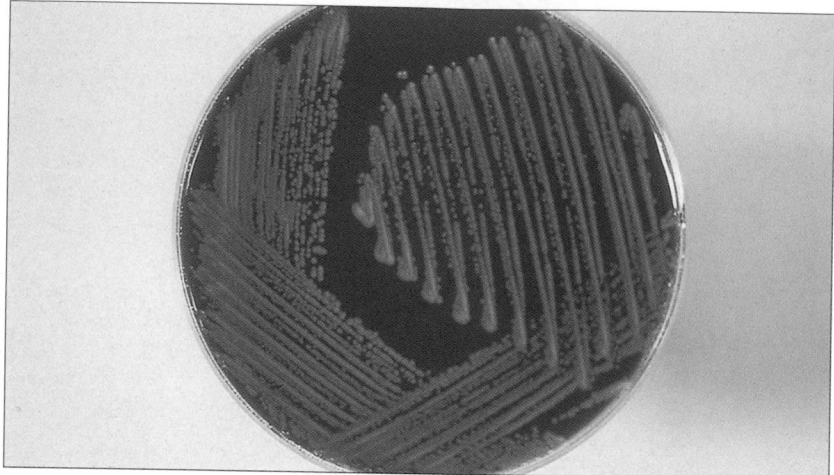

240 Culture of *Legionella pneumophila*. Specimens for *L. pneumophila* are cultured on buffered charcoal-yeast extract (BCYE) medium and incubated in air for up to 2 weeks. Colonies are glistening, grey-white and are Gram-negative bacilli. *(BCYE medium, 4 days at 37°C)*

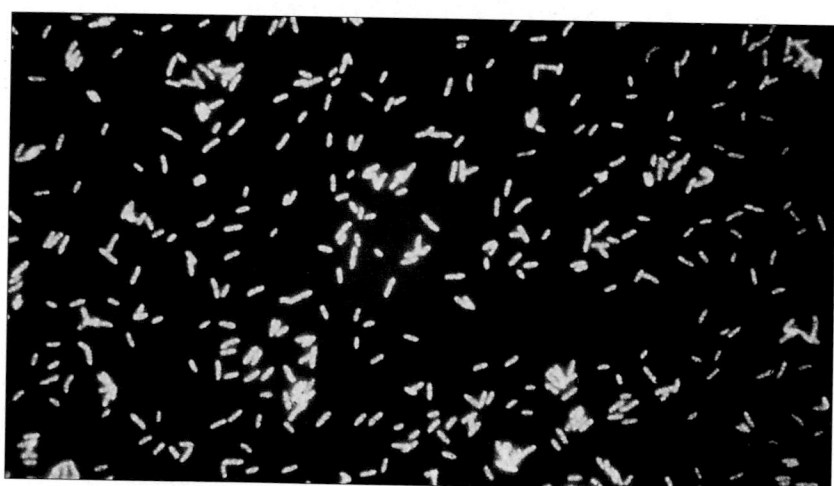

241 Fluorescence microscopy of *Legionella pneumophila*. *L. pneumophila* may be detected in respiratory secretions, by fluorescein labelled antibodies using fluorescence microscopy. *(Fluorescence microscopy, x1000)*

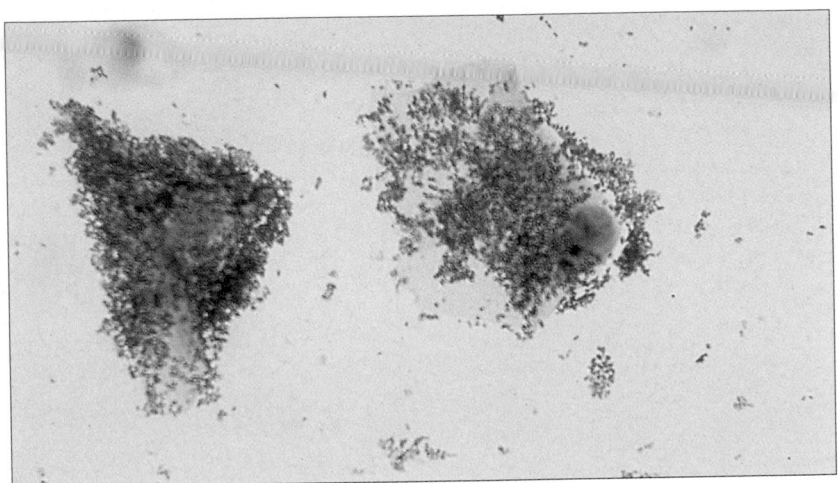

242 *Gardnerella vaginalis,* **Gram stain.** The Gram stain shows Gram-negative bacilli of *G. vaginalis* attached to the periphery of epithelial cells, sometimes called 'clue-cells'. *(Gram, x1000)*

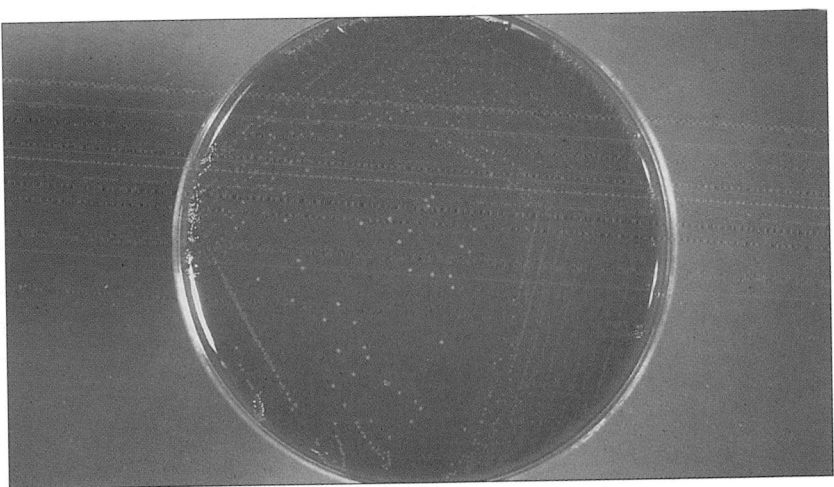

243 *Gardnerella vaginalis* **culture.** Culture of *G. vaginalis* showing small, grey colonies on *Gardnerella* medium, a Columbia agar base containing gentamicin, nalidixic acid and amphotericin. *(Gardnerella medium, 48 h in CO_2 at 37°C)*

PSEUDOMONADS AND OTHER NON-FERMENTATIVE GRAM-NEGATIVE BACILLI

Characteristics of these bacteria are summarised in (**244–246**).

Pseudomonas and related species include bacteria that are widely distributed in the environment, some of which are important human pathogens. *Pseudomonas* spp.are resistant to many of the commonly available antibiotics. *P. aeruginosa* causes a range of infections, including wound infections, urinary tract infections and septicaemia. **247** is a Gram stain of sputum showing the Gram-positive cocci

Pseudomonads and other non-fermentative Gram-negative bacilli Infections					
Organism	Major infection	Less common infection	Vaccine preventable	Incubation period	Period of infectivity
Pseudomonads					
P. aeruginosa	wound infections, urinary tract, septicaemia	pneumonia	No	—	—
Burkholderia cepacia	respiratory infections in cystic fibrosis	—	No	—	—
B. pseudomallei	meliodosis	—	No	up to several years	person-to-person unlikely
Stenotrophomonas maltophilia	—	bacteraemia	No	—	—
Eikenella					
E. corrodens	human bite wounds	meningitis, endocarditis	No	—	—
Flavobacterium					
F. meningosepticum	neonatal meningitis	wound infections	No	—	—
Kingella					
K. kingae	arthritis in children	bacteraemia	No	—	—
Dysgonic fermenters					
DF 3 (*Capnocytophoga canimorsus*)	Animal bites, septicaemia		No	—	—

244 Pseudomonads and other non-fermentative Gram-negative bacilli.
Infections.

of *S. aureus* and the Gram-negative bacilli of *P. aeruginosa*. *P. aeruginosa* is a non-lactose fermenter and is oxidase positive. *P. aeruginosa* often produces a green pigment (pyocyanin) on culture (**248**). Biochemically, *Pseudomonas* spp. can be distinguished from Enterobacteriaceae by oxidation–fermentation reactions (**249, 250**). *Burkholderia cepacia* (formerly *Pseudomonas cepacia*) is an important respiratory pathogen in patients with cystic fibrosis and can be detected by its resistance to colistin (**251**). *B. pseudomallei* causes the tropical human infection, meliodosis (**252–254**).

Eikenella corrodens occurs in human bite wounds. It produces white colonies on blood agar (**255**), which may 'pit' the agar. Flavobacteria include *F. meningosepticum*, a cause of neonatal meningitis and *F. odoratum*, an occasional pathogen in the immunocompromised. Flavobacteria produce yellow colonies on blood agar (**256**).

Pseudomonads and other non-fermenters
Sources and transmission of bacteria

Organism	Reservoir			Transmission					Comments
	Man	Animal	Env.	Insect	Faecal/oral	Droplet	Direct	Nosocomial	
Pseudomonas aeruginosa	+	–	+	–	–	+	+	+	
Burkholderia cepacia	+	–	+	–	–	+	+	+	
Stenotrophomonas maltophilia	–	–	+	–	–	–	+	+	
Burkholderia pseudomallei	–	±	+	–	–	–	+	–	Saprophytic in soil, occasional human infections in S.E. Asia.
Eikenella corrodens	+	–	–	–	–	–	+	–	
Flavobacterium meningosepticum	–	–	+	–	–	–	+	+	
Kingella kingae	+	–	–	–	–	–	+	+	
DF 3	–	+	–	–	–	–	+	–	

245 Pseudomonads and other non-fermenters. Sources and transmission of bacteria.

Pseudomonads and other non-fermenters
Identifying characteristics

Organism	Gram stain	Culture	Biochemical and other tests
Pseudomonas aeruginosa	negative bacilli	greenish pigment on blood agar	
Burkholderia cepacia	negative bacilli	grows on media with colistin	
Stenotrophomonas maltophilia	negative bacilli	rough colonies on blood agar	
Burkholderia pseudomallei	negative bacilli, often bipolar	wrinkled colonies on blood agar	
Eikenella corrodens	negative bacilli	pitting colonies on blood agar	
Flavobacterium meningosepticum	filamentous negative bacilli	yellow colonies on blood agar	
Kingella kingae	short, negative bacilli	'fried egg' colonies on blood agar	All are oxidase positive except *S. maltophilia*.
DF 3	negative cocco-bacilli	nutritionally fastidious oxidase negative	*Kingella* is an OF-fermenter (glucose); the remainder are non-fermenters

246 Pseudomonads and other non-fermenters. Identifying characteristics.

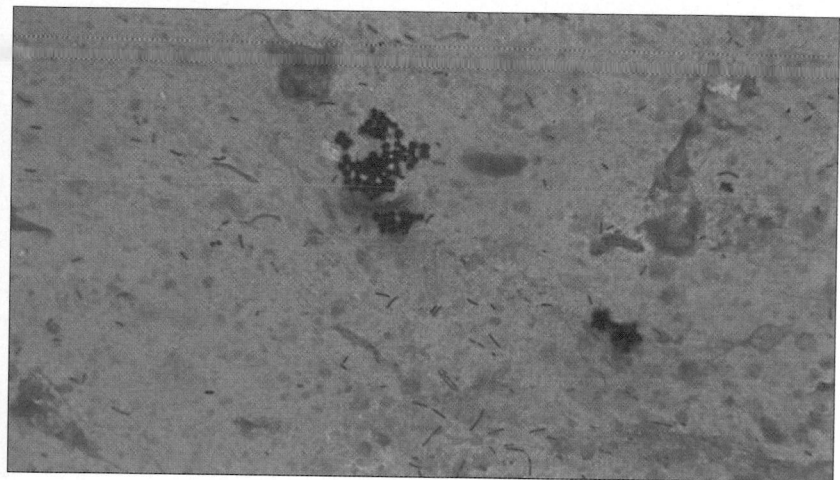

247   Gram stain of sputum containing *Pseudomonas aeruginosa.* Sputum
from patient with cystic fibrosis showing staphylococci and thin, Gram-negative bacilli of
Ps. aeruginosa. *(Gram, x1000)*

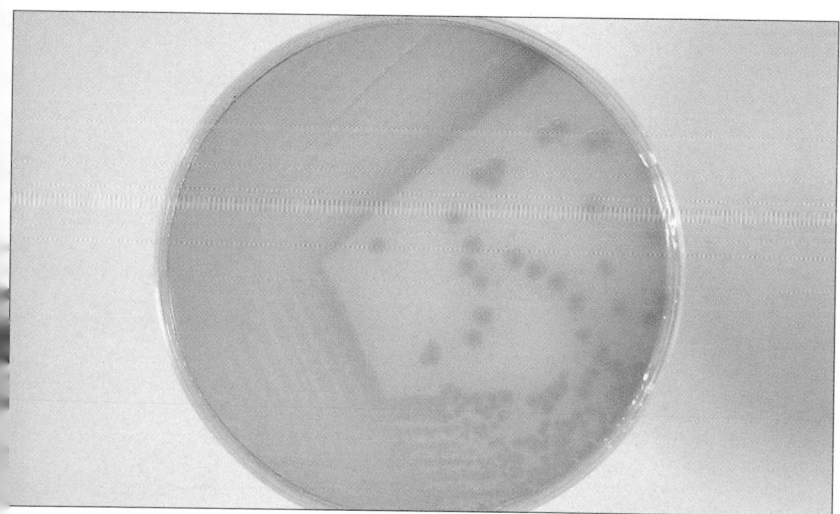

248   *Pseudomonas aeruginosa.* Culture on MacConkey medium. *Ps. aeruginosa*
s a non-lactose fermenter, and often produces a greenish pyocyanin pigment. *Ps.
aeruginosa* is oxidase positive. *(MacConkey agar, 18 h at 37°C)*

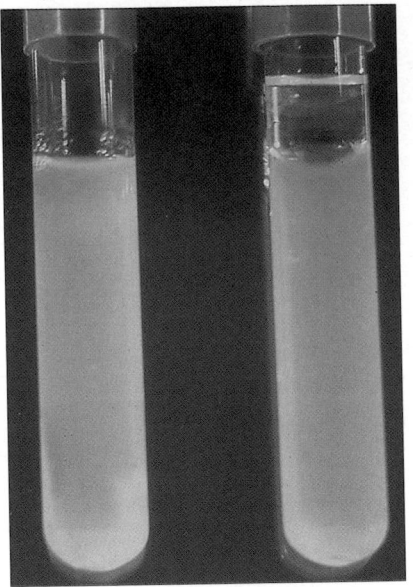

249, 250 Oxidation–fermentation reactions. The test organism is inoculated into two tubes of a tryptone agar medium containing glucose and the indicator bromothymol blue. The medium in one tube is sealed with a layer of liquid paraffin to exclude oxygen. The tubes are incubated for up to 7–14 days; acid production is indicated by a yellow colour. Bacteria that both oxidize and ferment glucose produce acid in both tubes, but oxidizers that do not ferment glucose produce acid in only the unsealed tube.

249 *Escherichia coli*, oxidation plus fermentation.

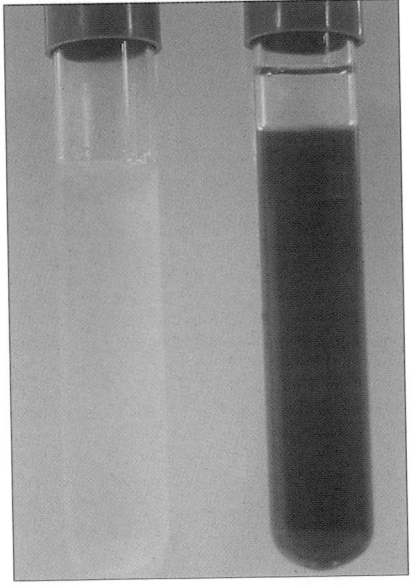

250 *Pseudomonas aeruginosa*. Acid is produced only in the oxidative tube (left), showing *Ps. aeruginosa* is a non-fermenter. *(Tryptone agar, 7 days at 37°C)*

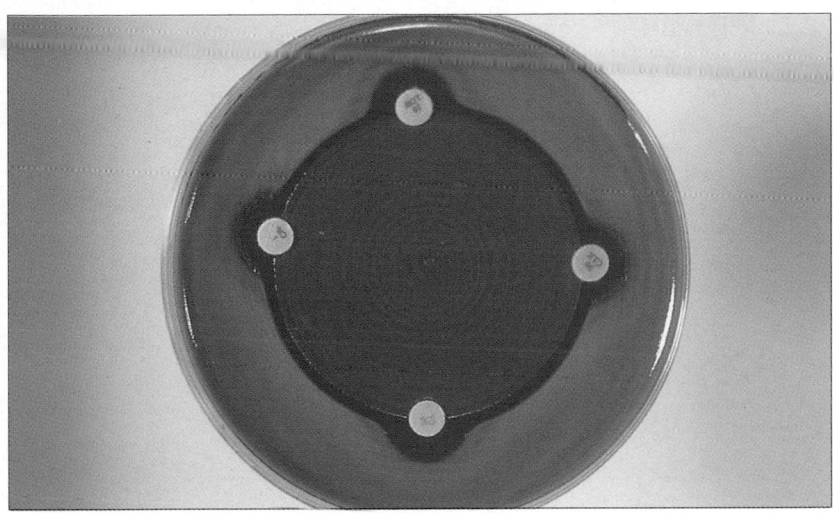

251 **Burkholderia cepacia.** *B. cepacia* (formerly *Pseudomonas cepacia*) is an increasingly important respiratory pathogen in cystic fibrosis patients. Most strains are multiply antimicrobial resistant. *B. cepacia* is inoculated centrally. A sensitive control is inoculated peripherally. *(Sensitivity test agar, 18 h at 37°C)*

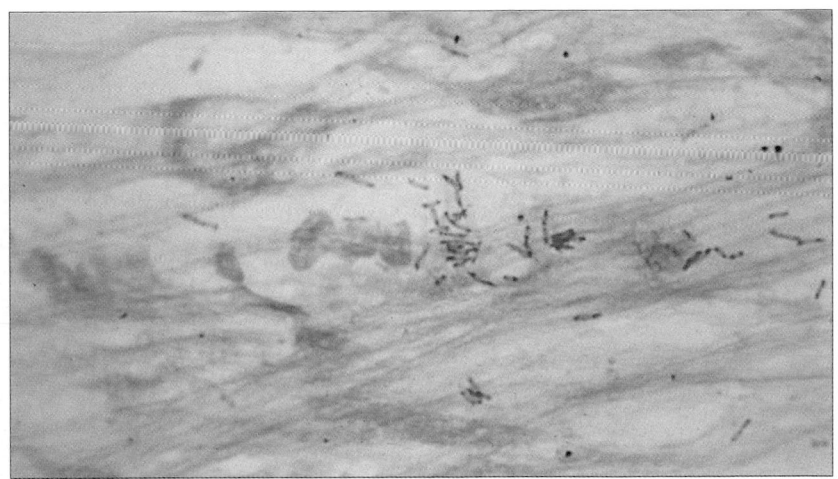

252 **Burkholderia pseudomallei.** Gram stain of *B. pseudomallei* in sputum. The organism is pleomorphic and may show bipolar staining. *(Gram, x1000)*

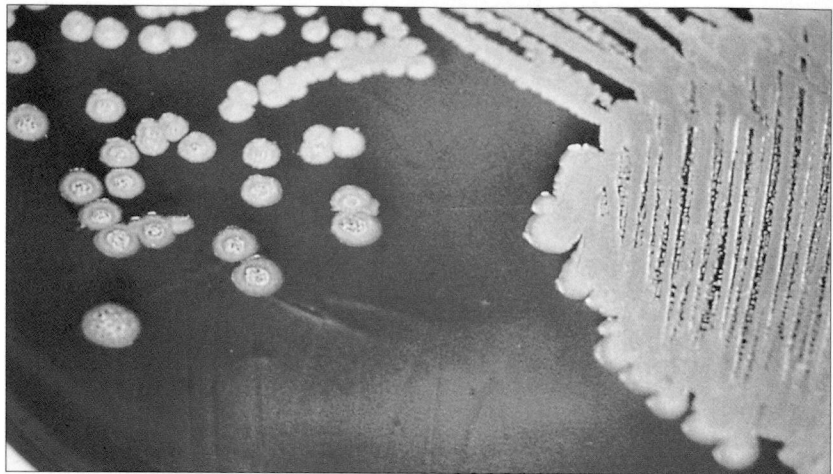

253 *Burkholderia pseudomallei*, blood agar. Culture after 72 h showing characteristic dry, wrinkled colonies. The cultures have a 'truffle' like odour. *(Blood agar, 72 h at 37°C)*

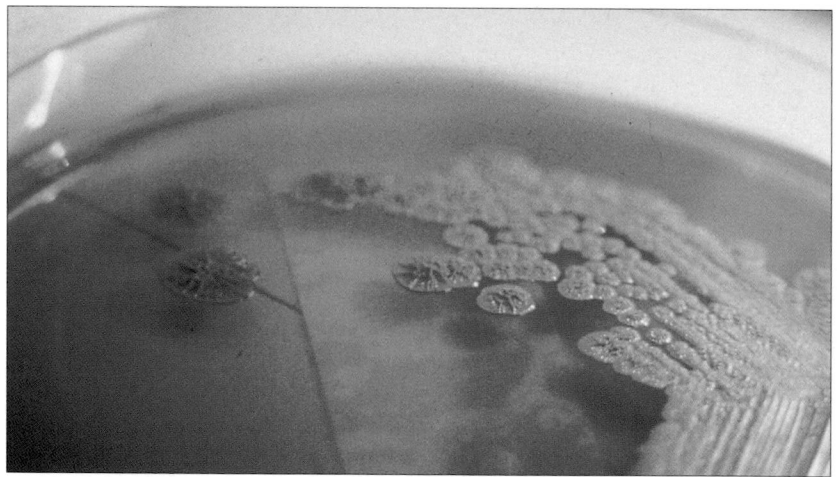

254 *Burkholderia pseudomallei*, Ashdown's medium. The medium is selective, containing crystal violet and gentamicin. The wrinkled morphology is enhanced by glycerol in the medium. *(Ashdown's medium, 72 h at 37°C)*

255 *Eikenella corrodens.* Culture on blood agar showing white colonies. When the colonies are scraped from the agar, the agar is often pitted. *(Blood agar, 18 h at 37°C)*

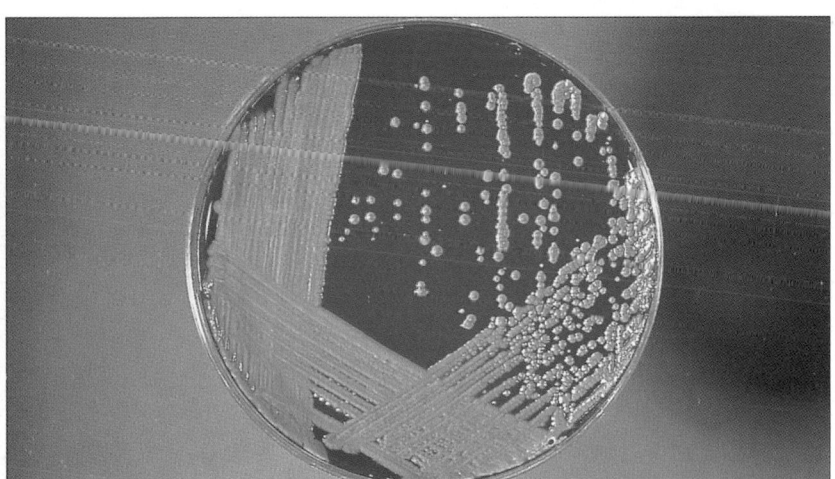

256 *Flavobacterium odoratum.* Culture on blood agar showing characteristic yellow colonies. Flavobacteria are widely disseminated in the environment and are occasional pathogens. *F. meningosepticum* is a cause of neonatal meningitis. *(Blood agar, 18 h at 37°C)*

OBLIGATE ANAEROBIC BACTERIA

Characteristics of anaerobic bacteria are summarized in (**257–259**)

ANAEROBIC GRAM-POSITIVE BACTERIA

Clostridia are spore-forming, Gram-positive bacilli including the causative agents of gas-gangrene, food poisoning, tetanus, botulism and antibiotic associated colitis. **260** is a Gram stain from gas-gangrene showing the brick-shaped Gram-positive bacilli of *C. perfringens*. **261** shows the bacilli of *C. tetani* with terminal spores. Clostridia will grow on blood agar, producing zones of haemolysis (**262** and **263**). Clostridia can be distinguished by their reactions in Robinson's cooked meat medium (**264**), on lactose egg yolk milk agar (**265**) and by the Nagler reaction (**266**). *C. difficile* is involved in antibiotic-associated colitis. On cycloserine-cefoxitin fructose agar (CCFA) it produces 'ground glass' colonies (**267** and **268**). Production of *C. difficile* toxin can be demonstrated by tissue culture cytotoxicity (**269**).

ANAEROBIC GRAM-NEGATIVE BACILLI

Bacteroides fragilis is frequently isolated from abdominal abscesses (**270**). *Bacteroides* species can be distinguished by their antimicrobial sensitivity patterns (**271**) and by the volatile fatty acids detected on gas-liquid chromatography (**272**). *B. melaninogenicus* (now *Prevotella melaninogenicus*) produces characteristic brown/black colonies on blood agar (**273**).

Fusobacterium spp. are a cause of chronic infections, including Vincent's angina, an infection of the jaw in which the spirochaete *Borrelia vincenti* is also involved with *F. nucleatum*. The latter are slender, Gram-negative rods, often with pointed ends (**274**). *F. necrophorum* is also a cause of infections in the head and neck and in severe cases can lead to septicaemia (**275** and **276**).

Organism	Major infection	Less common infection	Vaccine preventable	Incubation period	Period of infectivity
Obligate anaerobic bacteria **Infections**					
Gram-positive **Clostridium**					
C. tetani	tetanus		Yes	3–21 days	
C. perfringens (C. welchii)	gas gangrene, food poisoning, wound infections	puerperal sepsis, pig bel	No	6–24 h 12–36 h	
C. botulinum	botulism, infant botulism		No (antitoxin available)		
C. difficile	antibiotic associated colitis	—	No	—	up to 4 weeks
Propronibacterium					
P. acnes	prosthetic device infections	osteomyelitis, endocarditis	No	—	—
Gram-negative **Bacteroidaceae**					
B. fragilis	intra-abdominal sepsis, intra-cerebral abscess	pneumonia	No	—	—
B. melaninogenicus (Prevotella meluninogenicus)	abdominal wound infections		No	—	—
Fusobacterium					
F. nucloatum	Vincent's angina	tropical ulcer	No	–	—
F. necrophorum	head/neck infections	necrobacillosis	No	—	—

257 Obligate anaerobic bacteria. Infections.

Anaerobic bacteria
Sources and transmission of bacteria

| Organism | Reservoir | | | Transmission | | | | |
	Man	Animal	Env.	Faecal/oral	Droplet	Direct	Nosocomial	Comments
Clostridium tetani	–	–	+	–	–	+	–	
C. perfringens	–	+	+	+	–	–	–	
C. botulinum	–	–	+	+	–	–	–	
C. difficile	+	–	±	+	–	±	+	antibiotic associated diarrhoea
Propionibacterium acnes	+	–	±	–	–	+	+	
Bacteroides fragilis	+	–	–	–	–	+	+	
B. melaninogenicus	+	–	–	–	–	+	+	
Fusobacterium nucleatum	+	–	–	–	–	+	–	
F. necrophorum	+	–	–	–	–	+	–	

258 Anaerobic bacteria. Sources and transmission of bacteria.

Anaerobic bacteria
Identifying characteristics

Organism	Gram stain	Culture	Biochemical and other tests — Culture on lactose, egg-yolk, milk agar				Antibiotic tests		
			Lecithinase	Lipase	Lactose	Proteinase	Col.	Vanc.	Kan.(b)
Clostridium tetani	broad positive bacilli, spores rarely seen	film of growth on blood agar	–	–	–	–			
C. perfringens	positive bacilli	beta haemolytic on blood agar	+	–	+	–			
C. botulinum	positive bacilli with oval subterminal spores	large semitransparent colonies on blood agar	–	+	+	+			
C. difficile	positive bacilli	'ground glass' colonies on CCFA (a) agar							
Bacteroides fragilis	pleomorphic negative bacilli	grey, non-haemolytic colonies on blood agar					R	R	R
B. melaninogenicus	negative bacilli	brown/black haemolytic colonies on blood agar					S	R	R
Fusobacterium nucleatum	fusiform negative bacilli, pointed ends	bread crumb like colonies on blood agar					S	R	S
F. necrophorum	fusiform negative bacilli, rounded ends	pale colonies on blood agar					S	R	S

(a) CCFA: cycloserine-cefoxitin fructose agar. (b) Colistin, Vancomycin, Kanamycin; S= sensitive, R= resistant.

259 Anaerobic bacteria. Identifying characteristics.

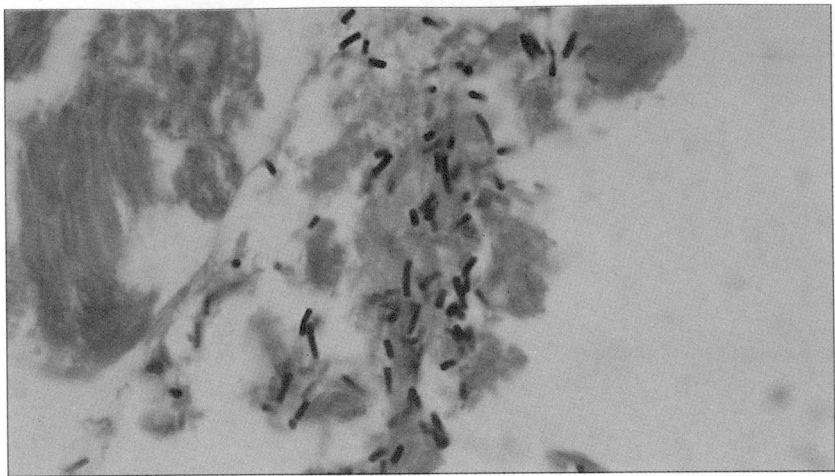

260 Clostridium perfringens (C. welchii). Gram stain from pus from gas gangrene showing thick, brick-shaped, Gram-positive bacilli. *(Gram, x1000)*

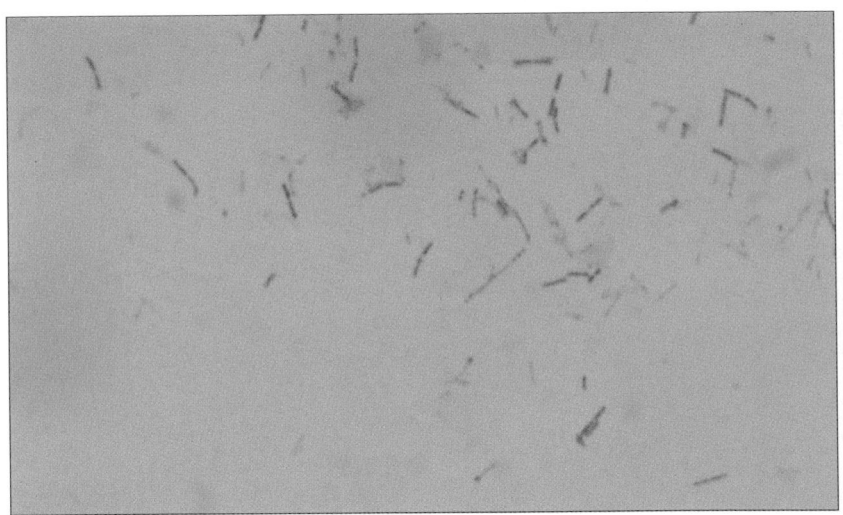

261 Clostridium tetani, Gram. *C. tetani* are thin, Gram-positive rods with terminal spores. The centres of the spores do not stain. *(Gram, x1000)*

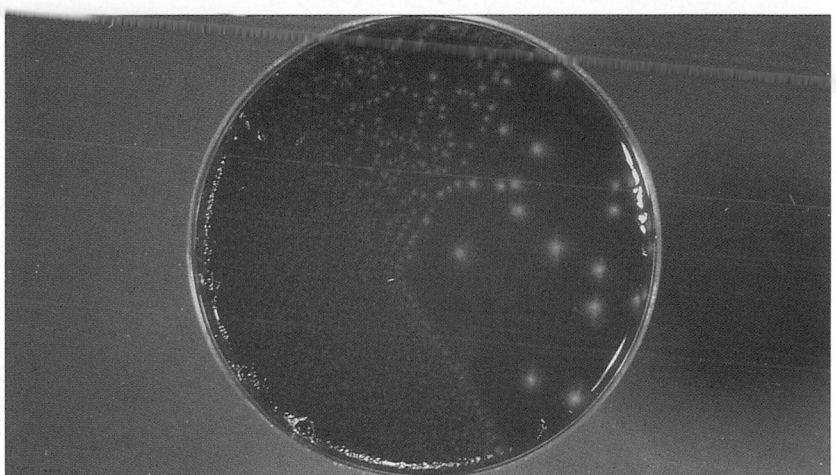

262 *Clostridium perfringens.* Culture on blood agar shows beta haemolysis. Some strains produce a double zone of haemolysis. *(Blood agar, 24 h anaerobically at 37°C)*

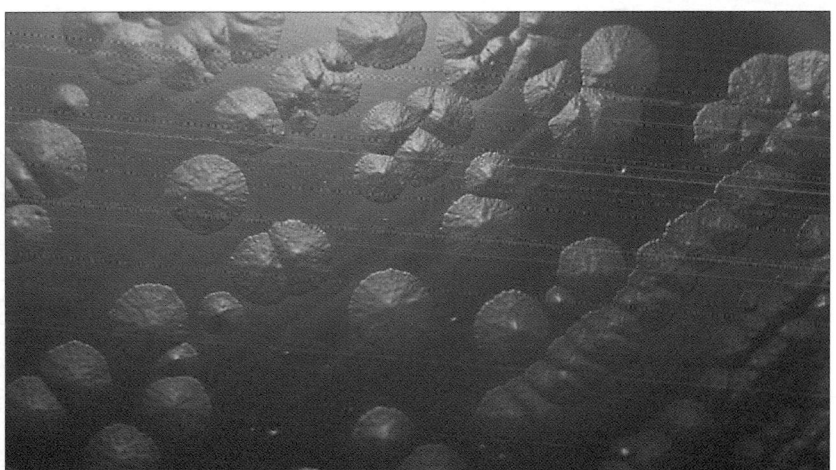

263 *Clostridium perfringens,* **blood agar.** The colonies show a halo of double haemolysis due to the different toxins present. *(Blood agar, 48 h, anaerobically at 37°C)*

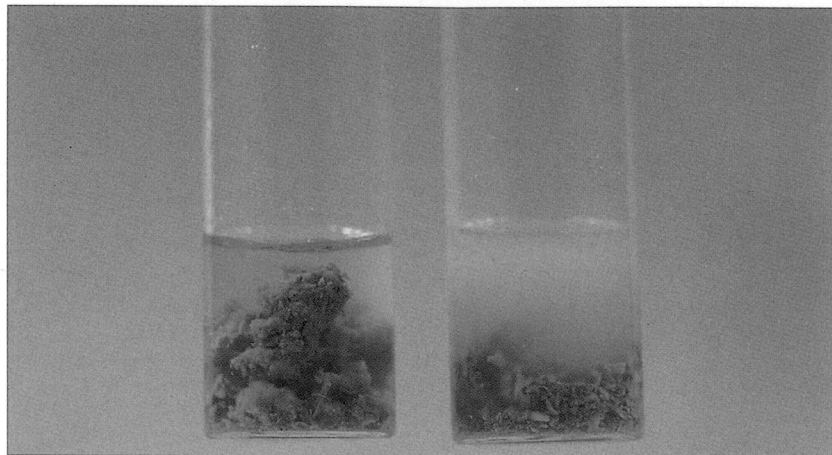

264 *Clostridium perfringens*, **Robertson's cooked meat medium.** Growth in Robertson's cooked meat medium (left) showing saccharolytic (reddening) and slight proteolytic (blackening) reactions. Gas is also produced. (Right, uninoculated). *(Cooked meat medium, 24 h at 37°C)*

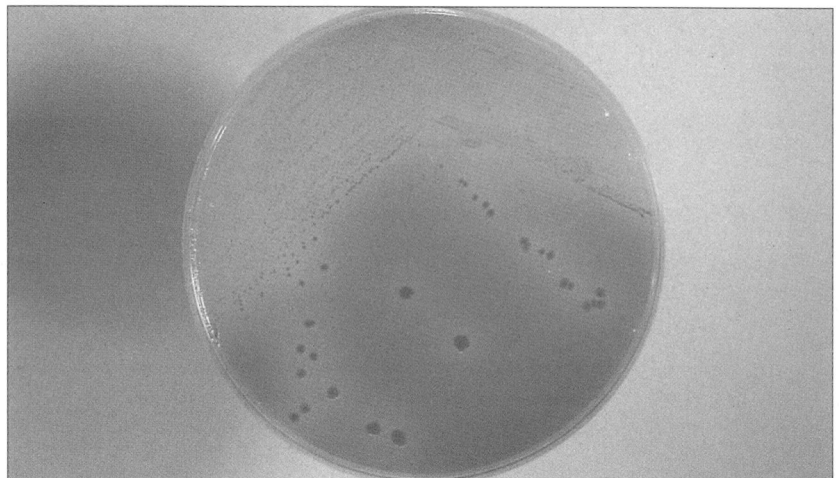

265 *Clostridium perfringens*, **lactose egg-yolk milk agar.** On lactose, egg-yolk, milk agar *C. perfringens* produce pink colonies due to lactose fermentation, surrounded by a zone of opacity due to the breakdown of lecithin. *(Lactose, egg-yolk, milk agar, 48 h anaerobically at 37°C)*

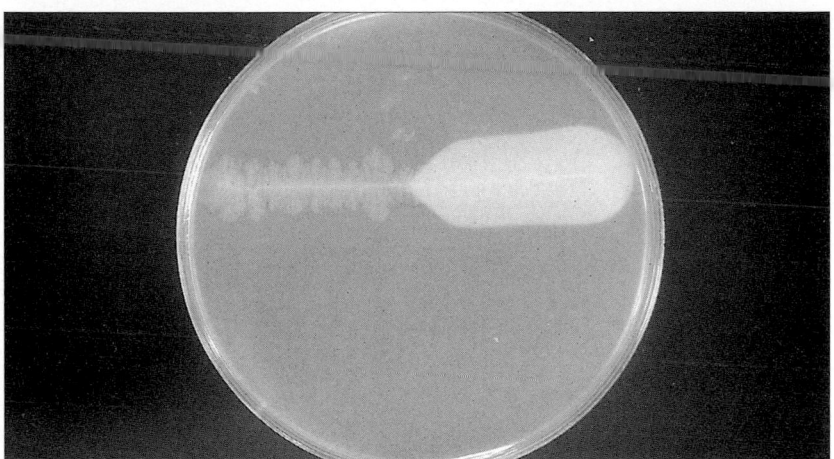

266 Nagler reaction. The Nagler plate contains an egg-yolk medium and half of the plate is covered with *C. perfringens* antitoxin. Organisms are streaked across the plate, so that inoculum passes from the antitoxin-free half of the plate to the antitoxin-covered part. After overnight anaerobic incubation, a positive result is shown by opacity in the medium surrounding the inoculum on the non-antitoxin half of the plate. Right side, no antitoxin. *(Nagler plate, 18 h anaerobically at 37°C)*

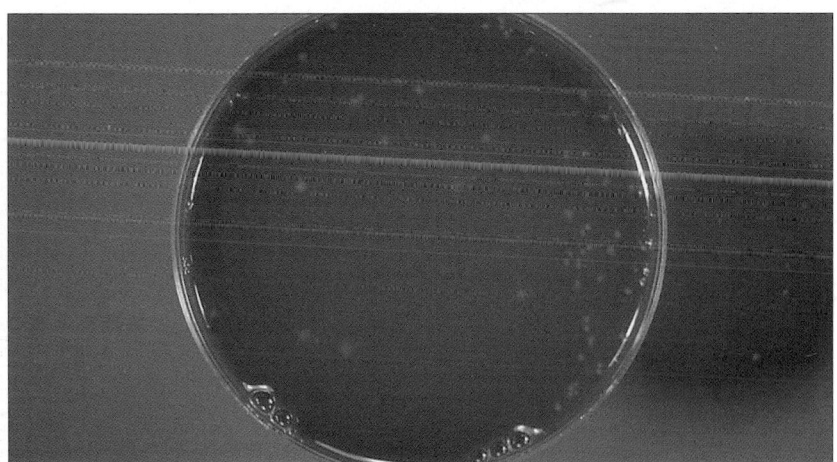

267 *Clostridium difficile*, cycloserine-cefoxitin, fructose agar (CCFA). *C. difficile* is associated with pseudomembranous colitis. On CCFA the colonies are a shiny, grey colour. *(Cycloserine-cefoxitin, fructose agar, 48 h anaerobically at 37°C)*

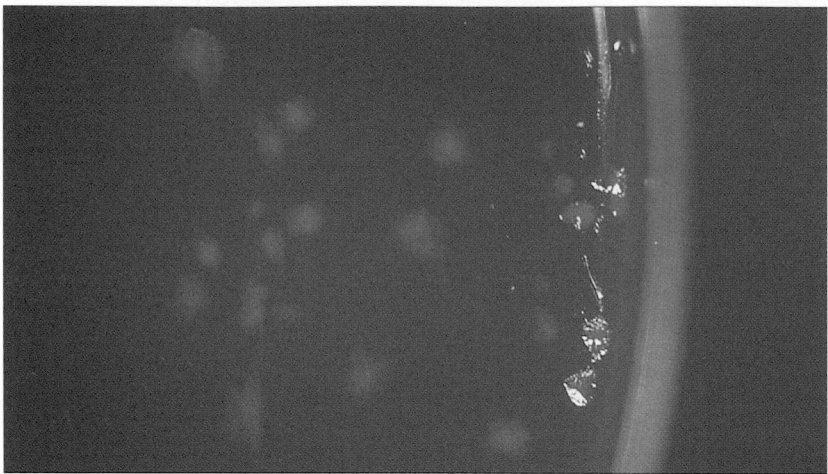

268   Clostridium difficile, CCBA agar, close-up of colonies. The 'metallic' shiny appearance of the colonies is demonstrated. *(CCB agar, 48 h anaerobically at 37°C)*

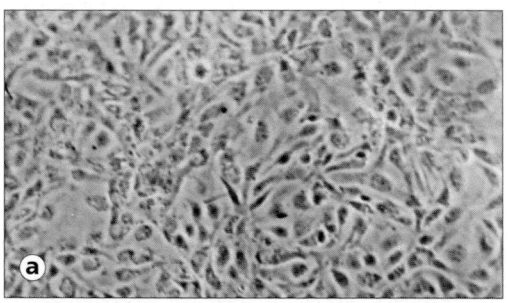

269   Tissue culture showing action of *Clostridium difficile* toxin
Colitis and diarrhoea are caused by toxin-producing strains of *C. difficile*. Toxin may be demonstrated by its effect on Vero cells after overnight incubation (**b**); uninoculated (**a**). *(Vero cells, 18 h at 37°C)*

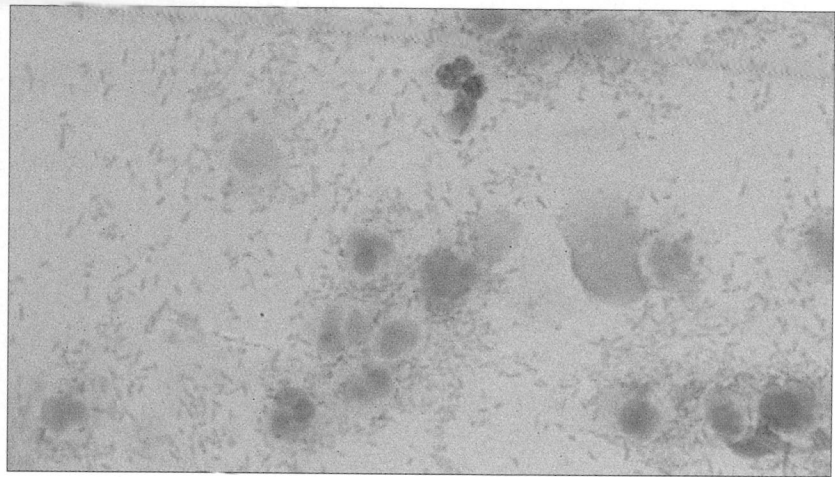

270 *Bacteroides fragilis,* Gram. *B. fragilis* are small, Gram-negative bacilli associated with intra-abdominal abscesses. *(Gram, x1000)*

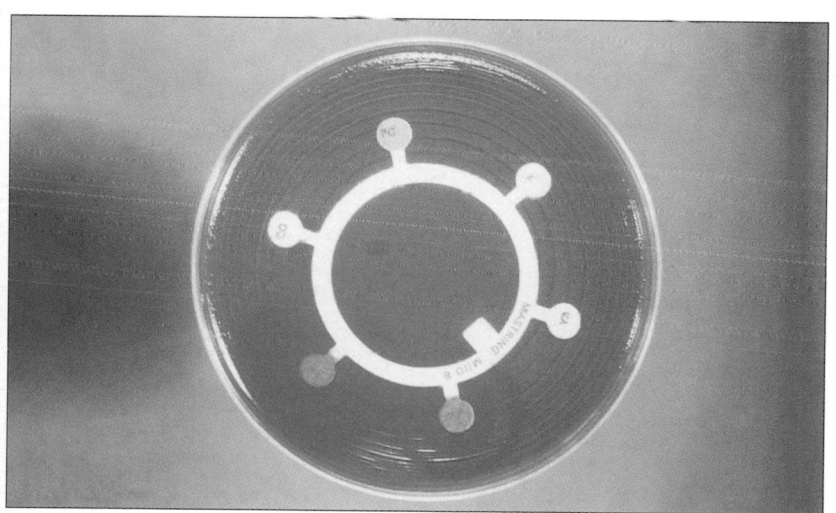

271 Identification of *Bacteroides* spp. by antimicrobial sensitivity.
Antimicrobial disk sensitivity can aid the identification of *Bacteroides* spp.
B. fragilis is resistant to colistin, penicillin, kanamycin and vancomycin, and sensitive to erythromycin and rifampicin.
(DST agar with 5% lysed blood, 48h anaerobically at 37° C)

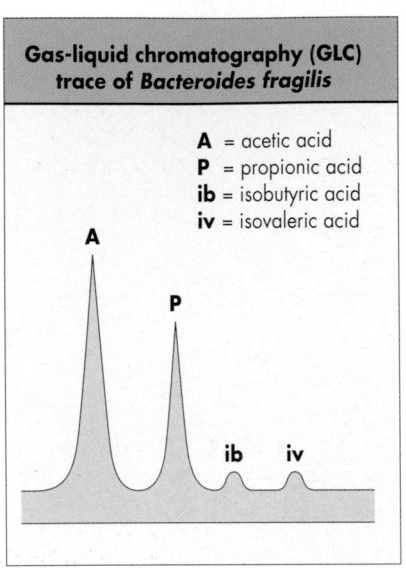

Gas-liquid chromatography (GLC) trace of *Bacteroides fragilis*

A = acetic acid
P = propionic acid
ib = isobutyric acid
iv = isovaleric acid

272 *Bacteroides* identification by gas–liquid chromatography. Trace of gas–liquid chromatograph (GLC) showing typical fatty acid peaks. *B. fragilis* gives peaks for acetic acid and propionic acid.

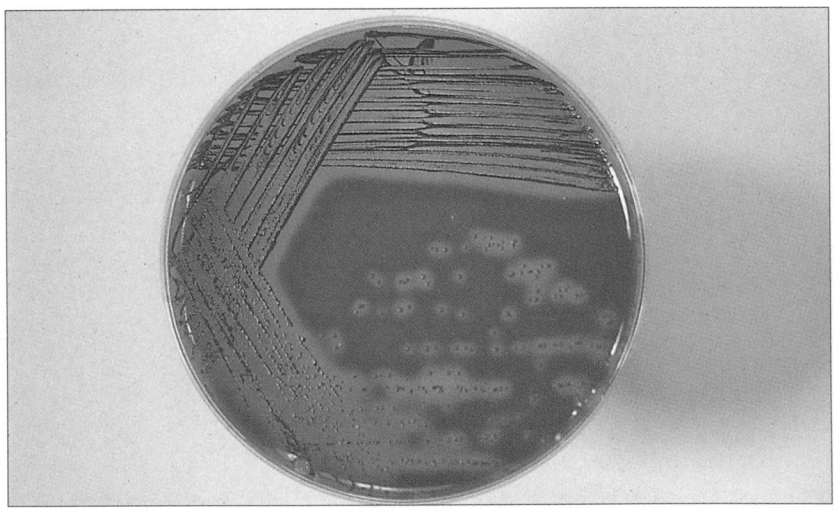

273 *Prevotella melaninogenicus* (formerly *Bacteroides melaninogenicus*). Culture on blood agar showing brown/black colonies after 5 days' incubation. *(Blood agar, 5 days anaerobically at 37°C)*

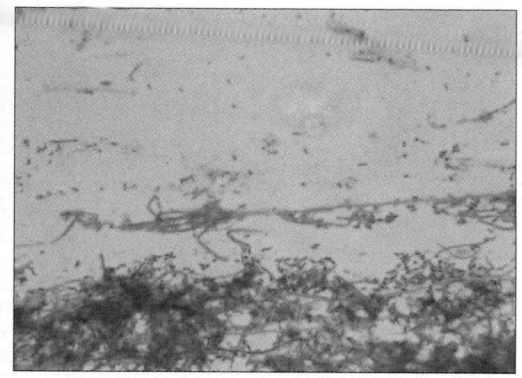

274 *Fusobacterium nucleatum*, Gram. Not all fusobacteria are fusiform. The Gram stain of *F. nucleatum* from a jaw infection shows Gram-negative bacilli, some with slender ends. *(Gram, x1000)*

275 *Fusobacterium necrophorum*. Gram stain from a blood culture of a patient with *F. necrophorum* septicaemia, originating from mastoiditis. *(Gram, x1000)*

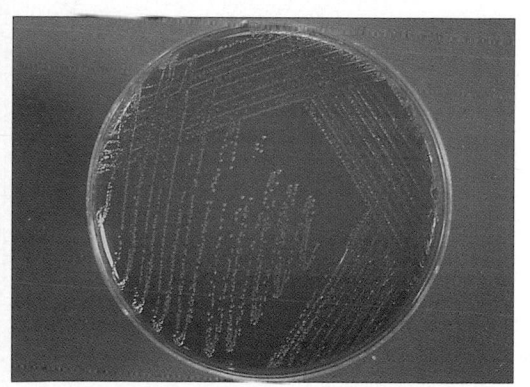

276 *Fusobacterium necrophorum*, blood agar. Culture of *F. necrophorum* on blood agar showing small, pale colonies. *(Blood agar, 48 h anaerobically at 37°C)*

UNCLASSIFIED BACTERIA

A number of bacteria, including an increasing number of newly described pathogens, do not fall neatly within standard classification. Characteristics of some of them are summarized in **277–279**. Many of them are difficult to cultivate or are relatively inert biochemically. *Bartonella bacilliformis* are Gram-negative coccoid bacteria that are the cause of bartonellosis, a febrile or chronic cutaneous disease restricted to parts of the Andean region of South America. It may be demonstrated by Giemsa staining from the blood of infected patients (**280**). *Bartonella henselae* has recently been described as the cause of cat scratch fever and bacillary angiomatosis, and is a Gram-negative bacillus (**281**).

'Unclassified' bacteria **Infections**				
Organism	Major infection	Less common infection	Vaccine preventable	Incubation period
Spirillum minus	rat-bite fever	–	–	1–3 months
Calymmatobacterium granulomatis	granuloma inguinale (donovanosis)	–	–	–
Bartonella henselae	bacillary angiomatosis, cat scratch fever	–	–	–
Bartonella bacilliformis	Oroya fever, verruga peruana	–	–	2 weeks – 4 months
Streptobacillus moniliformis	rat-bite fever, Haverhill fever	–	–	3–10 days

277 Unclassified bacteria. Infections.

'Unclassified' bacteria
Sources and transmission of bacteria

Organism	Reservoir			Transmission					Comments
	Man	Animal	Env.	Insect	Faecal/oral	Droplet	Direct	Nosocomial	
Spirillum minus	–	+ rats	–	–	–	–	–	–	
Calymmato-bacterium granulomatis	+	–	–	–	–	–	+	–	sexual transmission
Bartonella henselae	–	+	–	–	–	–	+	–	
Bartonella bacilliformis	+	–	–	+ sandfly	–	–	–	–	limited to Andean region of Peru and Ecuador
Streptobacillus moniliformis [a]	–	+	+	–	+	±	–	–	

(a) Infection by bite or from contaminated water or milk.

278 Unclassified bacteria. Sources and transmission of bacteria.

'Unclassified' bacteria
Identifying characteristics

Organism	Gram stain	Culture	Biochemical and other tests
Spirillum minus	thick, spiral, negative bacilli	Not cultured *in vitro*.	
Calymmatobacterium granulomatis	negative cocco-bacilli	Difficult to culture using egg-yolk based medium	
Bartonella henselae	negative bacilli		
Bartonella bacilliformis	negative cocco-bacilli	White colonies on blood agar after 7–14 days	Biochemically inert. Diagnosis usually by Giemsa stain from blood film
Stretobacillus moniliformis	pleomorphic, negative cocco-bacilli	non-haemolytic colonies on blood agar	Indole, oxidase, catalase, nitrate negative

279 Unclassified bacteria. Identifying characteristics.

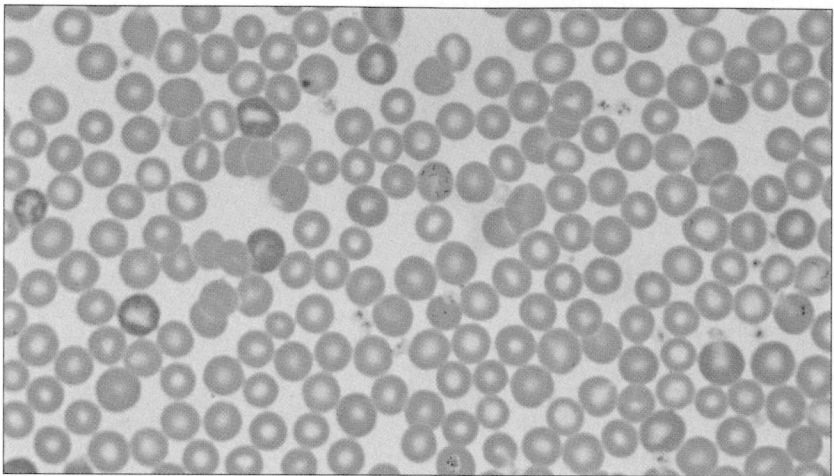

280 Giemsa stain of blood film showing *Bartonella bacilliformis* from patient with Oroya fever. The film shows the intracellular cocco-bacilli staining a deep purple. *Bartonella* multiplies in the red cells, causing their destruction and a subsequent anaemia. *(Giemsa, x1000)*

281 *Bartonella henselae*, Gram. Showing Gram-negative cocco-bacilli. *Bartonella henselae* is a cause of cat scratch disease and is associated with bacillary angiomatosis. *(Gram, x1000)*

MYCOBACTERIA

Features of Mycobacteria are summarized in **282–284**. Mycobacteria include the important pathogens of tuberculosis and leprosy and a large number of environmental strains that are opportunistic pathogens. Mycobacteria are stained by the Ziehl–Neelsen (ZN) method, showing pink, acid-fast bacilli (**285**). Auramine phenol staining may also be used (**286**). Mycobacteria have exacting nutritional requirements and will not grow on ordinary media. Lowenstein–Jensen (LJ) medium has ingredients including eggs, glycerol and malachite green. Most mycobacteria are slow-growing, taking 4–12 weeks to produce visible colonies. **287** shows *M. tuberculosis* after six weeks' culture on LJ medium, with a typical 'bread crumb like' appearance. *M. bovis* grows better on LJ slopes containing pyruvate rather than glycerol (**288**). **289** and **290** show the 'atypical' Mycobacteria, *M. kansasii* and *M. avium intracellulare*, grown on LJ slopes. Mycobacteria can be distinguished by the effect of temperature on growth, the production of pigment and the rate of growth. **291-293** show Mycobacteria with narrow and wide temperature growth ranges. Mycobacteria may be non-pigmented (non-chromogens), produce pigment in light only (photo-chromogens) or produce pigment in the dark and the light (scotochromogens). These are shown in **294** and **295**. **296** shows growth after 10 days of a slow-grower (*M. tuberculosis*) and a rapid grower (*M. fortuitum*). **297** shows a ZN stain of *M. leprae* from a slit skin smear.

Mycobacteria
Infections

Organism	Major infection	Less common infection	Vaccine preventable	Incubation period	Period of infectivity
Mycobacterium tuberculosis	tuberculosis	–	±	4–12 weeks	indefinite in untreated pulmonary infection
M. bovis	tuberculosis	–	±	4–12 weeks	–
M. ulcerans	Buruli ulcer	–	–		–
M. kansasii	pulmonary disease	–	–		–
M. marinum	'fish tank' ulcer	–	–		–
M. scrofulaceum	cervical lymphadenopathy	–	–		–
M. malmoense	cervical lymphadenopathy	–	–		–
M. avium-intracellulare	disseminated infection in immunocompromised	–	–		–
M. chelonei	occasional skin infections following minor trauma	–	–		–
M. gordonae	" " "	–	–		–
M. xenopi	" " "	–	–		–
M. fortuitum	abscesses	–	–		–
M. leprae	leprosy	–	–	4–8 years	indefinite if not treated

282 Mycobacteria. Infections.

Mycobacteria Sources and transmission of bacteria							
	Reservoir			Transmission			
Organism	Man	Animal	Env.	Faecal/oral	Droplet	Direct	Nosocomial	Comments
Mycobacterium tuberculosis	+	–	–	–	+	–	+	
M. bovis		+	–	+	±			
M. ulcerans			+			+		
M. kansasii	+		+		+			
M. marinum			+			+		
M. scrofulaceum			+	(+)	+	+		
M. malmoense			+			+		
M. avium-intracellulare	+	+			+			
M. chelonei			+			+		
M. gordonae			+			+		
M. xenopi			+			+		
M. fortuitum			+			+		
M. leprae	+	–	–	–	(+)	+	–	

283 Mycobacteria. Sources and transmission of bacteria.

Growth characteristics of mycobacteria								
	Rate	Temperature				Pigment production		
		25°C	32°C	36°C	44°C	N*	P*	S*
Mycobacterium tuberculosis	S	–	+	+	–	+	–	–
M. bovis	S	–	(+)	+		+	–	–
M. ulcerans	S	–	+	–	–	+	–	–
M. kansasii	S	+	+	+	–		+	–
M. marinum	S	+	+	±	–	–	+	–
M. scrofulaceum	S	+	+	+	–	–	–	+
M. malmoense	S	+	+	+	+	+	–	–
M. avium-intracellulare	S	+	+	+	+	+	–	+
M. chelonae	R	+	+	+	–	+	–	–
M. gordonae	S	+	+	+	–	–	–	+
M. xenopi	S	–	–	+	+	–	–	+
M. fortuitum	R	+	+	+	–	+	–	–
M. leprae	S(a)							

S = slow growth   R = rapid growth   S(a) = not cultivated on artificial media
N* = non-chromogen   P* = photochromogen   S* = scotochromogen

284 Growth characteristics of Mycobacteria.

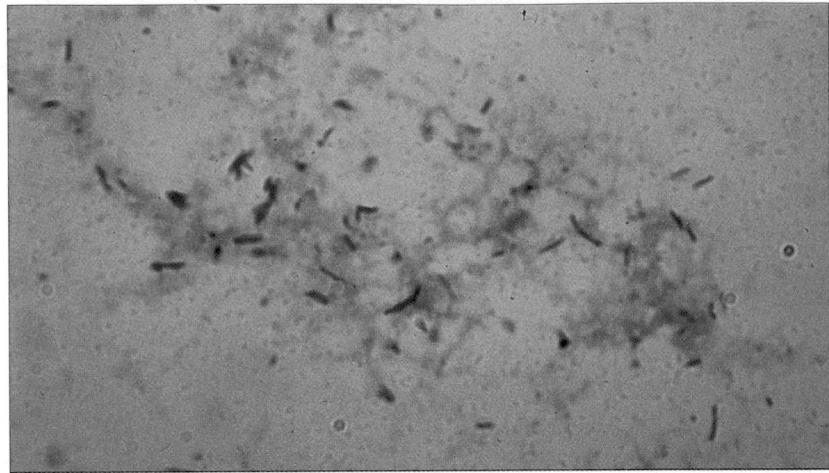

285 *Mycobacterium tuberculosis*. Ziehl–Neelsen staining of sputum from patient with tuberculosis, showing pink, acid-fast bacilli against a blue background of pus cells. *(Ziehl–Neelsen, x1000)*

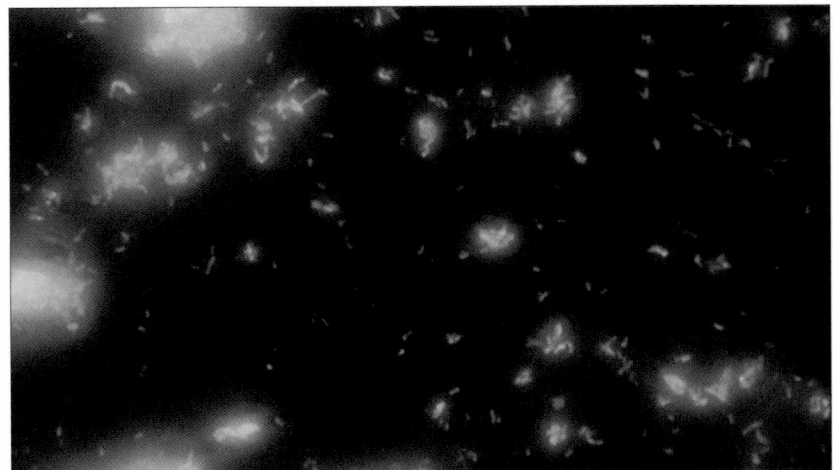

286 *Mycobacterium tuberculosis*, auramine-phenol fluorochrome. Auramine is a fluorochrome, a dye which fluoresces when illuminated by UV light. Tubercle bacilli fluoresce a white/yellow colour. *(Fluorochrome stain, x1000)*

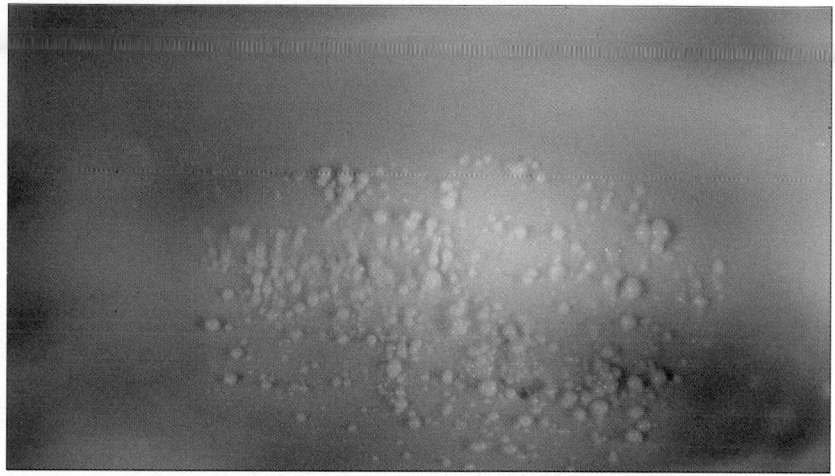

287 *Mycobacterium tuberculosis*, Löwenstein–Jensen (LJ) medium. Culture on Löwenstein–Jensen medium after 6 weeks. The mycobacteria produce creamy, breadcrumb like colonies. *(Löwenstein–Jensen medium, 6 weeks at 37°C)*

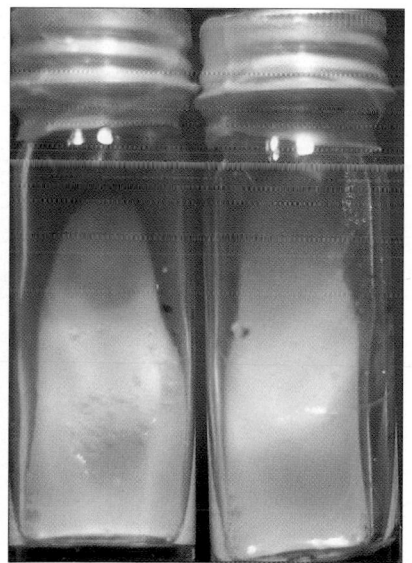

288 *Mycobacterium bovis*, LJ medium. Culture on LJ medium containing glycerol (right) and pyruvate (left). Growth of *M. bovis* is better on the pyruvate slope. *(Löwenstein–Jensen medium, 6 weeks at 37°C)*

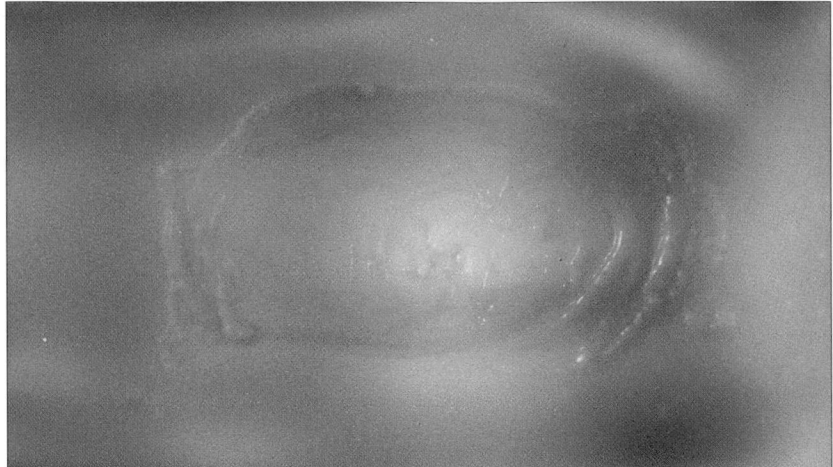

289 *Mycobacterium kansasii*, **LJ medium.** *M. kansasii* is an opportunistic mycobacterium and is an occasional cause of a tuberculosis-like pulmonary infection. *M. kansasii* is a photochromogen. *(Löwenstein–Jensen medium, 6 weeks at 37°C)*

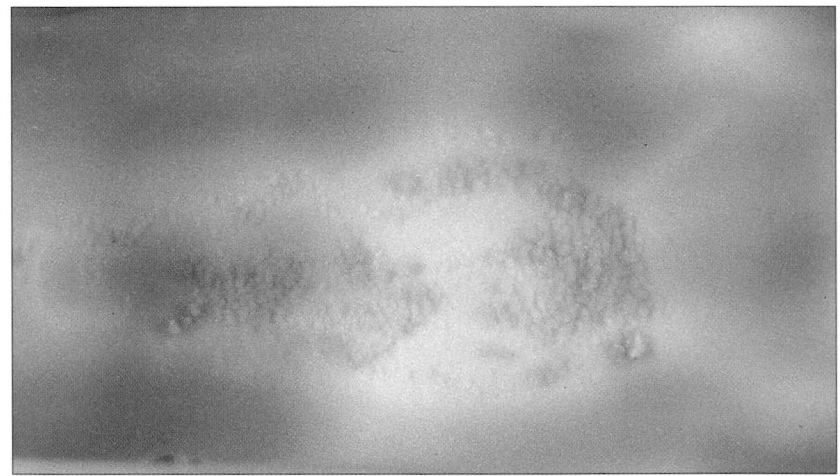

290 *Mycobacterium avium-intracellulare*, **LJ medium.** *M. avium-intracellulare* is a potential pathogen in the immunocompromised and is particularly associated with HIV infection. *(Löwenstein–Jensen medium, 6 weeks at 37°C)*

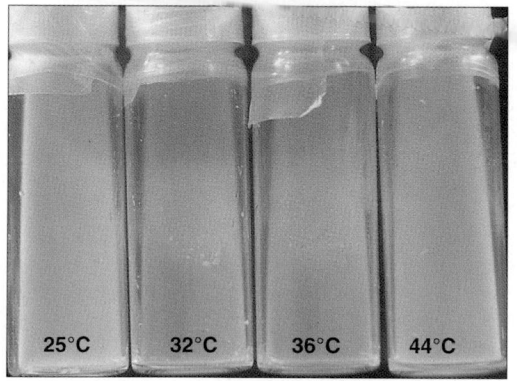

291–293 Effect of temperature on growth of mycobacteria. Different mycobacteria have different ranges of temperature for growth. The Löwenstein–Jensen slopes have been incubated at 25°C, 32°C, 36°C and 44°C. *(Löwenstein–Jensen medium, temperatures as indicated)*

291 *M. tuberculosis,* growth at 32° C and 36° C.

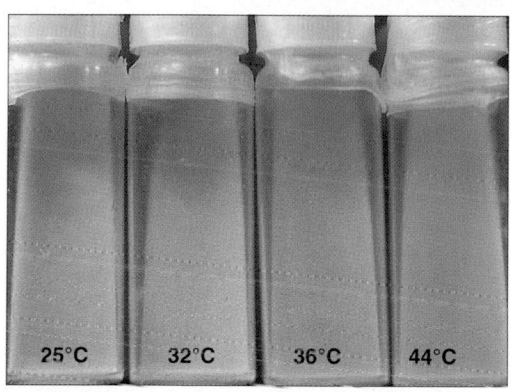

292 *M. kansasii,* growth at 25°C, 32°C and 36°C.

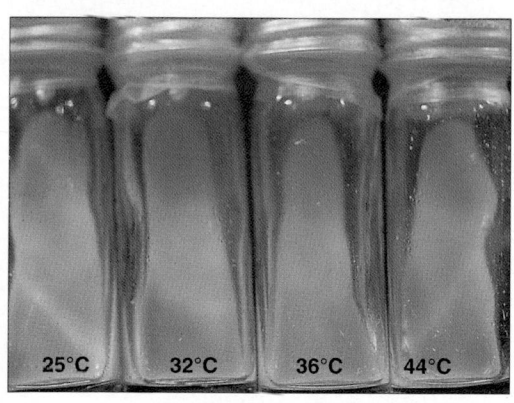

293 *M. malmoense,* growth at 25°C, 32°C, 36°C and 44°C.

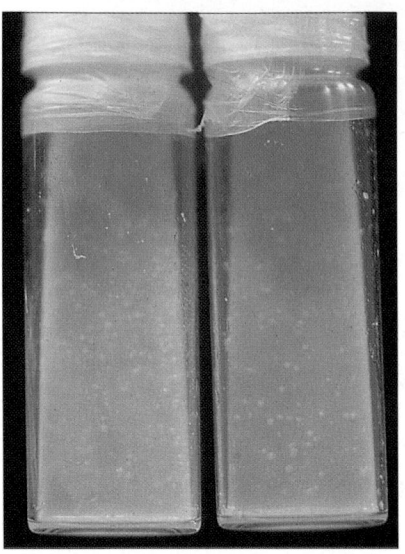

294, 295 Effect of light on mycobacteria. Mycobacteria that produce no pigment are non-chromogens. Those that produce pigment only in the light are photochromogens. Those that produce pigment in both light and dark are scotochromogens. In the figures, the left-hand slope was grown in the dark, and the right-hand slope in the light. *(Löwenstein–Jensen medium at 37°C)*

294 *M. kansasii*, photochromogen.

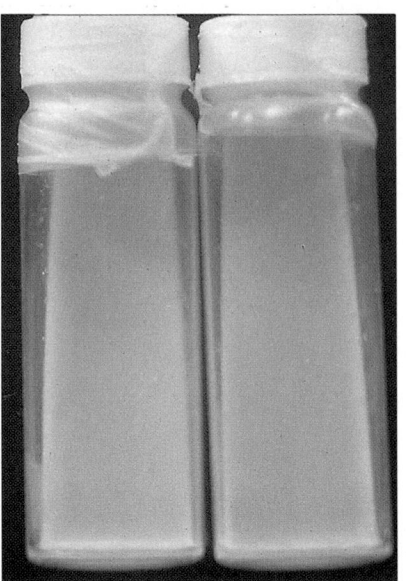

295 *M. gordonae*, scotochromogen.

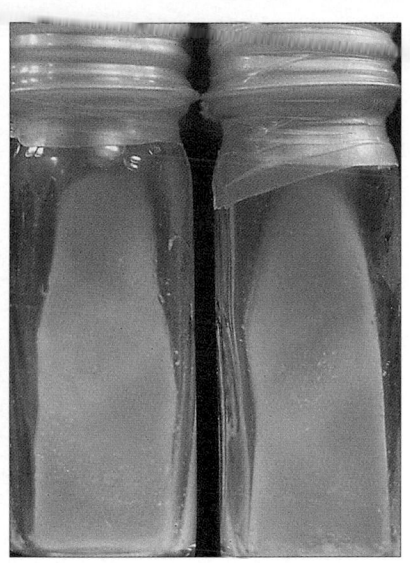

296 Rate of growth of mycobacteria. Mycobacteria may be divided into rapid and slow growers. Rapid growers will produce colonies in 3–4 days. Most mycobacteria require a minimum of 3–4 weeks before colonies are visible. The slopes have been incubated for 7 days. Right, *M. tuberculosis*, no growth; left, *M. fortuitum*, a rapid grower. *(Löwenstein-Jensen medium at 37°C)*

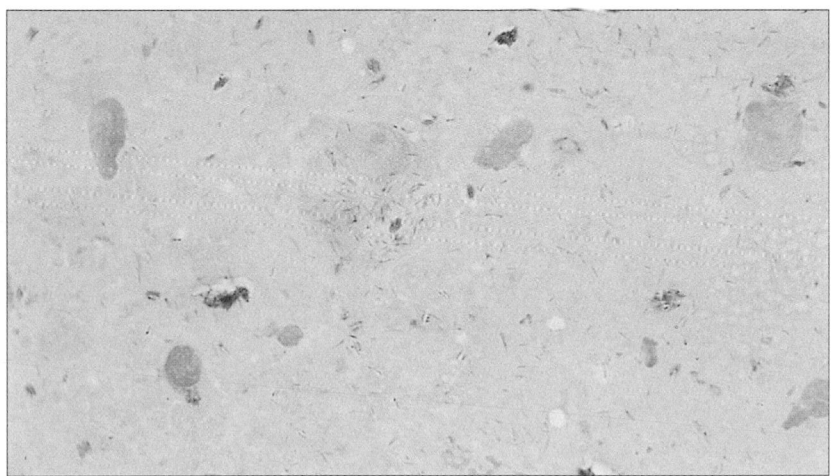

297 *Mycobacterium leprae*, Ziehl–Neelsen stain. *M. leprae* may be demonstrated by staining of slit skin smears by a modified ZN stain. *M. leprae* is only weakly acid-fast and a 1%, instead of 3%, acid-alcohol solution is used for decolorization. *M. leprae* appear as thin, pink bacilli, often within macrophage cells. *(Ziehl–Neelsen, x1000)*

MYCOPLASMA, SPIROCHAETES AND RICKETTSIAE

Characteristics of mycoplasmas and ureaplasmas are summarised in **298–300**, spirochaetes in **302–304** and *Rickettsia* and *Coxiella* in **309a–c**.

Mycoplasmas and ureaplasmas cannot be detected directly in stained specimens. They are slow-growing and produce small colonies after several days' incubation (**301**).

Spirochaetes are spiral, motile organisms that are not easily cultivated in the routine laboratory. The three genera of medical importance are *Treponema*, *Leptospira* and *Borrelia*. *Treponema pallidum*, the cause of syphilis, may be demonstrated as tightly wound spirochaetes using dark-field microscopy (**305**). Generally, serological tests are used in the investigation of syphilis. Both treponemal-specific antibodies and auto-antibodies (cardiolipin) from tissue damage are produced. The rapid plasma reagin test (**306**) is an example of a cardiolipin test.

Leptospira interrogans, the cause of leptospirosis, can be demonstrated by dark-field, silver staining and immunofluorescence (**307**). *Borellia recurrentis,* the cause of relapsing fever, can be seen in Giemsa stains of blood films from infected patients (**308**).

Rickettsia and *Coxiella* are obligate intracellular parasites and can only be cultured using embryonated egg or tissue culture techniques. Serological tests are used in the diagnosis of rickettsial infections. The Weil–Felix test is a nonspecific test based on the agglutination of certain *Proteus vulgaris* strains by antibodies to rickettsia (**310**). Q fever, caused by *Coxiella burnetii,* may be diagnosed by micro-titre complement fixation tests (**311**).

Organism	Major infection	Less common infection	Vaccine preventable	Incubation period	Period of infectivity
	Mycoplasma and Ureaplasma Infections				
Mycoplasma pneumoniae	Pneumonia, tracheobronchitis	myocarditis	–	6–21 days	up to 14 days
M. hominis	Urethritis, postpartum infection pelvic inflammatory disease	wound infection, neonatal meningitis	–	–	–
Ureaplasma urealyticum	Urethritis	–	–	–	–

298 Mycoplasma and Ureaplasma. Infections.

	Mycoplasma Sources and transmission of bacteria							
	Reservoir			**Transmission**				
Organism	Man	Animal	Env.	Faecal/oral	Droplet	Direct	Nosocomial	Comments
Mycoplasma pneumoniae	+	–	–	–	+	–	–	
M. hominis	+	–	–	–	–	+	–	
Ureaplasma urealyticum	+	–	–	–	–	+	–	

299 Mycoplasma. Sources and transmission of bacteria.

	Mycoplasma Identifying characteristics		
Organism	Microscopy	Culture	Other tests for identification
Mycoplasma pneumoniae *M. hominis* *Ureaplasma urealyticum*	Small, pleomorphic, non-motile organisms cannot be detected in stained specimens	Enriched media required Small colonies with 'fried egg' appearance after several days	Serological diagnosis by CFT and ELISA

300 Mycoplasma. Identifying characteristics.

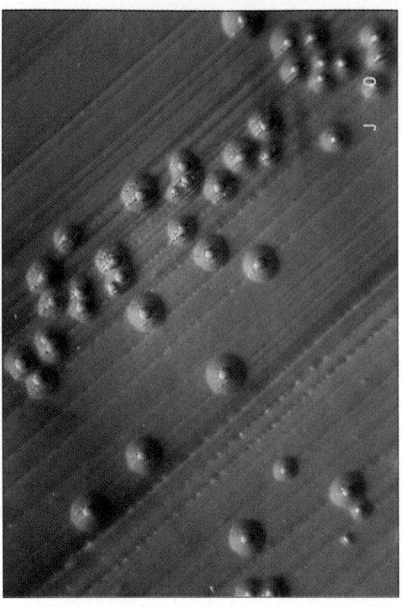

301 Culture of *Mycoplasma hominis*. Close-up of colonies, showing 'fried-egg' appearance, on mycoplasma enrichment ('pleuropneumonia-like organisms', PPLO) medium. *(PPLO medium, 5 days, at 37°C)*

		Spirochaetes Infections			
Organism	Major infection	Less common infection	Vaccine preventable	Incubation period	Period of infectivity
Treponema					
T. pallidum	syphilis		–	1–6 weeks	2–4 years if not treated
T. pertenue	yaws	–	–	2 weeks – 3 months	several years if not treated
T. carateum	pinta	–	–	2–3 weeks	several years if not treated
Leptospira					
L. interrogans	leptospirosis (Weil's disease)	–	–	4–20 days	person–to–person transmission rare
Borrelia					
B. vincenti	Vincent's angina	tropical ulcer	–	–	–
B. recurrentis	louse borne relapsing fever	–	–	5–15 days	–
B. duttoni	tick borne relapsing fever		–	5–15 days	–
B. burgdorferi	Lyme disease		–	3–30 days	–

302 Spirochaetes. Infections.

Spirochaetes Sources and transmission								
	Reservoir			**Transmission**				
Organism	Man	Animal	Env.	Insect	Faecal/oral	Droplet	Direct	Nosocomial	Comments
Treponema pallidum	+	–	–	–	–	–	+	–	
T. pertenue	+	–	–	–	–	–	+	–	
T. carateum	+	–	–	–	–	–	+	–	restricted to central and S. America
Leptospira interrogans	–	+	+	–	+	–	+	–	over 20 serogroups
Borellia vincenti	+	–	–	–	–	–	–	–	
B. recurrentis	+	–	–	+	–	–	–	–	
B. duttoni	–	+	–	+	–	–	–	–	
B. burgdorferi	–	+	–	+	–	–	–	–	

303 Spirochaetes. Sources and transmission.

Spirochaetes Identifying characteristics		
Organism	Microscopy	Other tests for identification
Treponema pallidum *T. pertenue* *T. carateum*	coiled, straight spirochaetes seen in dark field of specimen from ulcers	diagnosis usually by cardiolipin and trepanomal antibody tests
Leptospira interrogans	tightly coiled with hooked ends seen by dark-field microscopy of urine or CSF	diagnosis usually by serological tests
Borellia vincenti	Gram –ve wavy shape in smears	
B. recurrentis	wavy shaped spirochaetes seen in Giemsa blood stains	diagnosis usually from blood film and clinical symptoms
B. duttoni	" "	" "
B. burgdorferi	—	diagnosis usually by serological tests

304 Spirochaetes. Identifying characteristics.

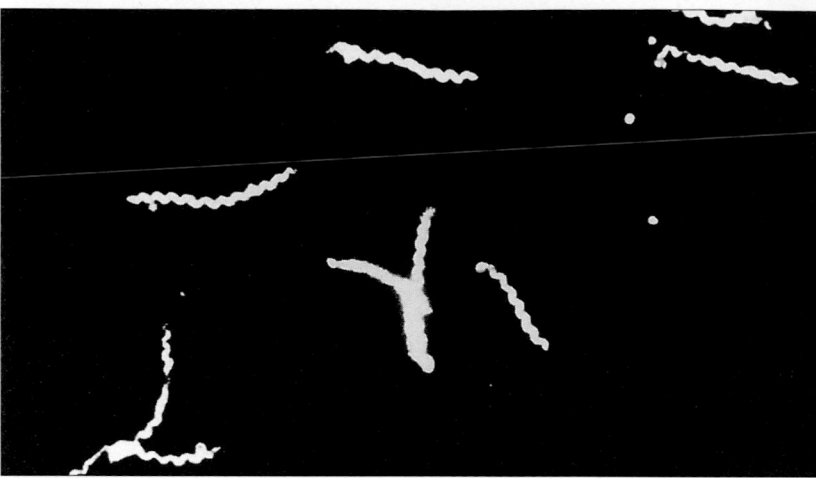

305 Dark-field microscopy of *Treponema pallidum*. *T. pallidum* appears as straight, tightly coiled spirochaetes on dark-field microscopy. *(Dark field, x1000)*

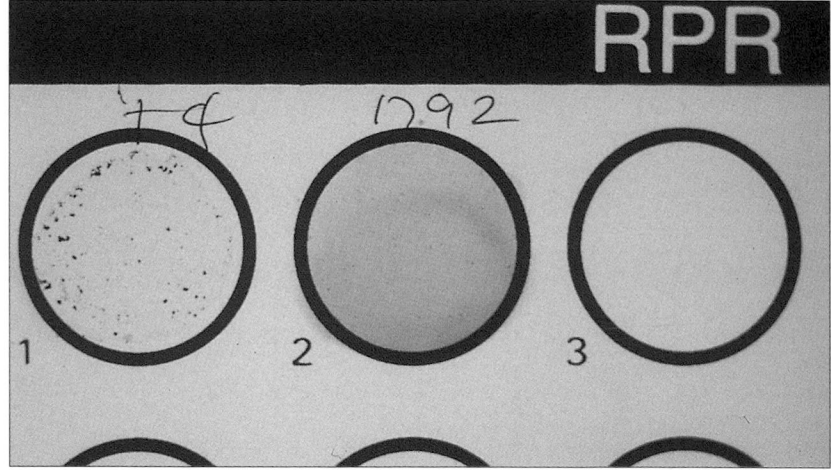

306 Rapid plasma reagin (RPR) test for syphilis. The RPR is a cardiolipin (non-treponemal) antibody test for syphilis, positive in the early stages of disease. Patient's serum is mixed with commercially prepared carbon-linked cardiolipin antigen. A positive serum shows clumping of the antigen particles. *(Clumping of particles observed after 4 min)*

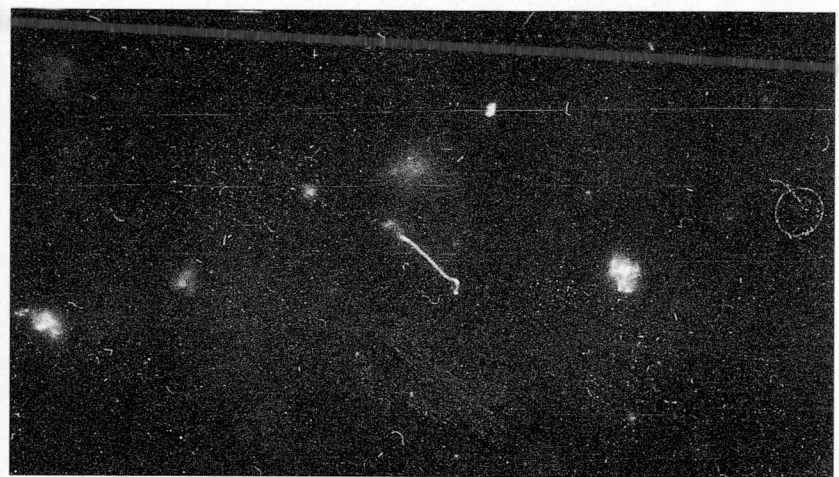

307   Dark-field microscopy of *Leptospira interrogans*. Leptospira are tightly coiled spirochaetes, characteristically with hooked ends. A zoonosis, they cause leptospirosis or Weil's disease in humans. *(Dark field, x1000)*

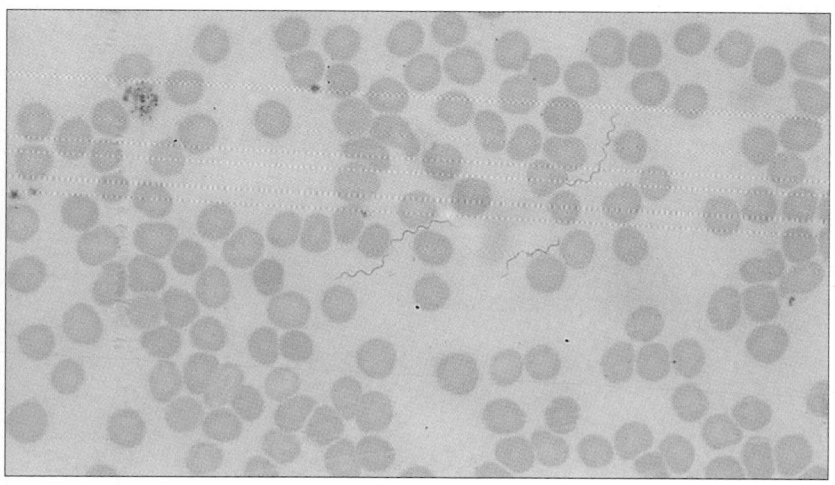

308   Giemsa stain of *Borrelia recurrentis* from the blood of a patient with relapsing fever. *Borrelia* are relatively large, wavy spirochaetes, appearing mauve-red by Giemsa staining. *(Giemsa, x1000)*

Rickettsia and *Coxiella* Infections					
Organism	Major infection	Less common infection	Vaccine preventable	Incubation period	Period of infectivity
Rickettsia typhi	flea borne (murine) typhus		–	1–2 weeks	not from infected cases
R. prowazekii	louse borne typhus	–	(+)	1–2 weeks	infective for lice in febrile period
R. tsutsugamushi	scrub (mite borne) typhus	–	–	6–21 days	not person-to-person
R. rickettsii	Rocky-mountain spotted fever	–	–	3–14 days	ticks up to 18 months
Coxiella burnetii	'Q fever', pneumonitis	endocarditis	±	2–3 weeks	–

309a   Rickettsiea and *Coxiella*. Infections.

Rickettsia and *Coxiella* Sources and transmission									
	Reservoir			Transmission					
Organism	Man	Animal	Env.	Insect	Ingestion	Droplet	Direct	Nosocomial	Comments
Rickettsia typhi	–	+	–	+ (flea)	–	–	–	–	
R. prowazeki	+	–	–	+ (louse)	–	–	–	–	
R. tsutsugamushi	+	+	–	+ (mite)	–	–	–	–	
R. rickettsii	–	+	–	+ (tick)	–	–	–	–	
Coxiella burnetii	–	+	–	–	±	+	–	–	

309b   *Rickettsia* and *Coxiella*. Sources and transmission.

Rickettsiae and *Coxiella* Identifying characteristics					
Organism	Microscopy	Serology	Weil–Felix reaction		
			OX-19	OX-2	OX-K
Rickettsia typhi	pleomorphic	diagnosis serological by	+	±	–
R. prowazekii	Gram-negative	CFT or Weil–Felix	+	±	–
R. tsutsugamushi	cocco-bacilli	reaction	–	–	±
R. ricketsii			+	+	–
Coxiella burnetii			–	–	–

309c   *Rickettsia* and *Coxiella*. Identifying characteristics.

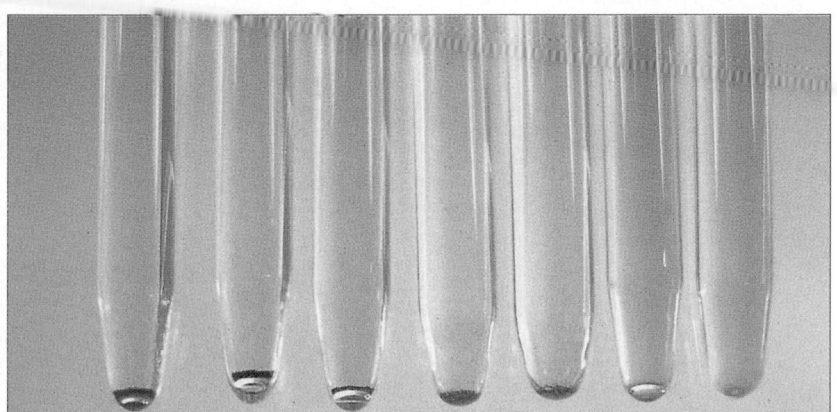

310   The Weil–Felix reaction in rickettsial infections. Antibodies to Rickettsiea cross-react with certain strains of *Proteus vulgaris* and *Proteus mirabilis*. The patient's serum is incubated with commercially prepared, stained, antigen suspensions and agglutination observed. Serial dilutions of serum are made from 1:20 to 1:1280. The patient's serum shows a positive reaction (in this case to *Proteus vulgaris* OX-19 antigen) at a titre of 1:320. *(4 h incubation at 50°C)*

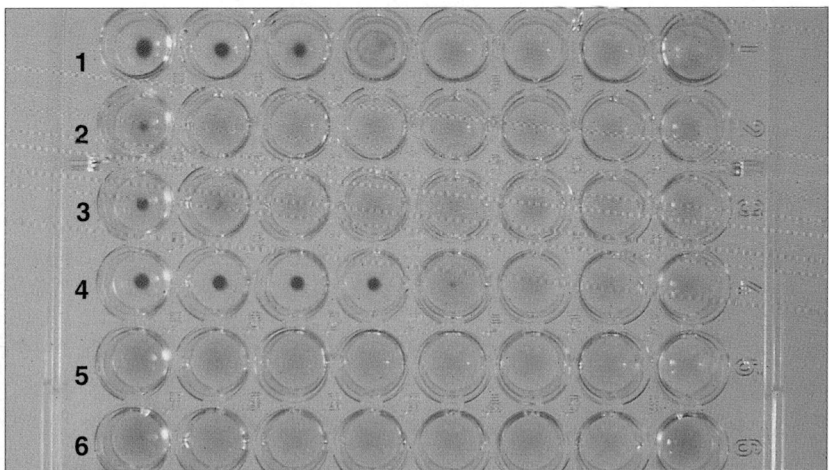

311   Micro-titre complement fixation test in the diagnosis of *a Coxiella burnetii* infection. Row 4 is a serial dilution of the patient's serum against the Phase I antigen of *Coxiella burnetii*, showing a positive result up to a titre of 1:64. (dilutions 1:8–1:512, control). *(18 h incubation at 4°C, red cells added and incubated for 30 min at 37°C)*

CHLAMYDIACEAE

Characteristics of the Chlamydiaceae are summarized in **312a,b** and **313**. These are obligate intracellular bacteria. They have both DNA and RNA, a cell wall and divide by binary fission. They enter their host cell by endocytosis and replicate within the endosome to form a large inclusion (**314**). They exist in two forms, the elementary body which is small and electron-dense and is the extracellular infective form, and the larger, more fragile reticulate body which is the replicating form found only in inclusions. There are three main species pathogenic for man.

Despite its name, *Chlamydia psittaci* infects a large variety of species as well as psittacine birds (parrots, budgerigars). *C. psittaci* is a cause of primary atypical pneumonia usually acquired from birds. Another serovar of *C. psittaci,* the ewe abortion agent, is a rare cause of early abortion, still-birth and fetal septicaemia. Diagnosis is by demonstration of the agent in tissue by immunofluorescence or by serology. Culture is by inoculation into the yolk sac of fertile hens' eggs and requires special containment facilities.

Chlamydia trachomatis strains A to C cause trachoma, which is the commonest infective cause of blindness in developing countries. *C. trachomatis* strains D to K cause a sexually transmitted infection throughout the world. Infection can be silent (especially in women) but can cause urethritis, cervicitis, epididymitis (in males) and ascend to cause pelvic inflammatory disease in women. It is the commonest sexually transmitted infection now that gonorrhoea has receded. If a neonate is born through an infected cervix it has a 50% chance of developing ophthalmia neonatorum, which may subsequently lead to pneumonia. Diagnosis can be by culture in epithelial cells (e.g. McCoy) but this takes up to 72 h for the characteristic inclusion to be visible (**315**). More rapid diagnosis is by ELISA and IFAT (**316**).

The recently discovered pathogen, *Chlamydia pneumoniae,* was originally called the TWAR (*Tai*w*an, A*cute *R*espiratory) agent. It is a cause of primary atypical pneumonia especially in adolescents and young adults. It has recently been associated with the development of coronary heart disease. Diagnosis is by serology, culture or genome detection by PCR.

Chlamydia
Infections

Organism	Major infection	Less common infection	Vaccine preventable	Incubation period	Period of infectivity
Chlamydia psittaci	psittacosis	infections in pregnancy (ovine strains)	–	4–15 days	person–to–person rare
C. trachomatis A–C	trachoma	–	–	5–12 days	years if not treated
C. trachomatis D–K	S.T.D. urethritis, P.I.D., neonatal pneumonia/ ophthalmia	–	–	7–14 days	?
C. trachomatis L1–L3	lymphogranuloma venereum	–	–	3–30 days	? years
C. pneumoniae (TWAR)	atypical pneumonia	otitis media	–	>10 days	? months

312a Chlamydia. Infections.

Chlamydia
Sources and transmission

Organism	Reservoir			Transmission					Comments
	Man	Animal	Env.	Insect	Faecal/oral	Droplet	Direct	Nosocomial	
Chlamydia psittaci	–	+	–	–	+	+	–	–	
C. trachomatis A–C	+	–	–	+	–	+	+	–	
C. trachomatis D–K	+	–	–	–	–	–	+	–	
C. trachomatis L	+	–	–	–	–	–	+	–	
C. pneumoniae	+	–	–	–	–	+	+	–	

312b Chlamydia. Sources and transmission.

Chlamydia
Identifying characteristics

Organism	Culture	Antigen/genome detection	Serology
Chlamydia psittaci	Fertile hens' eggs	IFAT/ELISA	CFT
C. trachomatis	McCoy cells	IFAT/ELISA	Micro-immune fluorescence (MIF)
C. pneumoniae	McCoy cells, but culture difficult	IFAT/PCR	MIF

313 Chlamydia. Identifying characteristics.

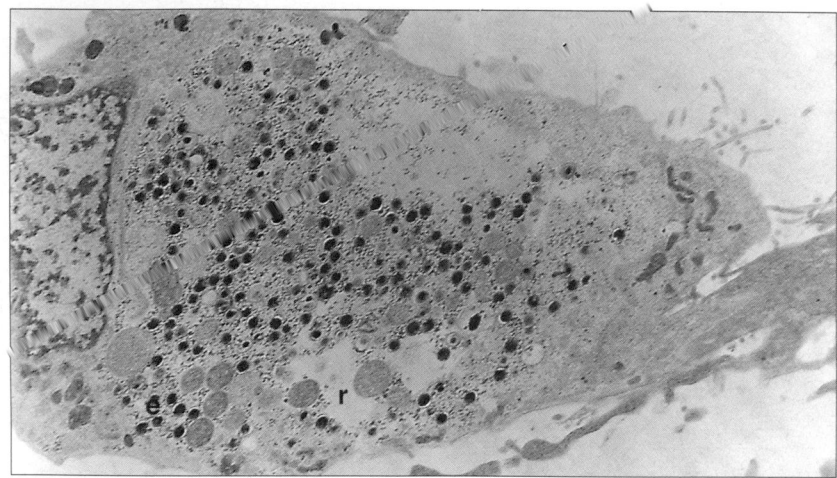

314 ***Chlamydia trachomatis* showing inclusion bodies.** Thin-section electron micrograph of a McCoy cell containing a large *C. trachomatis* inclusion. The small, electron-dense forms are elementary bodies (e) and the larger reticulate (r) bodies.

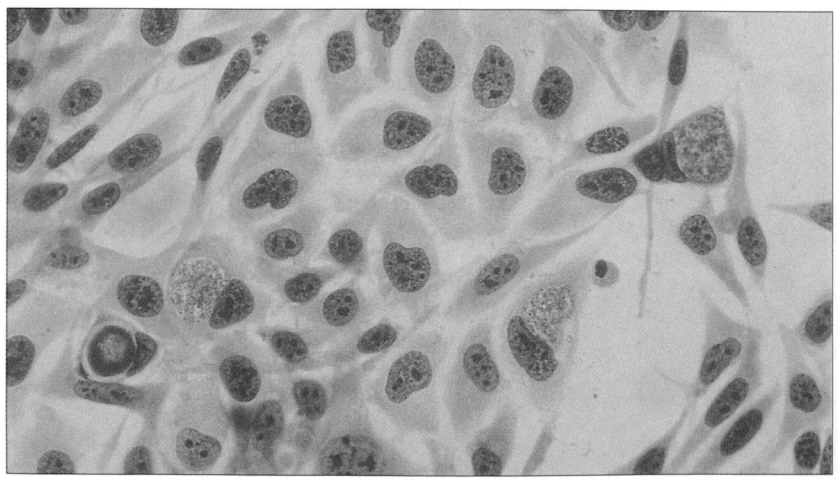

315 ***Chlamydia trachomatis* cultured on McCoy cells.** Giemsa-stained McCoy cells containing large chlamydial inclusions partially obscuring the nuclei. *(Giemsa, x1000)*

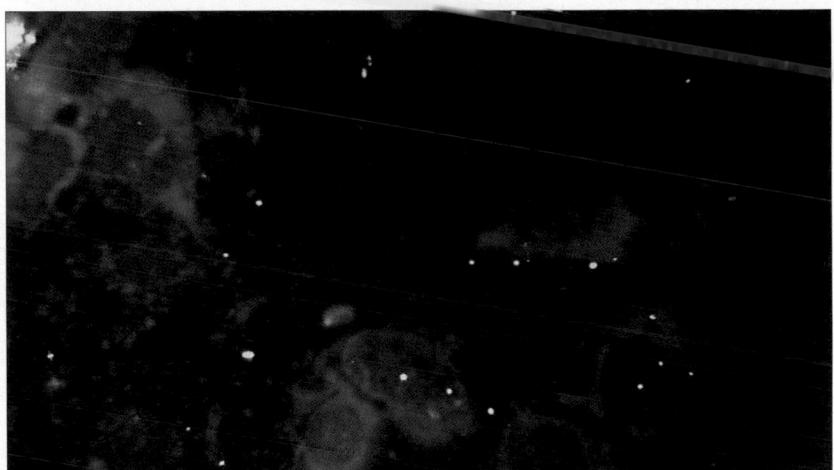

316 *Chlamydia trachomatis*, **immunofluorescence.** Indirect immunofluorescence of a cervical smear showing apple-green fluorescent *C. trachomatis*
elementary bodies. *(Fluorescence microscopy, x1000)*

ANTIMICROBIAL AGENTS AND ANTIMICROBIAL RESISTANCE

ABBREVIATIONS USED FOR ANTIBIOTICS

AMC	augmentin
MTZ	metronidazole
AML	amoxycillin
NA	nalidixic acid
C	chloramphenicol
OX	oxacillin
CAZ	ceftazidime
P	penicillin
CE	cefaclor
RD	rifampicin
CIP	ciprofloxacin
R	sulphamethoxazole
CN	gentamicin
T	tetracycline
CTX	cefotaxime
VA	vancomycin
F	nitrofurantoin
W	trimethoprim
MET	methicillin

Determining the antimicrobial sensitivity patterns of clinical bacterial isolates and the effectiveness of antimicrobial agents in therapy is an important role of the microbiology laboratory. The mechanisms by which important groups of antimicrobials inhibit bacterial growth are shown in **317**. Some bacteria may be intrinsically resistant to particular antibiotics, or they may acquire resistance through genetic transfer. Examples of bacterial resistance mechanisms are shown in **318**.

Within the laboratory, antimicrobial sensitivity testing is done most commonly by the disk diffusion method. Usually, plates are inoculated so that both the test isolate and a known, fully sensitive control organism can be compared. After inoculation of the plates, antimicrobial-containing disks are placed at the interface of the test and control inocula. The plates are incubated overnight and the growth inhibition zones compared between the test and control strains. In most cases, a resistant strain is defined as growing adjacent to a disk or having a zone radius of less than 2 mm. **319** shows the association between zone size and antibiotic

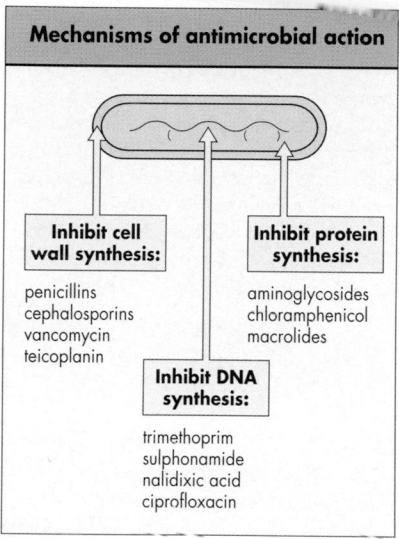

Mechanisms of antimicrobial action

017 Mechanisms of antimicrobial action against Lustoria.

Inhibit cell wall synthesis:

penicillins
cephalosporins
vancomycin
teicoplanin

Inhibit protein synthesis:

aminoglycosides
chloramphenicol
macrolides

Inhibit DNA synthesis:

trimethoprim
sulphonamide
nalidixic acid
ciprofloxacin

Mechanisms of antimicrobial resistance to antibiotics

Alternative metabolic pathway

trimethoprim
sulphonamides

Alternative DNA pathway

nalidixic acid
ciprofloxacin

Antibiotic modifying enzyme

aminoglycosides
chloramphenicol

Antibiotic destroying enzyme

beta-lactamases
penicillins
cephalosporins

Inhibit antibiotic uptake

tetracyclines

Altered cell wall binding sites

vancomycin
teicoplanin

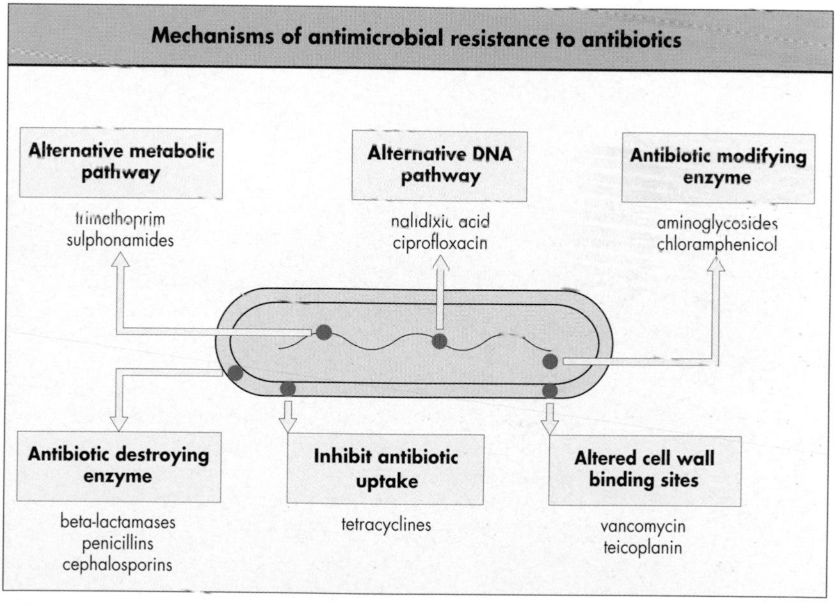

318 Mechanisms of bacterial resistance to antimicrobials.

Disk sensitivity: Relation between antibiotic concentration and zone size

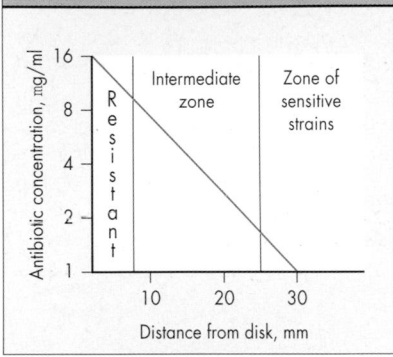

319 Regression line showing the association between distance from the antibiotic disk, antibiotic concentration and zone size for bacteria with different minimum inhibitory concentrations (MIC). The regression line represents the decreasing antibiotic concentration with distance from the disk. Zone size depends on the MIC and is usually compared to that of a known sensitive strain.

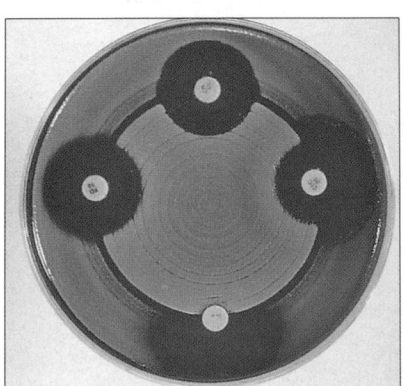

320 Disk sensitivity testing *Staphylococcus aureus*. The outer rim is a control *S. aureus* NCTC 6571 sensitive to P, F, CE and CN. Centrally *S. aureus* is resistant to P. It is sensitive to the other antimicrobials. *(DST agar with 5% lysed blood, 18 h at 37°C)*

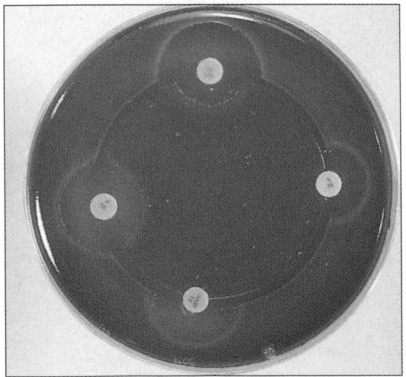

321 Sensitive and resistant *Escherichia coli* strains. The outer rim is a control *E. coli* NCTC sensitive to AML, W, F, and NA showing inhibition zones around each antimicrobial disk. An *E. coli* from a clinical specimen is plated centrally showing sensitivity to F and NA and resistance (no inhibition zones) to AML and W. *(DST agar with 5% lysed blood, 18 h at 37°C)*

concentration. Examples of disk sensitivity testing are shown for *S. aureus* (**320**) and *E. coli* (**321**). Resistance to penicillins and related antibiotics is often due to the production by the bacteria of beta-lactamase enzymes that destroy the beta-lactam ring. **322** shows an *E. coli* resistant to amoxycillin, due to beta-lactamase production, with no inhibition zone around the amoxycillin. The antimicrobial agent, augmentin, contains amoxycillin and the beta-lactamase inhibitor, clavulanic acid. The beta-lactamase is thus inhibited and the *E. coli* is rendered sensitive to the amoxycillin in the disk, resulting in a zone of inhibition. If a beta-lactamase producing organism fails to generate sufficient enzyme to destroy the concentration of antibiotic near the disk, an inhibition zone will occur but the colonies at the edge of the zone will be large, showing a 'heaped' appearance (**323**). Beta-lactamase production can be demonstrated by a simple colour test

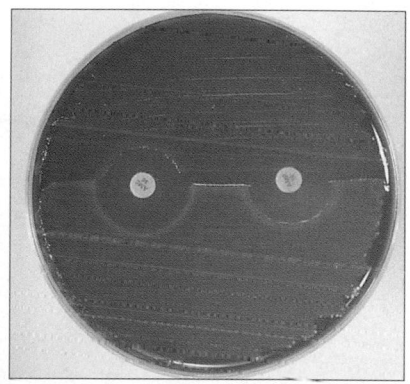

322 *Escherichia coli* **showing ampicillin resistance due to beta-lactamase production.** The plate is inoculated with an *E. coli* resistant to ampicillin. The strain is sensitive to augmentin. Augmentin is an agent containing ampicillin and the beta-lactamase inhibitor, clavulanic acid. *(DST agar with 5% lysed blood, 18 h at 37°C)*

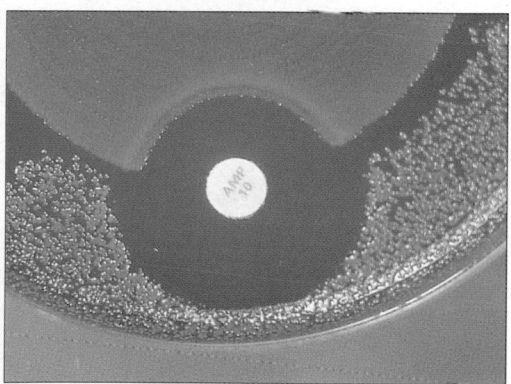

323 *Escherichia coli* **demonstrating amoxycillin resistance due to beta-lactamase production.** The outer rim is a fully sensitive *E. coli*. The resistant strain does show an inhibition zone, but it is smaller and the edge has a 'heaped' appearance. *(DST agar with 5% lysed blood, 18 h at 37°C)*

using the chromogenic cephalosporin, nitrocefin (**324**). Methicillin resistance among strains of *S. aureus* can be determined by placing a methicillin-impregnated (25 μg) strip across streaks of the test isolate and known methicillin and resistant strains, for comparison (**325**).

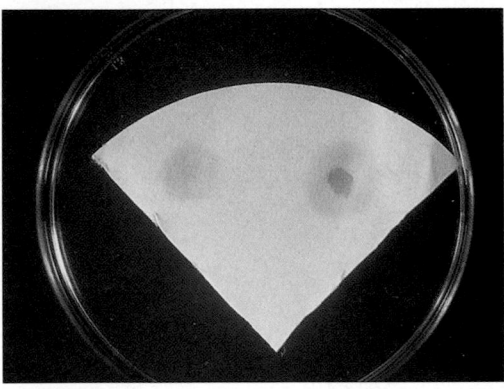

324 Chromogenic cephalosporin (nitrocefin) test to demonstrate beta-lactamase production. Nitrocefin changes colour from yellow to red in the presence of beta-lactamase. A beta-lactamase producing, ampicillin-resistant strain of *Haemophilus influenzae* has been scraped onto the strip, which shows the red colour after 60 sec.

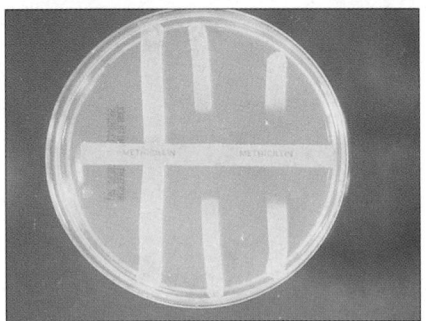

325 Methicillin resistant *Staphylococcus aureus.* The strip contains 25 μg methicillin. For sensitive strains there is a zone of no growth on either side of the strip. The methicillin resistant *S. aureus* (MRSA) grows up to the strip. *(Columbia agar, 18 h at 37°C)*

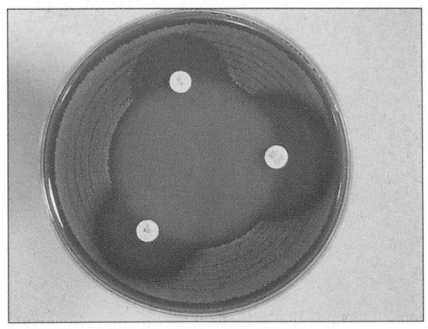

326 Penicillin resistant *Streptococcus pneumoniae.* The outer rim is inoculated with a sensitive control *S. aureus*. Penicillin resistant strains of *S. pneumoniae* are demonstrated using a 1 μg oxacillin disk. The *resistant S. pneumoniae* plated centrally is penicillin and erythromycin resistant. *(Chocolate agar, 18 h at 37°C)*

Penicillin resistance is an increasing clinical problem in *S. pneumoniae* and is due to alterations in penicillin-binding proteins. It has been shown that a 1 µg oxacillin disk gives the most reproducible in-vivo result (**326**). Disk sensitivity testing for *H. influenzae*, *N. meningitidis* and *N. gonorrhoeae* is shown in figures **327–329**.

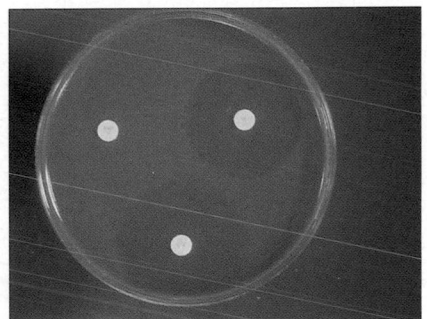

327 *Haemophilus influenzae,* ampicillin resistance. Disc sensitivity plate showing *H. influenzae* resistant to ampicillin but sensitive to chloramphenicol and cefotaxime. *(Chocolate agar, 18 h at 37°C)*

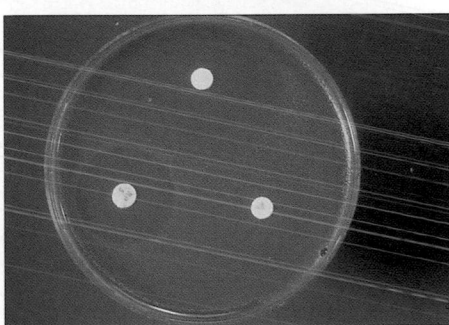

328 *Neisseria meningitidis* sensitivity. Disk sensitivity showing *N. meningitidis* sensitive to penicillin and rifampicin but resistant to sulphonamide. *(Chocolate agar, 18 h at 37°C)*

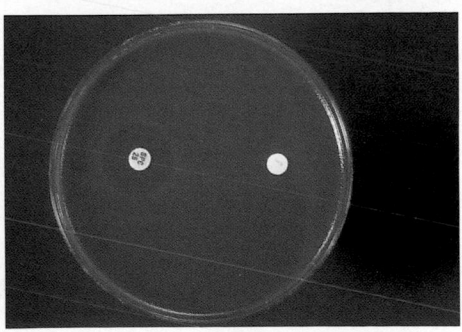

329 *Neisseria gonorrhoeae* resistant to penicillin. Disk sensitivity showing *N. gonorrhoeae* resistant to penicillin and sensitive to spectinomycin. *(Chocolate agar, 18 h at 37°C)*

Clinical isolates of *Ps. aeruginosa* are frequently resistant to multiple anti-microbials. **330** shows *Ps. aeruginosa* resistant to gentamicin and cefotaxime. There have been recent reports of *Enterococcus faecium* with low-level resistance to vancomycin (**331**). Where large numbers of isolates are to be tested for antimicrobial sensitivity, the use of agar plates with antibiotics of known concentrations incorporated is useful. The antibiotic concentration is chosen as a 'break point' below which sensitive strains will grow but above which only resistant strains will grow (**332**).

Disc sensitivity testing gives only a qualitative guide to the sensitivity or resistance of an isolate. More quantitative methods enable the determination of the minimum inhibitory concentration (MIC) and minimum bactericidal concentration (MBC) of an antimicrobial against a clinical isolate. These determinations are important in serious infections such as endocarditis and when using antimicrobials with a dose related toxicity. **333** and **334** show the tube method

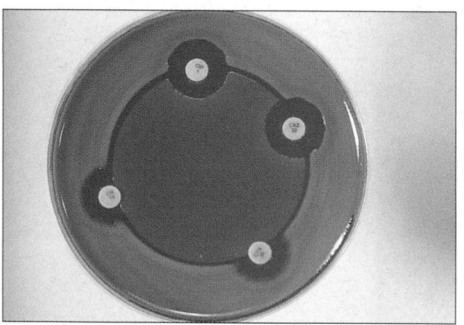

330 *Pseudomonas aeruginosa* sensitivity testing. The outer rim is a *Ps. aeruginosa* control (NCTC 10662) sensitive to CTX, CN, CIP, CAZ. The test sample shows resistance to cefotaxime and gentamicin. *(DST 5% lysed blood, 18 h at 37°C)*

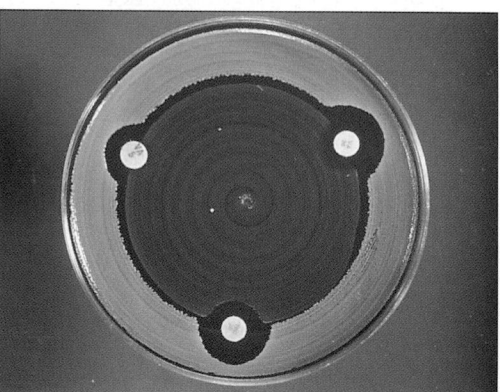

331 *Enterococcus faecalis* showing resistance to vancomycin. Some strains of *E. faecalis* show low level resistance to vancomycin. The strain is resistant to the 5 µg disk, but sensitive to the 30 µg disk and to teicoplanin. *(DST 5% lysed blood, 18 h at 37°C)*

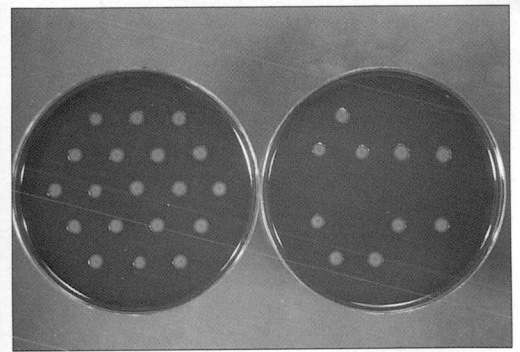

332 Break point sensitivity testing of *Escherichia coli* to amoxycillin. Test strains are inoculated onto media containing different concentrations of amoxycillin using a multipoint inoculator. After overnight incubation, presence or absence of growth is noted. *(DST agar with 5% lysed blood. Plate amoxycillin concentrations: left, 1 µg/ml; right, 8 µg/ml)*

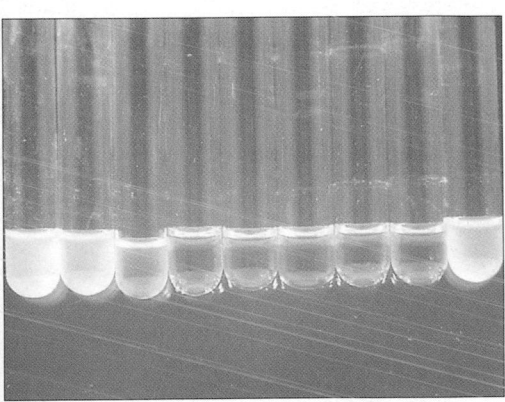

333

333, 334 Tube minimum inhibitory concentration of two *Escherichia coli* isolates to ampicillin. Serial dilutions of ampicillin from 0.5 µg/ml to 64 µg/ml are prepared. 1ml of the test organism suspension is added to each tube. After overnight incubation visual turbidity is noted. The MIC is the lowest antibiotic concentration in which there is no visible growth. In the upper row (**333**) the MIC is 2 µg/ml. In the lower row (**334**) the MIC is 32 µg/ml. *(Ampicillin concentrations (µg/ml) left to right: 0.5, 1, 2, 4, 8, 16, 32, 64, 0 (control))*

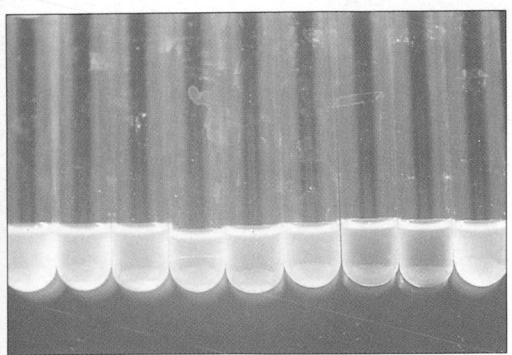

334

for determining MIC and **335** and **336**, the MBC determination. In clinical practice, knowledge of synergy and antagonism between antimicrobial agents is important. **337** demonstrates synergy between trimethoprim and a sulphonamide, two agents that work at different sites in bacterial nucleic acid synthesis. Antagonism between nalidixic acid and nitrofurantoin is shown in **338**.

Antagonism between antimicrobials may arise through the induction of class I betalactamase by one beta-lactam reducing the effect of a second beta-lactam (**339**).

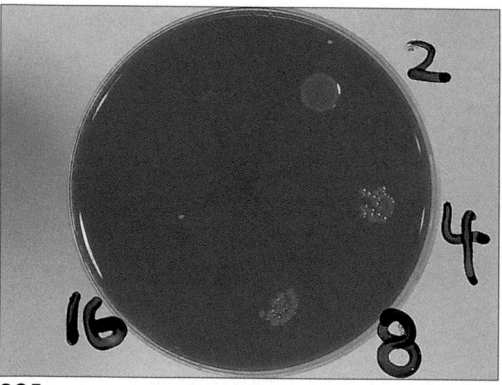

335

335, 336 Minimum bactericidal concentration (MBC) of *Escherichia coli* to ampicillin. From each of the non-turbid tubes of the MIC test, 20 μl is spotted on to a section of blood agar plate and incubated overnight. The lowest concentration giving no growth on the plate is the MBC. For the isolate with the MIC of 2 μg/ml, the MBC is 16 μg/ml (**335**). For the isolate with the MIC of 32 μg/ml the MBC is greater than 64 μg/ml (**336**). *(Blood agar, 18 h at 37°C)*

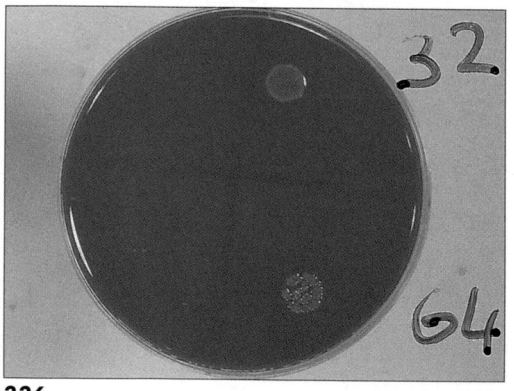

336

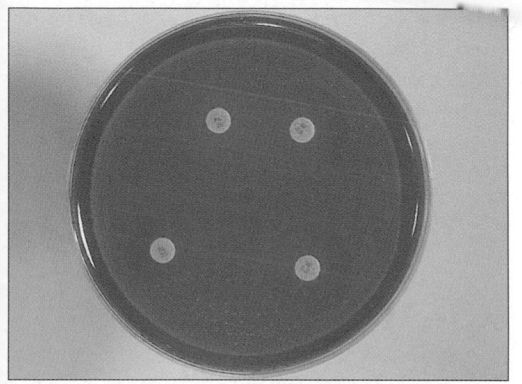

337 Demonstration of antimicrobial synergy.

The test shows synergy of action by trimethoprim and sulphamethoxazole. The zone size is increased in the area between the disks where both antibiotics are present. *(Escherichia coli on DST agar with 5% lysed blood, 18 h at 37°C)*

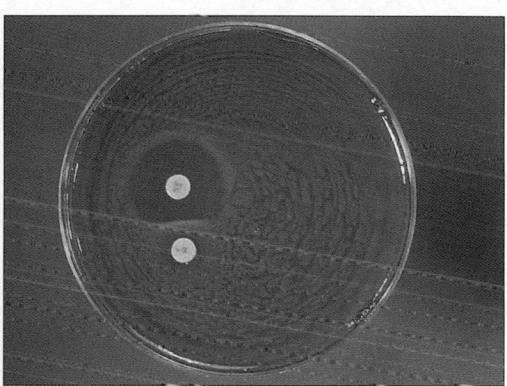

338 Demonstration of antimicrobial antagonism.

The test shows antagonism of antimicrobial action by nalidixic acid and nitrofurantoin. The zone size is decreased in the area between the disks where both antibiotics are present. *(Proteus vulgaris on CLED agar, 18 h at 37°C)*

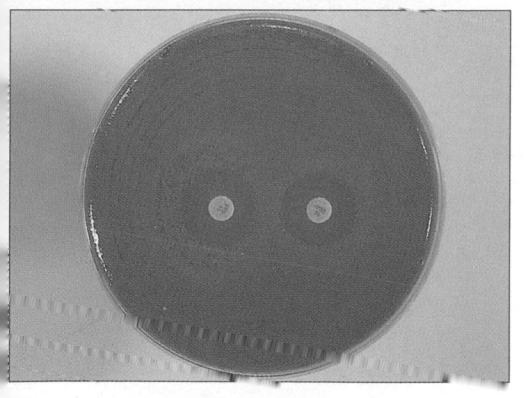

339 Induction of beta-lactamase production.

Imipenem induces beta-lactamase production in *Pseudomonas aeruginosa*, reducing the zone size to piperacillin. *(DST agar with 5% lysed blood, 18 h at 37°C)*

Synergistic activity is important in clinical practice, where a combination of antimicrobials may allow a lower dose of a potentially toxic agent to be used. **340** and **341** demonstrate the synergistic effects of gentamicin and penicillin.

In severe infections, it is useful to determine the serum bactericidal activity against the patient's clinical isolate. Serum samples are taken pre-dose and generally 1 h post-dose and the maximum serum dilution giving inhibitory and bactericidal activity is determined (**342–344**). A minimum bactericidal dilution of 1:8 in the peak serum sample is regarded as adequate, though some studies suggest a dilution in excess of 1:32 may be necessary for cure.

Effect of antibiotics in combination						
Rows	Gentamicin µg/ml	Penicillin µg/ml				
		2	1	0.5	0.12	0
A	32	–	–	–	–	–
B	16	–	–	–	–	+
C	8	–	–	–	–	+
D	4	–	–	–	+	+
E	2	–	–	+	+	+
F	0	+	+	+	+	+
		1	2	3	4	5
+ = Growth				Columns		

340

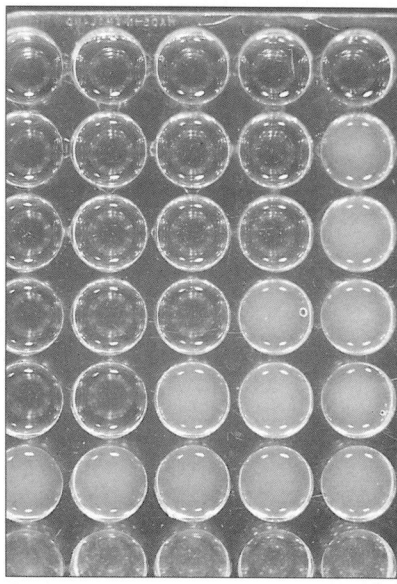

341

340, 341 Antimicrobial agents in combination. Each well in the plate contains different combinations of penicillin and gentamicin, shown in **340**. Row F shows growth at all concentrations of penicillin in the absence of gentamicin. Column 5 shows growth at all concentrations of gentamicin, except at 32 µg/ml, in the absence of penicillin. The two antimicrobials work synergistically, growth being inhibited at a gentamicin concentration of 2 µg/ml in the presence of 1 µg/ml of penicillin (**341**).

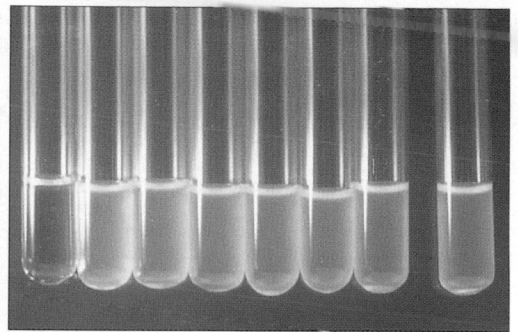

342

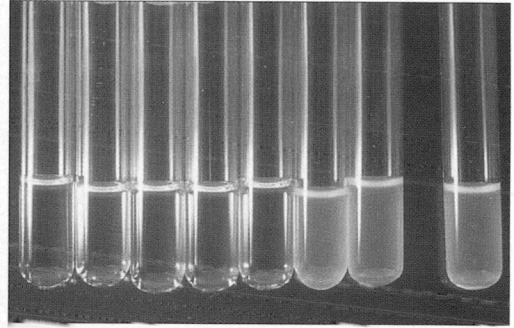

343

342, 343 Back titration to determine anti-microbial activity in serum. Pre- and post-dose blood samples are taken from the patient during antimicrobial therapy. The serum is serially diluted and inoculated with 1 ml of a broth culture of the patient's isolate and the tubes are incubated overnight. **342** and **343** show that the pre-dose minimum inhibitory dilution (MID) is 1:2 and the post-dose, 1:32. *(Broth dilutions, left to right – 1:2, 1:4, 1:8, 1:16, 1:32, 1:64, 1:128, control)*

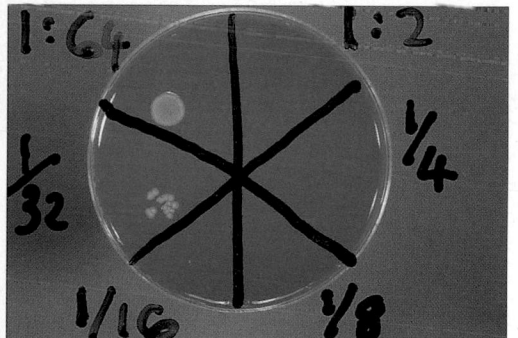

344 Minimum bacteriocidal dilution (MBD). For the post-dose, 20 µl samples from tubes with no growth have been spotted onto blood agar and incubated overnight to determine the MBD, which is 1:16. *(Blood agar, 18 h at 37°C)*

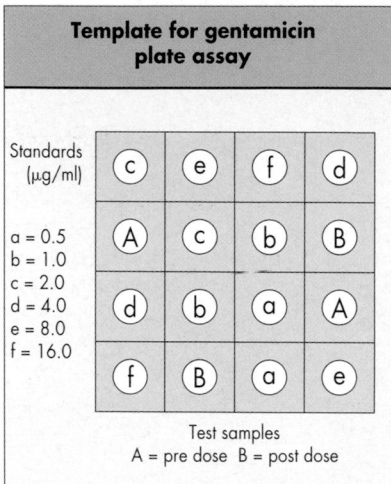

Template for gentamicin plate assay

Standards (μg/ml)

	c	e	f	d

a = 0.5
b = 1.0
c = 2.0
d = 4.0
e = 8.0
f = 16.0

A	c	b	B
d	b	a	A
f	B	a	e

Test samples
A = pre dose   B = post dose

345

345, 346, 347 Plate assay to determine blood concentration of gentamicin. The plate is poured with isosenitest agar, which after setting, is inoculated with 1:50 dilution of an overnight broth culture of *Klebsiella edwardsii*. The wells are cut and gentamicin standards and the test sample added as in **345**. After overnight incubation (**346**), the inhibition zones are measured and a standard curve drawn (**347**). The concentration of gentamicin in the test samples is determined from the graph. Sample A concentration is 1 μg/ml and sample B is 10 μg/ml.

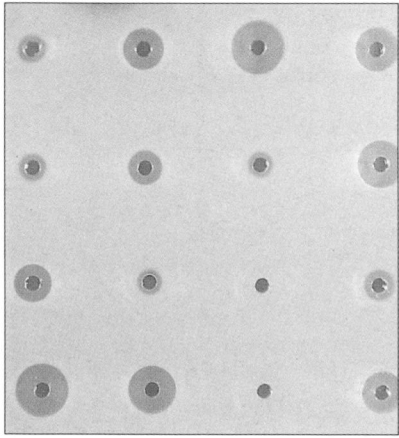

346

Calibration curve for gentamicin assay

Zone diameter, mm

Calibration curve from standards

Post dose

Pre dose

16   Gentamicin,   8   4   2 1
μg/ml

Pre dose zone =
9.6 mm = 1 μg/ml

Post dose zone =
20 mm = 10 μg/ml

347

An additional investigation to determine the likely in vivo activity of an antimicrobial and to monitor toxic levels, is to assay the antimicrobial concentration in the serum. **345–347** show microbiological plate assays to determine the pre- and post-dose levels of gentamicin.

The remaining figures in this section describe the transfer of antimicrobial resistance determinants. **348** describes the principle of plasmid-mediated transfer of resistance genes. In the laboratory, exponential cultures of a multiply resistant donor and a suitable recipient, containing a chromosomally located resistance marker, are incubated overnight and plated to a medium containing the recipient marker antibiotic and one of the antibiotics to which the donor is resistant. Transconjugants (the recipient strain now containing plasmid-borne genes from the donor) will grow on the selective plate. **349–351** demonstrate resistance transfer in *E. coli*. **352** is a gel showing the plasmid profiles of donors and recipients, demonstrating the transferred plasmids.

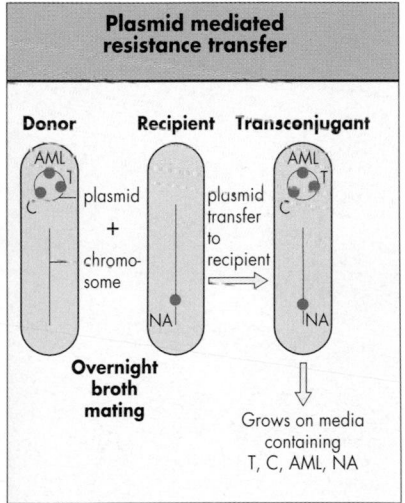

348 Plasmid mediated transfer of antimicrobial resistance genes. The donor is resistant to ampicillin, tetracycline and chloramphenicol, and sensitive to nalidixic acid. The recipient *E. coli* K12 is resistant only to nalidixic acid. The transconjugant is resistant to all four antimicrobial agents.

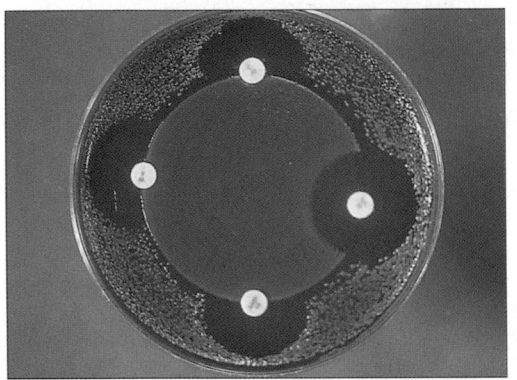

349

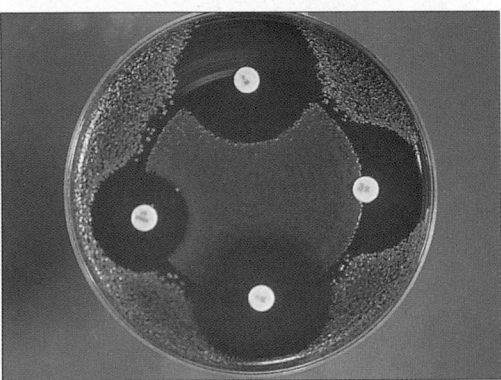

350

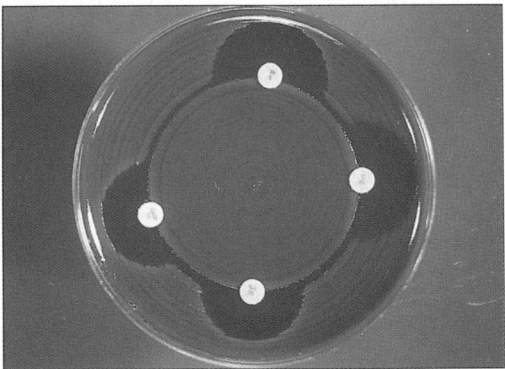

351

349, 350, 351 Transfer of resistance by bacterial conjugation. The donor *Escherichia coli* isolate (**349**) is sensitive to NA and resistant to AML, T and C. The recipient is a laboratory strain (*E. coli*, K12, NA^R) sensitive to AML, T and C with chromosomally located NA resistance (**350**). **351** shows the transconjugant, which is resistant to all four antibiotics.

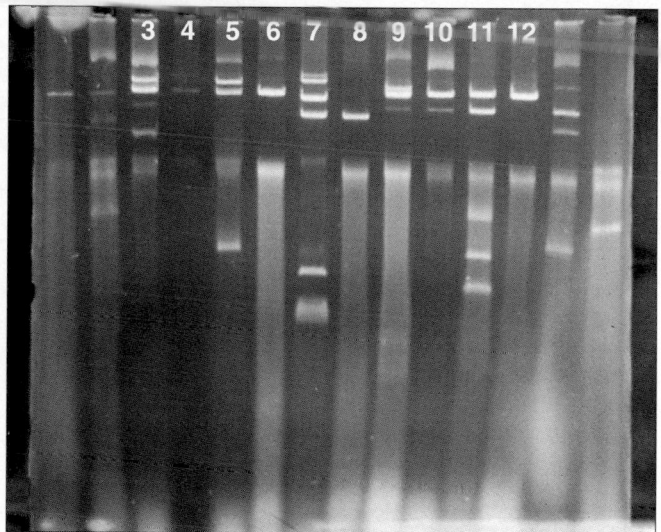

**352 Agarose gel electrophoresis showing transfer of
antimicrobial resistant plasmids.** Lanes 3 to 12 show alternate
donors and transconjugants demonstrating plasmid transfer. As an
example, lane 3 is a donor with four plasmids (above the broad
band of chromosomal DNA). Lane 4 is the transconjugant that has
one plasmid from the donor. *(DNA extraction by SDS lysis and
ethanol precipitation. 0.7% agarose gel electrophoresis. Stained with
ethidium bromide.)*

EPIDEMIOLOGICAL TECHNIQUES

In the investigation of disease outbreaks and hospital cross-infection, typing of the pathogens to further than species level is often necessary to identify the 'outbreak strain'. In this section, examples of particular typing techniques are shown. More general methods (such as biochemical properties, antimicrobial resistance patterns and serotyping) may also be used. Such techniques are illustrated elsewhere in this book.

353 shows bacteriophage typing of *S. aureus*. The phage type of the strain is given by the reference number of the phages that produce lysis on the plate. **354** illustrates pyocin (bacteriocin) typing of *Pseudomonas aeruginosa*. Bacteriocin typing has also been used for *Shigella* spp. and other Enterobacteriaceae. It is a labour intensive method and is rarely used now that more specific and reproducible molecular techniques are available. **355** demonstrates Dienes typing of swarming *Proteus* strains. Differing strains produce a 'ditch' of no growth between the swarming edges.

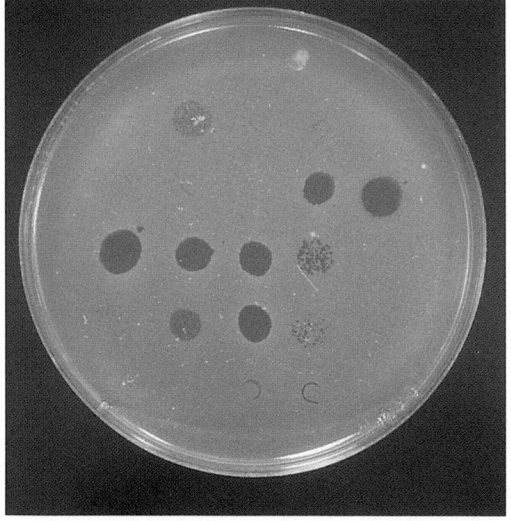

353 Bacteriophage typing of *Staphylococcus aureus*. A broth culture of *S. aureus* is seeded on to the plate, and specific phages spotted on a grid system. After overnight incubation, lysis indicates the phage type of the *S. aureus* strain. *(Nutrient agar, 18 h at 37°C)*

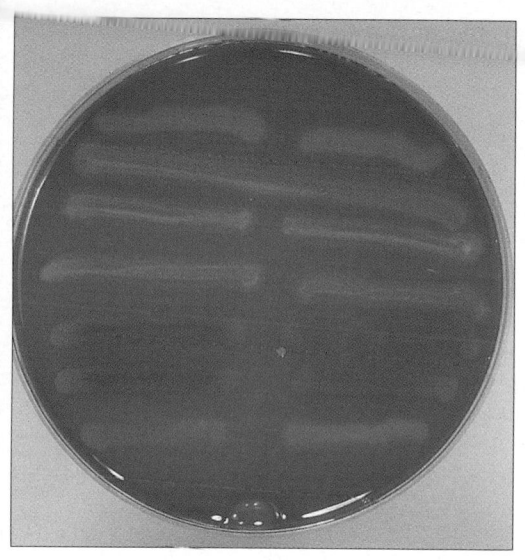

354 Pyocin typing of *Pseudomonas aeruginosa.*
The test strain is streaked down the centre of the plate. The growth is removed from the plate which is then exposed to chloroform vapour to kill remaining growth. Typing strains are streaked across the plate, which is again incubated. Inhibition of typing strains demonstrates the pyocin type of the test strain. *(Blood agar, 18 h at 37°C)*

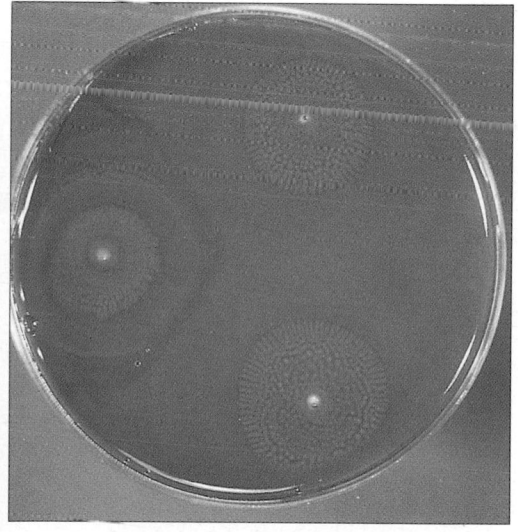

355 Dienes typing of *Proteus strains.* Three
strains are spotted equidistantly around the periphery of the plate and incubated overnight. The two identical strains show no line of separation where the growth merges. The third, different strain shows the line of separation. *(Blood agar, 18 h at 37°C)*

Molecular and related methods that are increasingly used in epidemiological studies include whole cell and outer membrane protein typing, plasmid profiling and plasmid chromosomal DNA restriction endonuclease typing.

356 shows whole cell protein typing in the investigation of *B. cepacia* isolates from cases of cystic fibrosis. Additional non-DNA based techniques include outer membrane protein analysis and lipopolysaccharide typing (**357**).

Rapid methods for small-scale DNA extraction have led to a new range of typing techniques that have a wide scope of applicability, are reproducible and provide good discrimination between strains. **358** shows plasmid profiles of *Sh. sonnei* strains isolated from different clusters of infection and demonstrates how the profiles can distinguish different strains.

The spread of multiply antimicrobial resistant Gram-negative bacteria is an increasing problem in hospital infection. Restriction endonuclease digests of plasmids from strains with common resistance patterns can help in defining the particular outbreak strain (**359**). Restriction endonucleases can also be used to

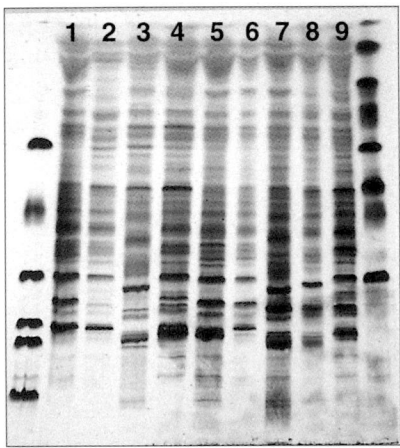

356 Whole cell protein typing of B. cepacia. After cell lysis, whole cell proteins are separated by polyacrylamide gel electrophoresis and stained with coomassie blue. The outer lanes are molecular weight standards. The protein profiles show similarity of the strains on lanes 1–5 and lane 9.

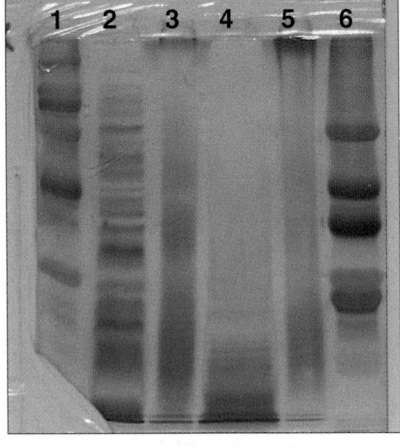

357 Demonstration of whole cell protein (WCP), outer membrane protein (OMP), and lipopoly-saccharide (LPS) typing of Legionella. Lanes 1 and 6 are molecular weight markers. Lane 2 shows the WCP profile. Lane 3 shows OMP profile. Lane 4 shows LPS profiles. *(Polyacrylamide gel electrophoresis with silver stains)*

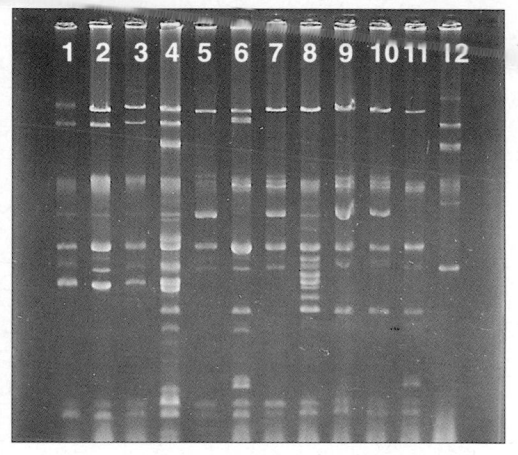

358 Plasmid profile typing of *Shigella sonnei.* Lane 12 shows plasmid molecular weight markers. The lanes demonstrate groups of strains with identical plasmid profiles (e.g. lanes 1–3, lanes 5 and 7, lanes 9 and 10) and others with distinct and separate profiles. *(DNA extraction by SDS lysis and ethanol precipitation. 0.7% agarose gel electrophoresis. Stained with ethidium bromide.)*

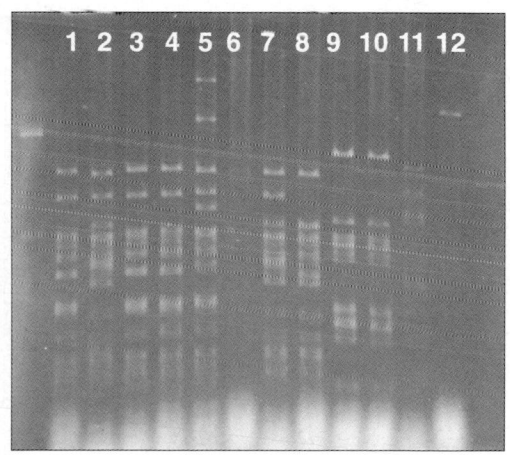

359 Restriction endonuclease characterization of antimicrobial resistance plasmid from *Escherichia coli.* The gel shows digests of single plasmids all of molecular weight 62 Md, using the enzyme *Pst*1. Restriction profiles of plasmids in lanes 1, 2, 3, 4 and 7 appear identical. The plasmids in lanes 9 and 10 have a common restriction pattern, but are distinguishable from the other patterns. *(DNA extraction by SDS lysis and ethanol precipitation. Enzyme digest at 37°C for 2 h 0.7% agarose gel electrophoresis. Stained with ethidium bromide.)*

produce chromosomal DNA profiles. Because of the large number of fragments produced, pulsed field electrophoresis, with varying time/voltage parameters, is used to improve discrimination (**360**).

Disease outbreak investigations may also require environmental microbiological studies. **361** shows an example of the investigation of water quality. Faecal coliforms will grow at 44°C and this is used to demonstrate faecal contamination.

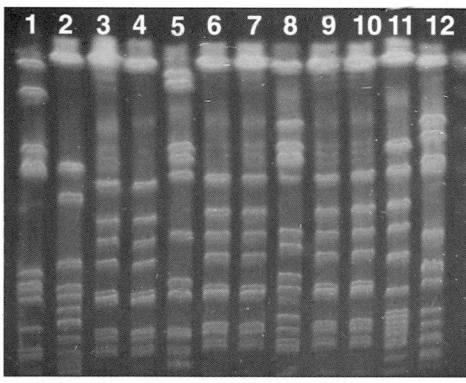

360 Pulsed field gel electrophoresis (PFGE) of chromosomal DNA from different isolates of methicillin resistant *Staphylococcus aureus* (MRSA). The gel shows chromosomal DNA from different MRSA isolates which have been digested with the restriction endonuclease *SmaI* and run by pulsed field electrophoresis. The isolates in lanes 3, 4, 6, 7, 9 and 10 had identical profiles and were identified as an 'outbreak strain'. *(DNA extraction by cell lysis and proteinase K treatment. Electrophoresis on 1% agarose gel, angle 120°, 6 volts/cm, initial switch time 5.3 sec, final switch time 34.9 sec)*

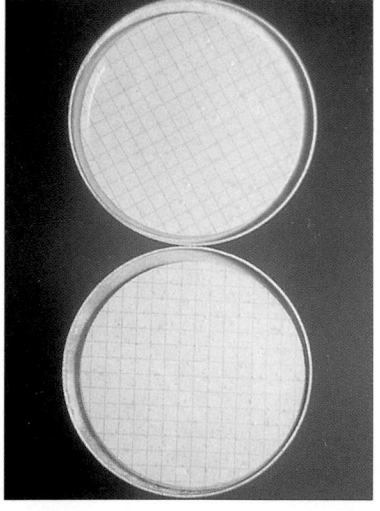

361 Membrane filtration technique for microbiological testing of water quality. 100 ml water samples are passed through 0.45 μm membrane filters, which are soaked in lauryl sulphate medium and incubated at 44°C for 16 h. Faecal coliforms produce yellow colonies and the count/100 ml is determined. Top, low coliform count; bottom, high coliform count, suggesting considerable faecal contamination.

5.
Medically Important Fungi

Fungi form an extremely large kingdom but only a small number are pathogenic for man. Fungi are eukaryotic, possessing a nucleus and a cell wall composed of chitin. The major groups of pathogenic fungi are outlined in **362**. Fungi may grow in a unicellular mode (e.g. yeasts) or in a multicellular form when cells elongate to form filaments called hyphae. The four major taxa of the true fungi (Eumycetes) are delineated by their methods of reproduction. The Zygomycetes reproduce sexually and zygotes form by fusion of hyphal tips. Pathogenic members of this genus include *Mucor* and *Absidia* spp. The Basidiomycetes carry sexual spores externally on club-shaped cells called basidia. Ascomycetes produce sexual spores within an ascus and pathogens include *Piedraia hortae*. Most human

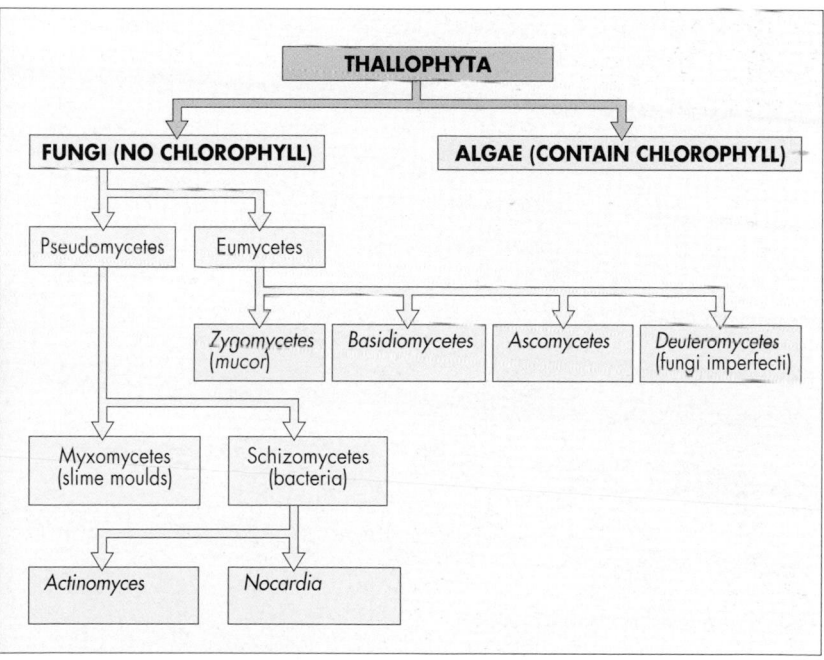

362 Taxonomy of fungi.

pathogens are in the taxon Deuteromycetes. They are also called imperfect fungi since they do not reproduce sexually but produce asexual spores or conidia. Pathogenic *Fungi Imperfecti* include *Epidermophyton, Candida* and *Pityrosporum* spp. However, a more useful classification is based on disease associations, namely superficial mycoses, subcutaneous mycoses and systemic mycoses (**363**). Although *Actinomyces* spp. and *Nocardia* spp. are branching bacteria they are more conveniently covered here.

Fungi and Human Disease		
Superficial mycoses	Dermatophytes (tinea capitis, tinea cruris, tinea pedis, endothrix, ringworm). *Epidermophyton floccosum.* *Microsporum audouinii (M. gypseum, M. canis).* *Trichophyton rubrum (T. terrestre, T. mentagrophytes, T. verrucosum, T. violaceum, T. schoenleinii, T. tonsurans).* Pityriasis versicolor – *Malassezia (Pityrosporum) furfur.* Black piedra – *Piedraia hortae.* Tinea nigra – *Cladosporium werneckii.*	
Subcutaneous mycoses	Sporotrichosis –	*Sporothrix schenckii.*
	Chromomycosis –	*Phialophora verrucosa, Phialophora (Fonsecaea) pedrosi. Cladosporium carrionii.*
	Mycetoma –	*Actinomadura madurae, Nocardia asteroides, N. brasiliensis, Streptomyces somaliensis.*
	Rhinosporidiosis –	*Rhinosporidium seeberi.*
	Zygomycosis –	*Basidiobolus haptosporus, Conidiobolus coronatus.*
Systemic mycoses primary pathogens	Histoplasmosis –	*Histoplasma capsulatum*
	Coccidiomycosis –	*Coccidiodes immitis*
	Blastomycosis –	*Blastomyces dermatitidis*
	Paracoccidiomycosis –	*Paracoccidioides brasiliensis*
	Cryptococcosis –	*Cryptococcus neoformans*
opportunistic pathogens	*Aspergillus fumigatus* *Candida albicans* *Pneumocystis carinii* *Mucor* spp.	

363 Fungi and human disease.

ACTINOMYCETACEAE

These are branching bacteria (**364**) that can be part of the normal flora. The major pathogen is *Actinomyces israelii* which is Gram-positive, non acid-fast and anaerobic or microaerophilic. It produces abscesses in the jaw, chest or abdomen and is also associated with infections of plastic intrauterine contraceptive devices. Diagnosis is by Gram film of pus, which may contain sulphur granules (**365**) and

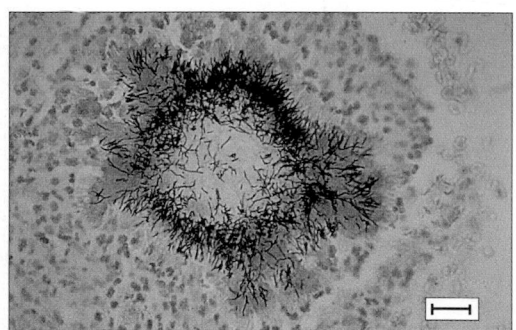

364 Gram-positive *Actinomyces israelii* pus.
A Gram film of pus from a patient with abdominal actinomycosis. Branching Gram-positive *Actinomyces israelii* is visible. (bar = 10 μm)

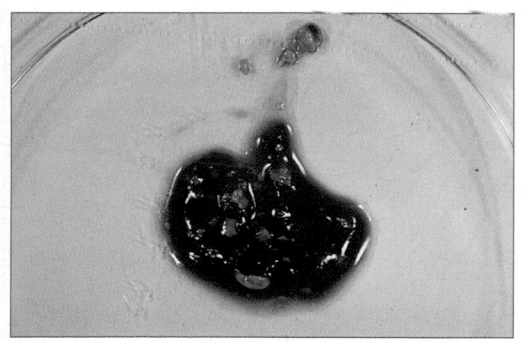

365 Actinomycosis.
Sulphur granules from a case of abdominal actinomycosis.

culture in liquid or solid media. On solid media it produces white-grey colonies with an irregular surface resembling the surface of a tooth (**366**). Treatment is effected by draining the abscess and administering penicillin.

NOCARDIACEAE

These, too, are filamentous and Gram-positive (**367**) but are only partially acid-fast bacteria with, unlike *A. israelii*, bacillary and coccoid forms. *Nocardia asteroides* is found world-wide and causes deep abscesses. *N. brasiliensis* and *N. caviae* are a cause of mycetoma (Madura foot). On blood agar *N. asteroides* produces colonies with an irregular surface. Treatment requires surgical drainage and long-term administration of sulphonamides, or cotrimoxazole.

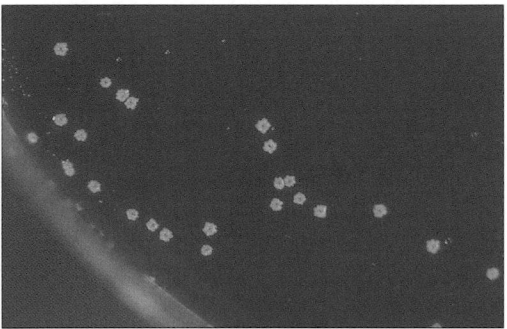

366 *Actinomyces israelii* colonies. Colonies of *Actinomyces israelii* on blood agar. These had been incubated at 37°C under micro-aerophilic conditions for 4 days. Note the irregularly shaped (dentate) colonies.

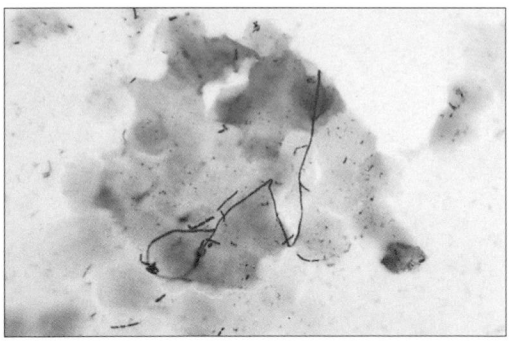

367 Gram-positive *Nocardia asteroides* pus. A Gram stain of pus containing *N. asteroides*.

SUPERFICIAL MYCOSES

The dermatophytes are a group of fungi (**368**) that can utilize keratin as a source of nutrition. In tissues they are present as hyphae or may divide into arthrospores. On solid culture medium (e.g. Sabouraud's dextrose agar) they produce fluffy or powdery colonies (**369–371**) and their characteristic macro- or microconidia, which permit speciation. Biochemical properties are not used frequently for speciation. *Epidermophyton* spp. have rough-walled pyriform macroconidia (**372**), *Microsporum* spp. rough-walled fusiform macroconidia (**373**) and *Trichophyton* spp. smooth-walled cylindrical macroconidia. The production of macroconidia by *Trichophyton* spp. is poor even when cultured on Sabouraud's malt agar. The diagnostic feature of *T. mentagrophytes,* in particular, is the production of spiral hyphae (**374**). Infections are termed ringworm or tinea followed by reference to

The dermatophytes		
Anthropophilic	Zoophilic	Geophilic
Epidermophyton floccosum	Microsporum canis	Microsporum fulvum
Microsporum audouinii	M. distortum	M. gypseum
M. ferrugineum	M. equinum	Trichophyton ajelloi
M. rivalieri	M. nanum	T. terrestre
Trichophyton concentricum	M. persicolor	
T. gourvilii	Trichophyton equinum	
T. interdigitale	T. erinacei	
T. megninii	T. gallinae	
I. rubrum	T. mentagrophytes	
T. schoenleinii	T. quinckeanum	
T. soudanense	T. simii	
T. tonsurans	T. verrucosum	
T. violaceum		
T. yaoundii		

368   The dermatophytes.

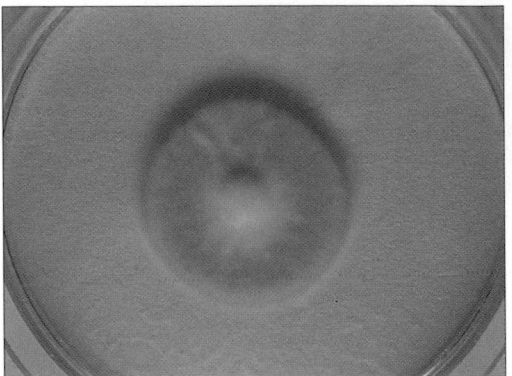

369 *Trichophyton rubrum* culture. *T. rubrum* cultured for 10 days on Sabouraud's dextrose agar.

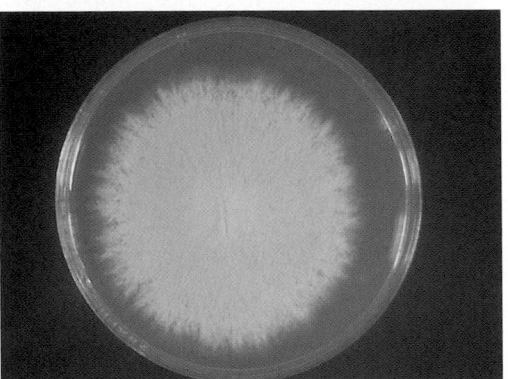

370 *Microsporum gypseum* culture. *M. gypseum* cultured for 10 days on Sabouraud's dextrose agar.

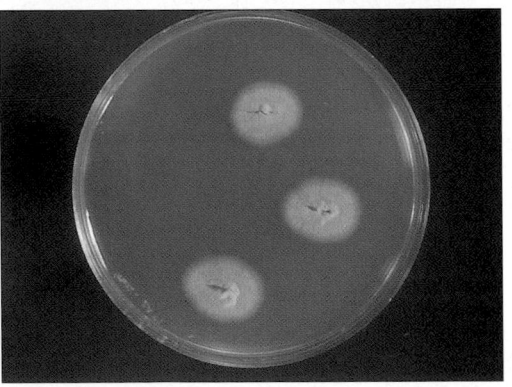

371 *Epidermophyton floccosum* culture. *E. floccosum* cultured for 10 days on Sabouraud's dextrose agar.

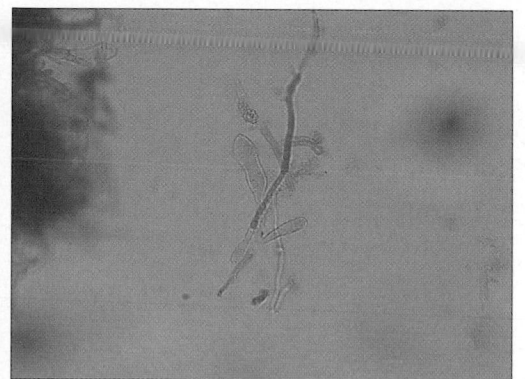

372 *Epidermophyton floccosum* culture. Lactophenol cotton blue stained preparation of *E. floccosum* cultured on Sabouraud's agar showing the typical pyriform macroconidia.

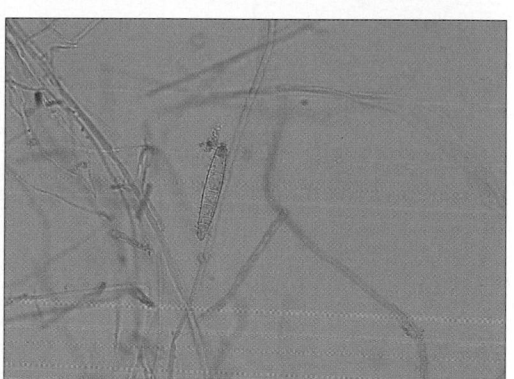

373 *Microsporum canis* culture. Lactophenol cotton blue stained preparation of *M. canis* cultured on Sabouraud's agar showing the rough-walled macroconidia.

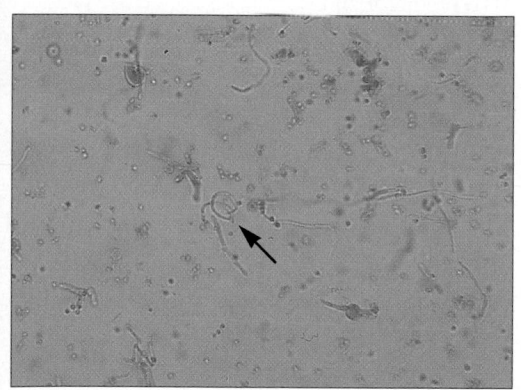

374 *Trichophyton mentagrophytes* culture. Lactophenol cotton blue stained preparation of *T. mentagrophytes* cultured on Sabouraud's agar showing spiral hyphae (arrow).

the site. Thus tinea capitis is scalp ringworm; tinea corporis, body ringworm (**375**); tinea cruris, groin ringworm; tinea pedis, foot ringworm or athlete's foot; tinea manum, hand ringworm; tinea barbae, ringworm of facial hairs; and tinea unguium, ringworm of the nails (**376**). Tinea imbricata is due to *T. concentricum* and is characterized by concentric rings on the skin (**377**). Dermatophytes may

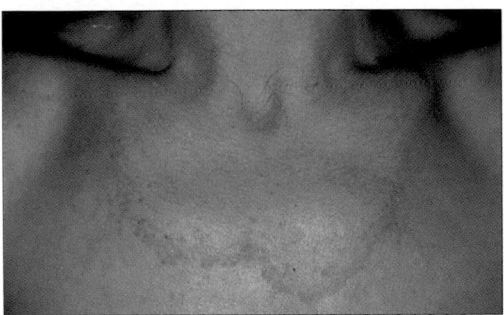

375 Tinea corporis. A case of ringworm (tinea corporis).

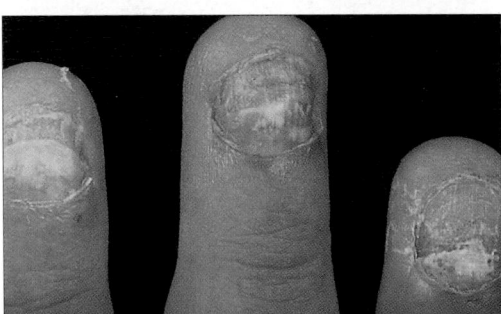

376 Tinea unguium. A case of tinea unguium.

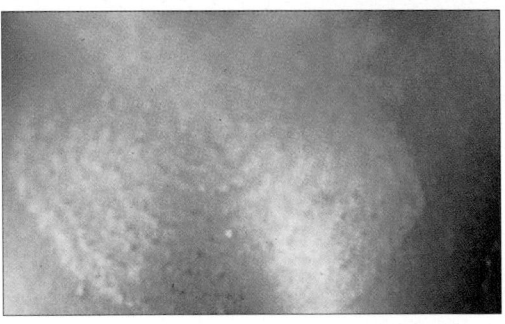

377 Tinea imbricata. A case of tinea imbricata due to *Trichophyton concentricum.*

also invade hairs. When present on the outside surface, the condition is termed ectothrix and inside, endothrix (**378**). Zoophilic dermatophytes tend to produce a much more florid response and may cause a kerion (**379**). Diagnosis is by taking skin or nail scrapes or hair samples and placing them in potassium hydroxide (KOH, 30%) on microscope slides. The slide is then examined for fungal hyphae

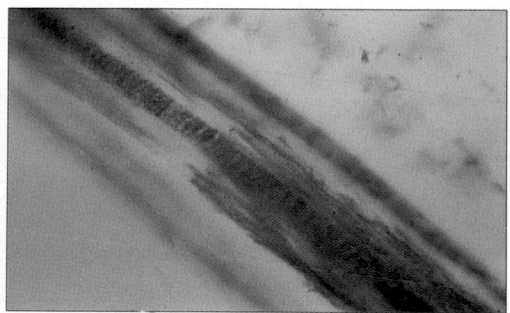

378 Endothrix showing fungal hyphae inside a hair shaft.

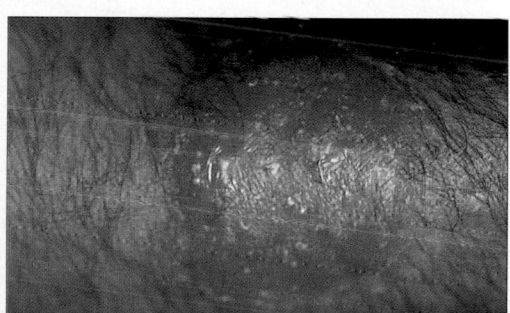

379 A kerion which is an excessively florid reaction to a zoophilic dermatophyte (*Microsporum canis*).

380 KOH technique showing fungal hyphae. A potassium hydroxide treated skin scraping showing fungal hyphae and arthrospores.

and arthrospores (**380**). Some dermatophyte lesions (e.g. due to *M. audouinii, M. canis* or *T. schoenleinii*) fluoresce when exposed to long-wave ultraviolet light (365 nm; Wood's lamp). For precise diagnosis samples are cultured at room temperature (better still at 26–28°C) for up to 2 weeks on Sabouraud's dextrose agar. A small portion of the colony is placed on a microscope slide and spread in lactophenol cotton blue solution. This allows microscopic visualization of the spore arrangements (**372–374**). Treatment, if needed, is by oral griseofulvin.

SUBCUTANEOUS MYCOSES

These infections are caused by a variety of fungi (and even bacteria) but tend to be found in tropical or sub-tropical regions. Most often the fungi are present in soil and are introduced into subepidermal tissues by trauma.

MYCETOMA

This presents as a destructive localized lesion, most often on the feet (**381**) or hands, with discharging sinuses. Actinomycetoma is due to bacteria such as *Actinomadura madurae* and *Nocardia asteroides*. Eumycetomata are due to fungi

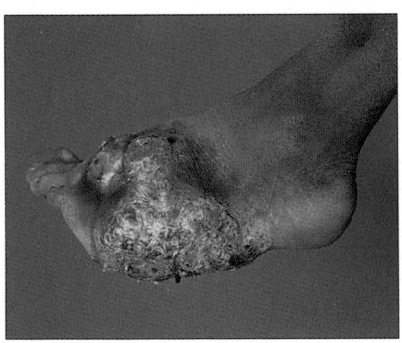

381 Mycetoma of the foot, due to *Fusarium* spp.

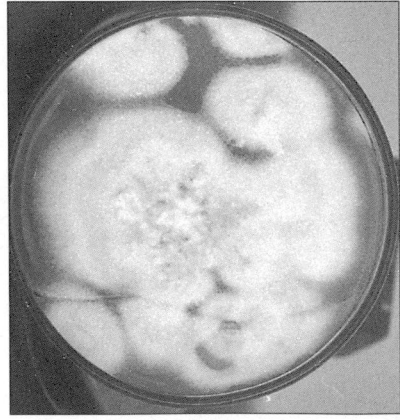

382 *Fusarium* spp. growing on Sabouraud's dextrose agar.

such as *Madurella mycetomatis, Acremonium, Aspergillus* and *Fusarium* (**382**) species. Diagnosis is by microscopic examination of sinus fluid or skin scrapings (in KOH). However, examination of a biopsy and culture (3–4 weeks) on Sabouraud's agar (without cycloheximide) provides definitive diagnosis. Treatment involves surgery and appropriate antifungal or antibacterial drugs.

CHROMOMYCOSIS

This disease occurs in Africa and Latin America and is characterized by the appearance of warty nodules. Pathogens include *Phialophora (Fonsecaea) pedrosi, P. verrucosa* and *Cladosporium carrionii*.

SPOROTRICHOSIS

This is the one subcutaneous mycosis that can occur in temperate countries, albeit rarely. The causative agent is *Sporothrix schenckii*, which is a dimorphic fungus. In human tissues it is present as the yeast form. It begins as a nodular lesion which may ulcerate. Secondary nodules arise along the lymphatic vessels draining the primary lesion (**383**).

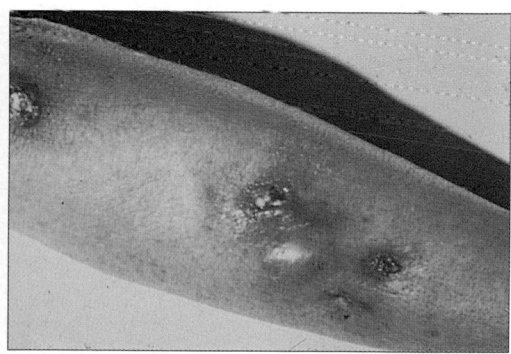

383 Sporotrichosis. A case of sporotrichosis showing secondary lesions along the distribution of the lymphatics.

SYSTEMIC MYCOSES

Most of these infections result from inhalation of fungal spores although *Candida albicans* can be acquired from the gastro-intestinal tract or via intravascular lines. Several, such as histoplasmosis and paracoccidiomycosis, are limited to certain geographical regions where climatic conditions are optimal for their growth. Some affect previously fit individuals but many are opportunistic pathogens.

ASPERGILLOSIS

Asperigillus fumigatus, A. flava and *A. niger* are the major pathogens. They are predominantly opportunistic pathogens. They can colonize pre-existing lung cavities to cause an aspergilloma (**384**) or may invade lung tissue and elsewhere

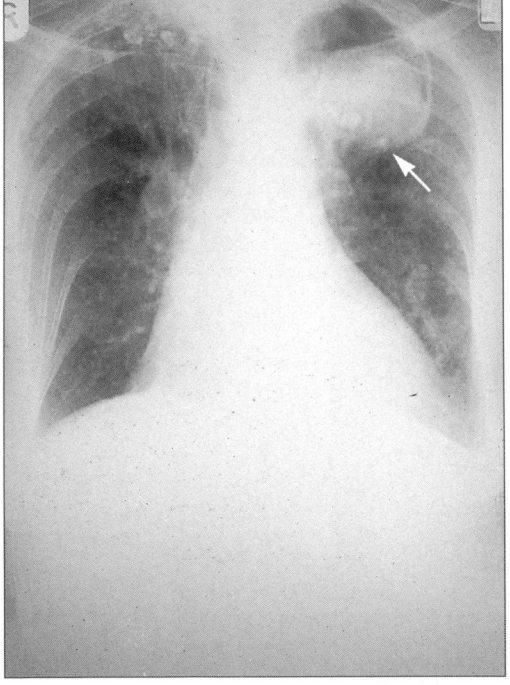

384 Chest X-ray showing aspergilloma. A chest radiograph showing a lung cavity containing an aspergilloma (arrow).

when the patient is immunocompromised. They are ubiquitous in the environment. Recently, increases in infection rates in, for example, bone marrow transplant units have been associated with building, excavations or refurbishment in the vicinity of the hospital. *A. fumigatus* produces smoky green colonies with a velvety texture (**385**) and conidia produce a columnar mass in the axis of the stalk of the conidiophore (**386**).

BLASTOMYCOSIS

This infection was thought to be restricted to North America but cases have been reported from Africa and Asia. *Blastomyces dermatitidis* is a dimorphic fungus, the source of which is unknown. Primary lesions occur in the lung but patients usually present with skin lesions.

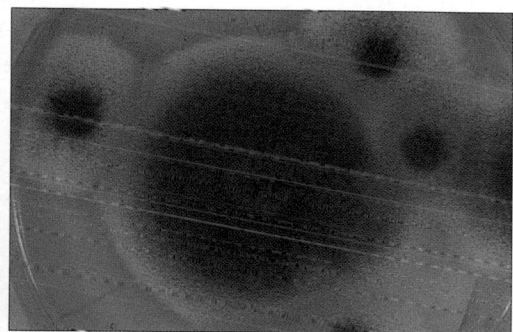

385 Aspergillus fumigatus culture.
Aspergillus fumigatus growing on Sabouruud's dextrose agar.

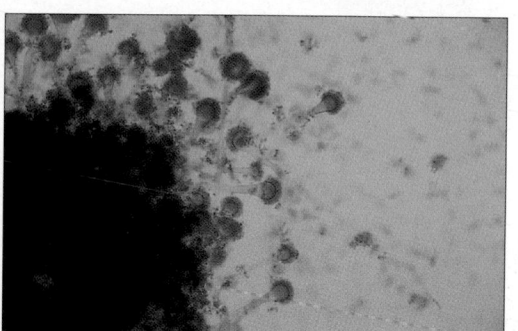

386 Aspergillus fumigatus culture.
Lactophenol cotton blue stained preparation of Aspergillus fumigatus cultured on Sabouraud's agar showing a conidiophore and microconidia.

CANDIDOSIS

The major pathogen is *Candida albicans* but *C. parapsilosis* and *C. tropicalis* may also cause disease. *C. albicans* can cause superficial as well as systemic infection, but the latter only occurs in the immunocompromised individual. *C. albicans* is part of the normal flora of the intestine. Superficial infection includes thrush (oral (**387**) and

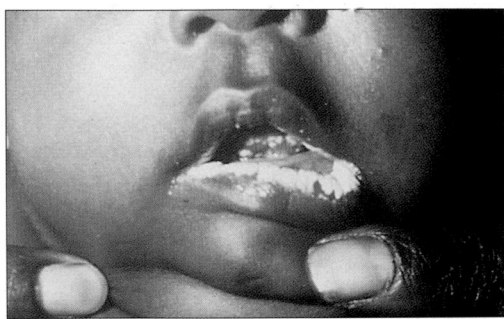

387 *Candida albicans* on oral mucosa. Oral thrush showing a white patch of *C. albicans* on the oral mucosa. Removal of the lesion reveals an inflamed area beneath it.

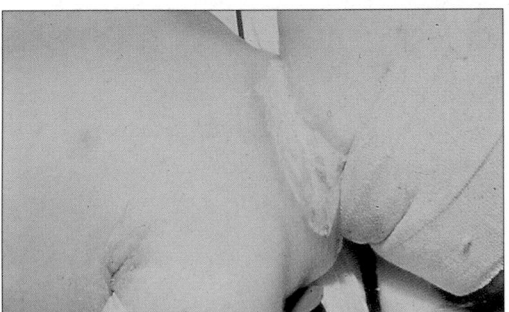

388 Intertrigo.

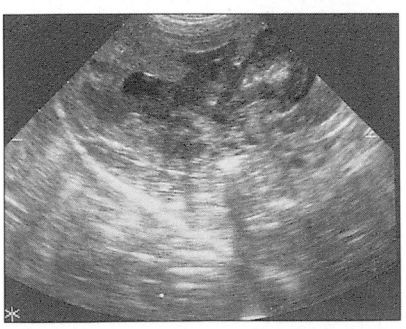

389 Fungus ball on kidney. An abdominal ultrasound of a neonate's kidney showing a fungus ball in the renal calyx. *Candida albicans* was obtained on urine culture.

vaginal), intertrigo (**388**) (moist skin) and nail involvement. Disseminated infection can occur in any part of the body. Premature neonates, in particular, are prone to develop urinary tract infection which ascends to produce a fungal mass in the kidney (**389**). In tissues when invading, it produces pseudohyphae (**390**). On Gram film large, Gram-positive pleomorphic blastospores are visible (**391**). *Candida* spp. grow well on Sabouraud's (**392**) or blood agar. To differentiate *C. albicans* from other species the

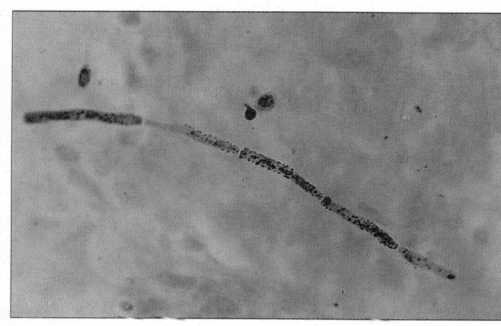

390 *Candida albicans* pus. A Gram stained preparation of pus from a skin abscess due to *C. albicans* showing pseudohyphae.

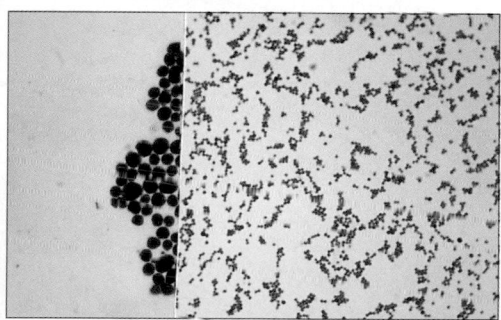

391 *Candida albicans* film compared with *Staphylococcus aureus*. A Gram stained film of *C. albicans* (left) compared with *S. aureus* (right). *C. albicans* blastospores are two or three times larger than *S. aureus* cocci.

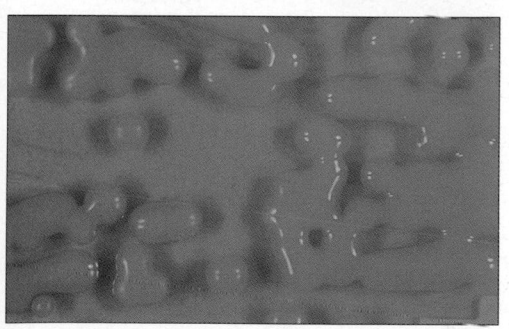

392 *Candida albicans* culture. *C. albicans* growing on Sabouraud's dextrose agar.

yeast is incubated at 37°C in serum. *C. albicans* produces a germ-tube (**393**). Nystatin is used for topical therapy and amphotericin B (liposomal or in combination with 5-flucytosine) or fluconazole is used for systemic infection.

COCCIDIOMYCOSIS

The fungus (*Coccidiodes immitis*) is endemic in dry desert regions of south-western USA, Mexico and Central America and is present in soil. Infection is primarily in the lungs but dissemination can occur. Primary infection limited to the lungs often resolves spontaneously. Treatment is with amphotericin B or an imidazole.

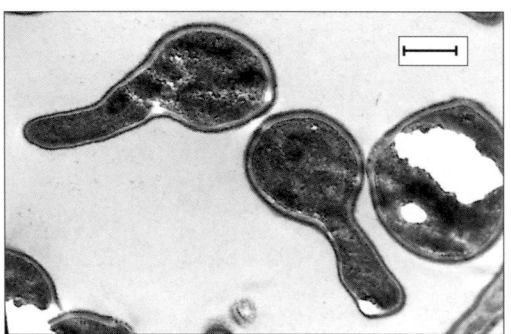

393 *Candida albicans* electron micrograph. A thin-section electron micrograph of *C. albicans* showing a germ tube. *(bar = 5 μm)*

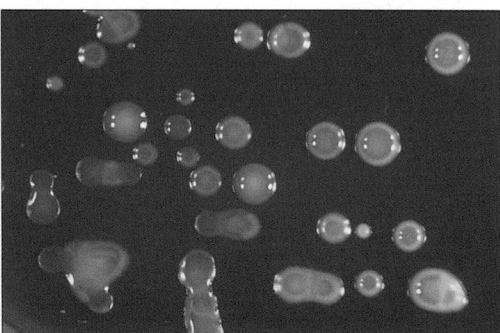

394 *Cryptococcus neoformans* culture. Mucoid *C. neoformans* growing on blood agar. The glistening surface of the colony is due to the profuse polysaccharide capsule produced by the yeast form.

CRYPTOCOCCOSIS

Cryptococcus neoformans is a dimorphic yeast, which is usually associated with opportunistic infection but which may also be a primary pathogen. At ambient temperatures it produces hyphae but at body temperature it is a yeast. It gains access through the lungs but is rapidly disseminated to the central nervous system to cause cryptococcal meningitis. It grows well on Sabouraud's or blood agar (**394**) where it produces mucoid colonies. The mucoid character is imparted by a thick polysaccharide capsule (**395**) which can be seen using India ink stain either directly on cerebrospinal fluid (**396**) or from colonies. A latex particle agglutination test is also available for rapid diagnosis. Treatment is as for disseminated candidosis.

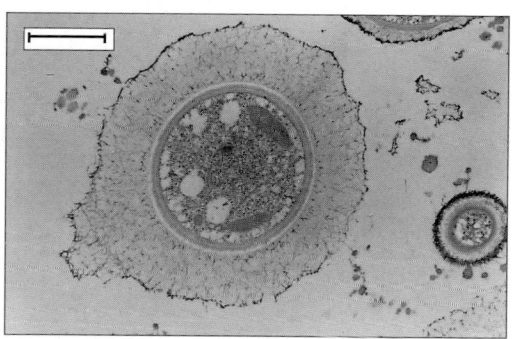

395 *Cryptococcus neoformans* electron micrograph. Thin-section electron micrograph of *C. neoformans* stained by ruthenium red to demonstrate the capsule. *(bar = 5 μm)*

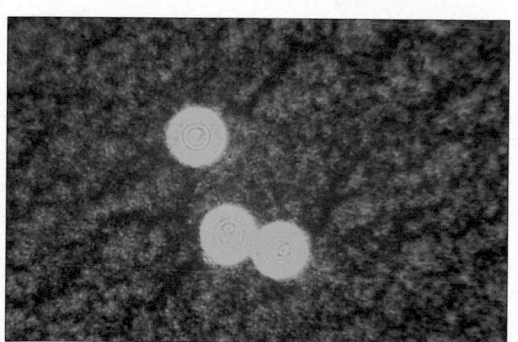

396 Cerebrospinal fluid in cryptococcal meningitis. India ink stain of CSF from a patient with cryptococcal meningitis.

HISTOPLASMOSIS

Histoplasma capsulatum causes an acute or chronic pulmonary infection which rarely disseminates. It is found in soil containing bird droppings and is a particular cause of infection in Mississippi and surrounding US states.

PARACOCCIDIOMYCOSIS

Paracoccidiodes brasiliensis causes oral and pulmonary infection (granulomas). It is restricted to South and Central America.

ZYGOMYCOSIS (SYNONYMS PHYCOMYCOSIS, MUCORMYCOSIS)

This is a rapidly evolving infection in immunocompromised patients. Pulmonary infection is the hallmark of immunocompromise due to cytotoxic drug therapy, gastric disease of malnutrition and rhinocerebral infection of diabetes mellitus. Pathogens include *Mucor pusillus* (**397**), *Absidia corymbifera* and *Fusarium* spp. For mucormycosis, amphotericin B is the only antifungal agent to show efficacy *in vitro*.

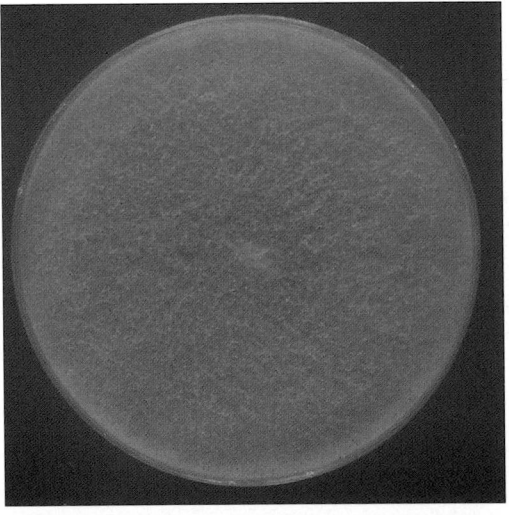

397   *Mucor pusillus* culture. *M. pusillus* growing on Sabouraud's dextrose agar.

PNEUMOCYSTIS CARINII

There is some controversy over the kingdom to which this respiratory tract pathogen belongs. Originally, on the basis of morphology and antimicrobial susceptibility, it was classified as a protozoan. However, recent analysis of gene sequences encoding its 16S ribosomal RNA, places it much closer to fungi such as *Candida* and *Saccharomyces* spp. Furthermore, its dihydrofolate reluctase (which is inhibited by trimethoprim) and thymidylate synthetase genes are not linked, whereas in protozoa they are encoded on a single gene. Unfortunately *P. carinii* has not been grown in artificial culture. In immunocompetent individuals infection is asymptomatic. In the immunocompromised (by AIDS, cytotoxic drugs or even malnutrition) it causes pneumonia. Most evidence suggests that a large number of individuals are exposed at an early age and that the cysts remain in the lungs until immunity is impaired, when it reactivates. Diagnosis is by examination of broncho-alveolar lavage by methenamine silver or immuno-fluorescence (**398**). Lung biopsy may also be of value when trophozoites and cysts can be demonstrated by electron microscopy (**399**) or by silver impregnation stains (**400**). Recently PCR detection of *P. carinii* genome has been used to demonstrate the organism in nasopharyngeal aspirates. Treatment is with high dose co-trimoxazole, dapsone or pentamidine. Co-trimoxazole is used also for prophylaxis in the immunocompromised individual.

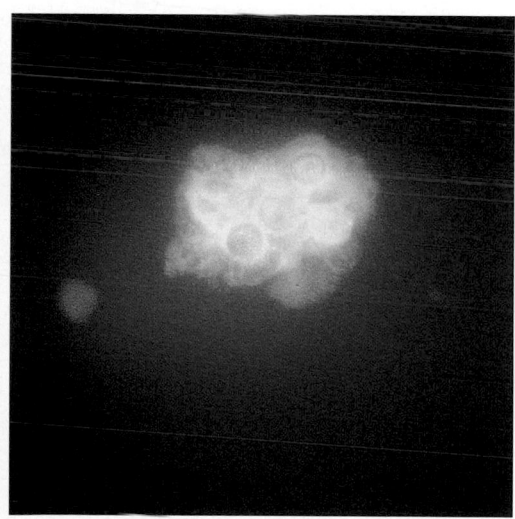

398 *Pneumocystis carinii* **by immunofluorescence.** *P. carinii* demonstrated in a broncho-alveolar lavage by immunofluorescence.

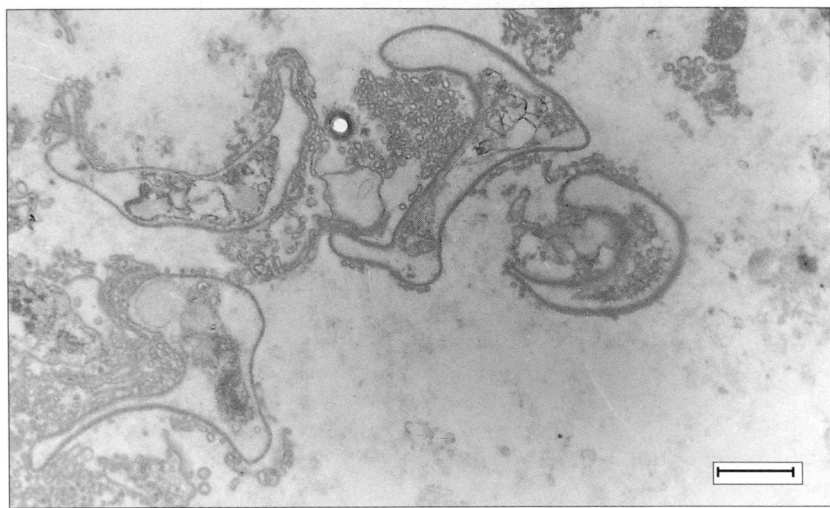

399   *Pneumocystis carinii* electron micrograph of lungs. Thin-section electron micrograph of lung showing cysts of *P. carinii. (bar = 5 μm)*

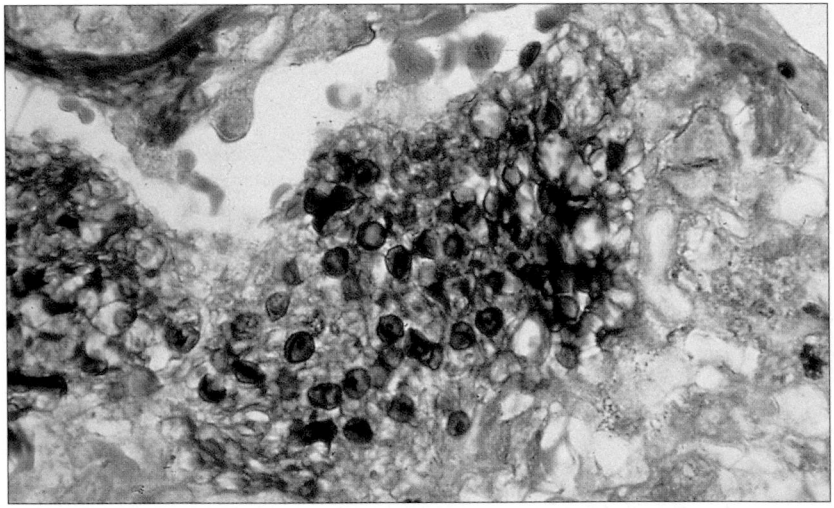

400   *Pneumocystis carinii* cysts. Silver impregnation stain of lung showing cysts of *P. carinii.*

6.
Medically Important Parasites

This section covers the protozoa (unicellular parasites) and helminths (multi-cellular parasites) that are encountered in medical microbiology.

PROTOZOA

Many different protozoa can be found in the animate and inanimate environment; some are even commensals of man (e.g. *Entamoeba coli, Endolimax nana*). Only a small number of protozoa are pathogenic for man (**401**). Classification of protozoa is by appearance and biological properties but a more useful classification is to divide them into mucosal pathogens and tissue and bloodstream pathogens (**402**).

MUCOSAL PATHOGENS

Microsporidia
Microsporidia, and specifically *Enterocytozoon bieneusii*, can cause diarrhoea in immunocompromised patients, particularly those with AIDS. In such patients, conjunctivitis may also result. The definitive diagnosis is by demonstration of the organisms in biopsy samples of upper or lower intestine (**403**). They may also be demonstrated by trichrome stain of faeces. Treatment is with co-trimoxazole or albendazole but relapse is frequent.

Entamoeba histolytica
This amoeba exists as a series of different strains or zymodemes (based on isoenzyme profiles), only some of which cause disease. It causes amoebic dysentery and can invade beyond the large intestine to cause liver abscesses. It is spread faeco-orally by ingestion of food or water contaminated by cysts (**404**). Specific diagnosis can be by examination of fresh stools, looking for trophozoites containing ingested erythrocytes (**405**). Trophozoites may also be seen in samples scraped from colonic ulcers and on histological examination of biopsy samples (**406**). Treatment is with metronidazole.

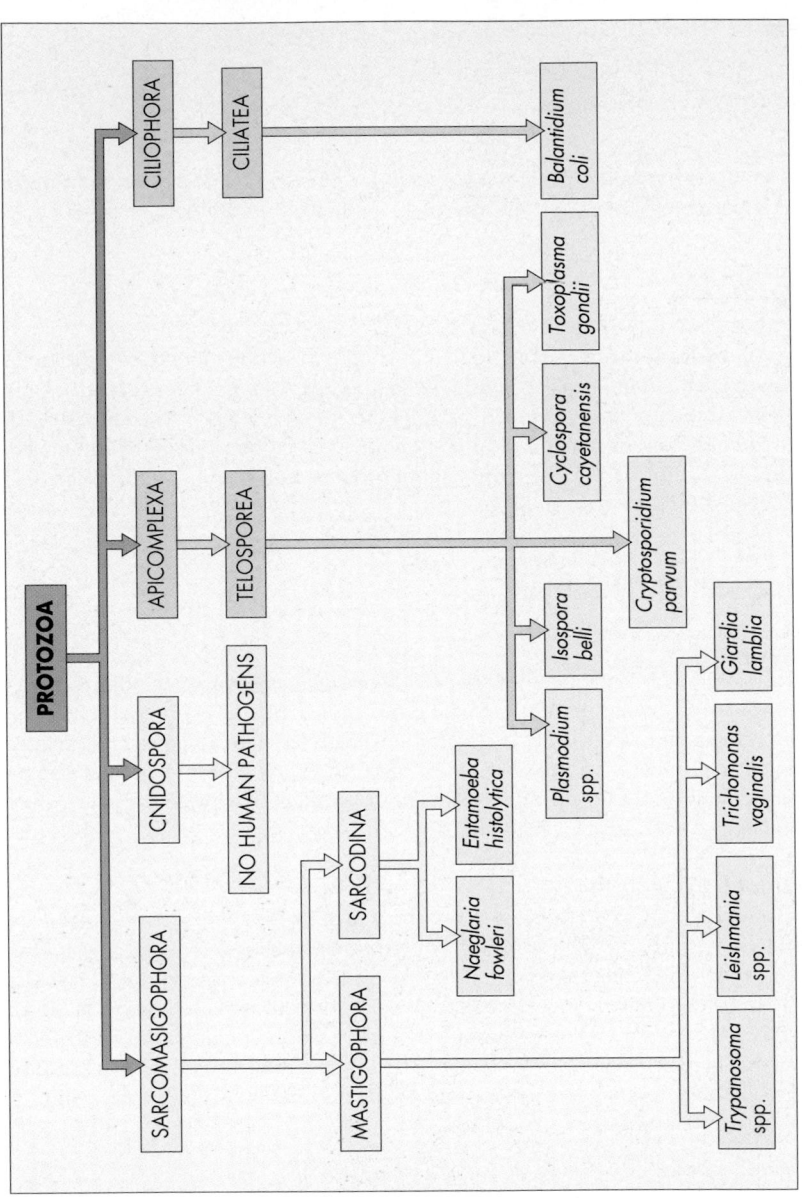

401 Medically important protozoa.

Pathogenic protozoa

MUCOSAL PATHOGENS	BLOOD AND TISSUE PATHOGENS
Enterocytozoon bieneusi – diarrhoeal disease	*Entamoeba histolytica* – liver abscess
Entamoeba histolytica – dysentery	*Naegleria fowleri* – meningitis
Giardia lamblia (intestinalis) – diarrhoeal disease	*Trypanosoma brucei* – sleeping sickness
Trichomonas vaginalis – vaginitis	*Trypanosoma cruzi* – Chaga's disease
Isospora belli – diarrhoeal disease	*Leishmania donovani* – kala-azar
Cryptosporidium parvum – diarrhoeal disease	*Leishmania tropica* – oriental sore
Cyclospora cayetanensis – diarrhoeal disease	
Balantidium coli – dysentery	
	Plasmodium falciparum – malignant tertian malaria
	Plasmodium ovale – ovale tertian malaria
	Plasmodium malariae – quartan malaria
	Plasmodium vivax – benign tertian malaria
	Toxoplasma gondii – encephalomyelitis, retinitis

402 Pathogenic protozoa.

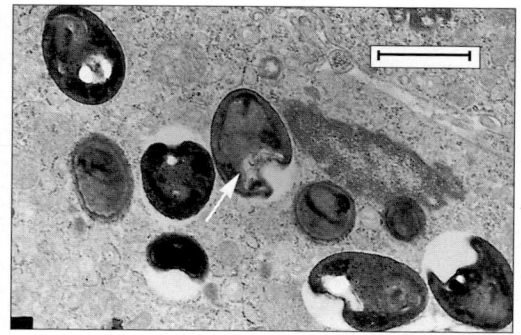

403 *Enterocytozoon bieneusii* electron micrograph. Thin-section electron micrograph of duodenal enterocytes infected with *Enterocytozoon bieneusii* (microsporidiosis). The spirally coiled polar filament (arrow) used for impaling the cell to be infected has been cut in section. *(bar = 100 nm)*

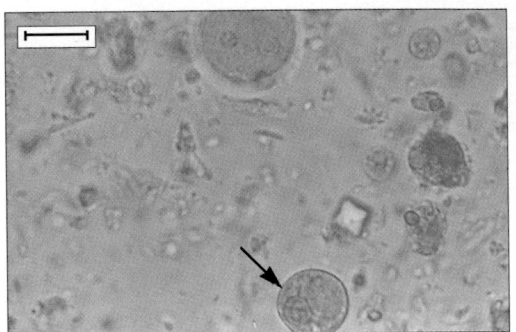

404 Entamoeba histolytica cysts and Entamoeba coli. Iodine-stained wet preparation of stool showing cysts of *E. histolytica* (arrow) and the non-pathogenic *E. coli*. (bar = 10 μm)

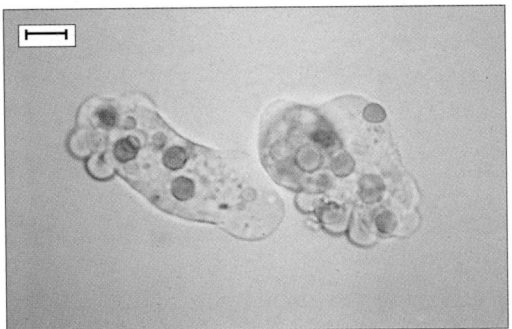

405 Entamoeba histolytica trophozoites. Trophozoites of *E. histolytica* which have engulfed erythrocytes. This is pathognomonic of *E. histolytica*. (bar = 10 μm)

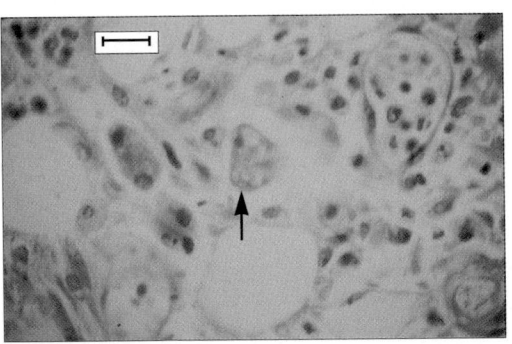

406 Entamoeba histolytica found at biopsy. Section of a rectal biopsy stained by haematoxylin and eosin. The section shows an amoebic ulcer with an infiltrate of inflammatory cells and *E. histolytica* (arrow). (bar = 30 μm)

Giardia intestinalis (lamblia)

This is a ubiquitous protozoan parasite with flagella and a characteristic pear-shaped outline (**407**). It is spread faeco-orally and can survive in water for long periods. It is excreted as cysts which are the infective form (**408**). *Giardia* infects the proximal small intestine, causing diarrhoeal disease. Not all infected patients are symptomatic but infection may also be chronic. Diagnosis is by examination of stools (at least three samples) for cysts or examination of duodenal juice (collected by gastroscopy or string) for trophozoites. Treatment is with metronidazole.

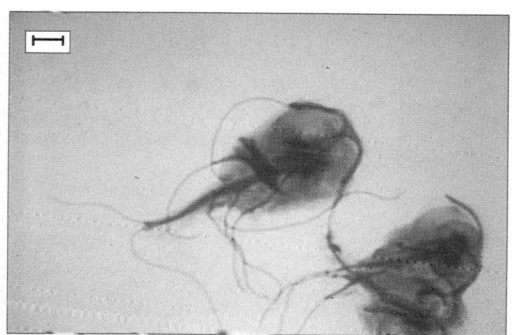

407 Giardia intestinalis (lamblia) trophozoites. Trophozoites of *G. intestinalis (lamblia)*. The flagella are clearly visible. *(bar = 5 μm)*

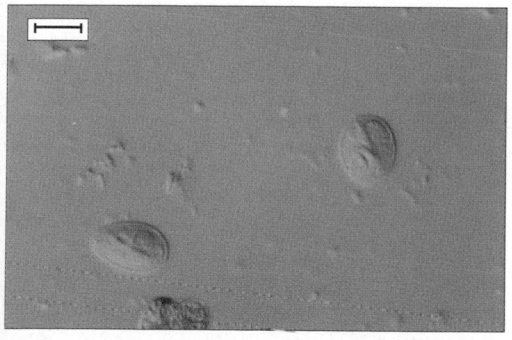

408 Giardia intestinalis (lamblia) cysts. Cysts of *G. intestinalis (lamblia)* in faeces, viewed by Normarski phase-contrast microscopy. *(bar = 5 μm)*

Trichomonas vaginalis

This flagellate protozoan parasite can reach a length of 30 µm but is most often in the range 5–15 µm (**409**). As its name implies, it causes vaginitis with vaginal discharge as the commonest presenting feature. The discharge is profuse and can result in perineal inflammation. On colposcopy the vaginal mucosa is seen to be inflamed, with punctate lesions. There may also be dysuria and frequency. Infection in males is normally asymptomatic but may rarely cause prostatitis or epididymitis. Diagnosis is by examination of vaginal discharge by phase-contrast microscopy. Treatment is with metronidazole.

Isospora belli

This is usually an asymptomatic infection but may cause severe diarrhoeal disease in the immunocompromised patient, in particular those with AIDS. It is spread faeco-orally and the infective form is the oocyst (about 30 µm × 12 µm) which contains two sporocysts (**410**). The oocyst is immature when excreted and

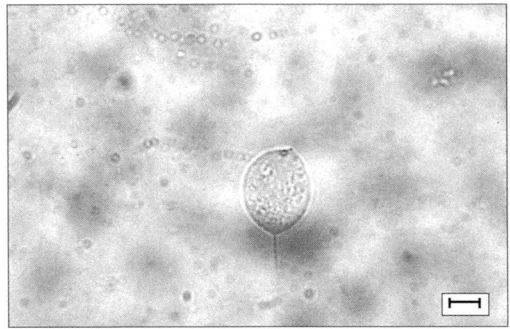

409 Trichomonas vaginalis. Wet preparation of *T. vaginalis* by phase-contrast microscopy. The flagellum which imparts motility is visible. *(bar = 5 µm)*

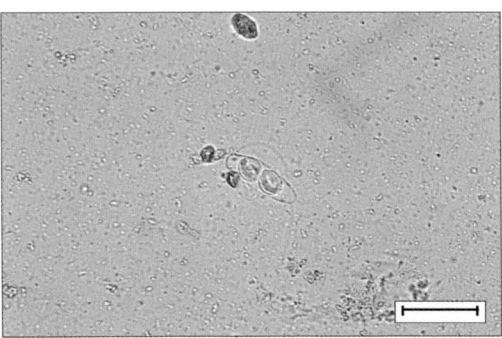

410 Isospora belli oocyst and sporocysts. Iodine-stained wet preparation of faeces showing an oocyst of *I. belli*. The two sporocysts are visible inside the oocysts. *(bar = 20 µm)*

matures in the stool to become infective. Diagnosis is by modified Ziehl–Neelsen or safranin-methylene blue stains of faecal smears (**411**). Co-trimoxazole is the treatment of choice.

Cryptosporidium parvum

This small coccidian parasite is a major cause of diarrhoeal disease in children (2–19% of cases) and a life-threatening pathogen in the immunocompromised host. It is spread faeco-orally and the first reported cases were zoonotic. However, person-to-person spread is at least as important. The oocyst is the infective form (**412**), which is fully infective when excreted and is excreted in large quantities. The oocyst is small (4–5 µm) and its thick wall renders it resistant to many disinfectants. As a result, large water-borne epidemics of diarrhoeal disease (up to 250,000 patients) have occurred in USA and UK. The oocyst contains four sporozoites which attach to and penetrate the enterocytes. They develop to form trophozoites (**413**) which are described as being intra-enterocytic but extracytoplasmic, since they are kept

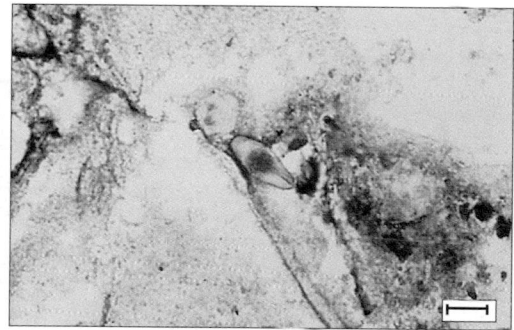

411 Isospora belli oocyst and sporocyst. An oocyst of *I. belli* stained by safranin-methylene blue. The immature sporocyst has retained the safranin (pink) and the cyst wall, the methylene blue. *(bar = 10 µm)*

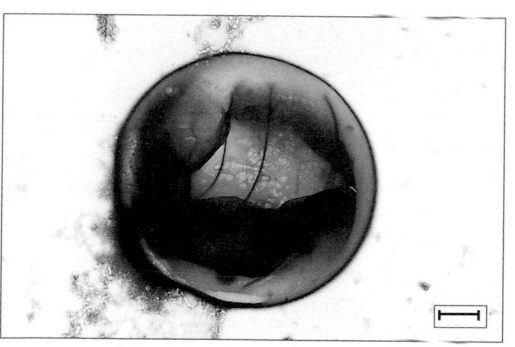

412 Cryptosporidium parvum oocyst electron micrograph. Negative-stain electron micrograph of an oocyst of *C. parvum*. *(bar = 1 µm)*

from the main part of the enterocyte by a so-called feeder organelle. How they produce diarrhoea is unclear. Diagnosis is by examination of faecal smears by modified Ziehl–Neelsen, safranin-methylene blue (**414**) or auramine-phenol (**415**) stains. IFAT and ELISA tests are also available for detection of antigen or of serological response. There is no safe and effective therapeutic agent.

Cyclospora cayetanensis

This recently described protozoan is a cause of prolonged diarrhoeal disease. It is spread faeco-orally and water-borne outbreaks have occurred in developing countries. The infective form is the thick-walled oocyst which is up to 8 μm in diameter (**416**). Diagnosis is by microscopic examination of suitably strained faecal smears (**417**). Treatment is with co-trimoxazole.

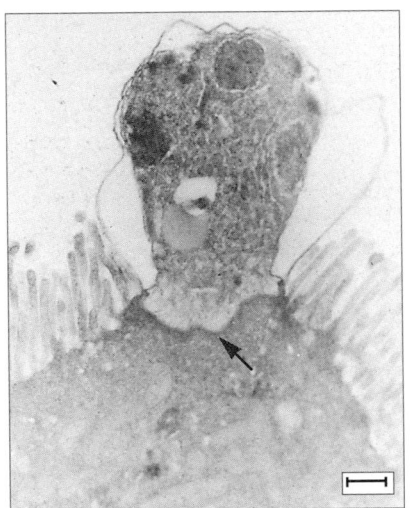

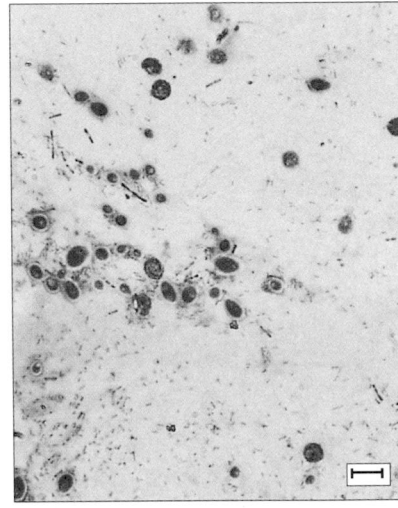

413 *Cryptosporidium parvum* **trophozoite found at biopsy.** Thin-section electron micrograph of a duodenal biopsy from a patient with crypto-sporidiosis. A trophozoite of *C. parvum* is within the enterocyte but separated from the rest of the cytoplasm by the so-called feeder organelle (arrow). *(bar = 5 μm)*

414 *Cryptosporidium parvum* **oocysts.** A smear of faeces stained by safranin-methylene blue. The *C. parvum* oocysts stain pink whereas all other components of faeces stain blue. *(bar = 10 μm)*

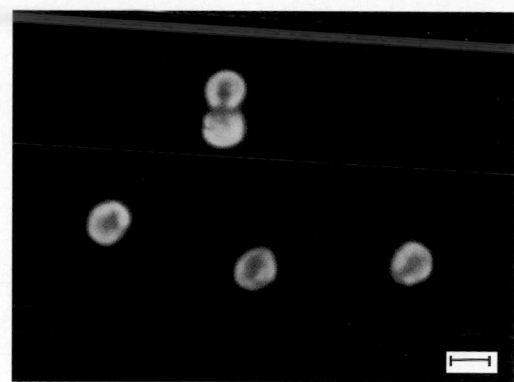

415 Fluorescent microscopy of *Cryptosporidium parvum*. A faecal smear stained by auramine phenol and viewed by fluorescence microscopy. The *C. parvum* oocysts retain auramine-phenol, which causes them to fluoresce. *(bar = 5 μm)*

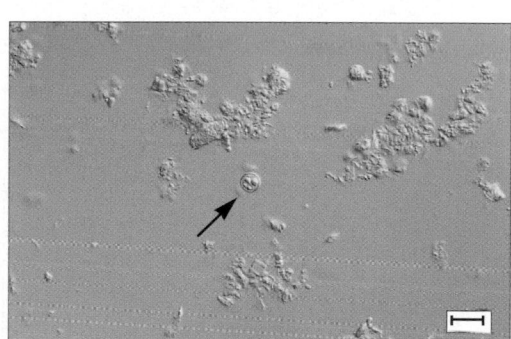

416 *Cyclospora cayetanensis* cysts. A wet preparation of faeces containing cysts of *C. cayetanensis* (arrow) viewed by Normarski phase-contrast microscopy. *(bar = 5 μm)*

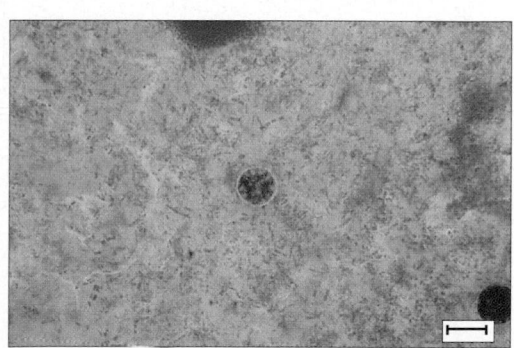

417 *Cyclospora cayetanensis*. Faeces containing *C. cayetanensis* stained by safranin-methylene blue. *(bar = 5 μm)*

Balantidium coli

This is the only ciliate to infect man (**418**). It is a rare cause of diarrhoeal disease. Treatment is with oxytetracycline.

BLOOD AND TISSUE PATHOGENS

Naegleria fowleri

This is an amboeboflagellate which in tissue is in the amoeboid form. It is a rare cause of meningitis and occurs when soil contaminates swimming pools. Cases have been described in individuals swimming in the Roman baths in Bath (warm water is insufflated through the nose). Diagnosis is by microscopic examination of CSF. (The pathogen produces a purulent meningitis.) Treatment is with amphotericin B which might be potentiated by tetracyclines.

Trypanosoma spp.

Two distinct forms of disease due to trypanosomes occur in man. African sleeping sickness is due to *Trypanosoma brucei (gambiense* or *rhodesiense)*. It is transmitted by the bite of the tsetse fly (most frequently *Glossina palpalis* for *T. b. gambiense* and *G. morsitans* for *T. b. rhodesiense*). The East African variety (*T. b. rhodesiense*) is more virulent but both can lead to meningoencephalitis. The reservoir for *T. b. rhodesiense* is game or domestic cattle. No animal reservoir for *T. b. gambiense* has been identified. Diagnosis is by identification of trypomastigotes in blood films (**419**). Treatment is with suramin, melarsoprol or pentamidine.

   T. cruzi is spread via the faeces of reduviid bug (*Panstrongylus megistus*). The trypanosome develops in the hindgut of the reduviid bug which defecates on man when it bites. The *T. cruzi* is then introduced into the tissue, producing a chagoma

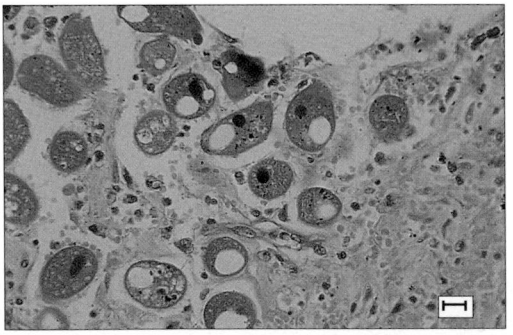

418 Balantidium coli found at biopsy. A rectal biopsy showing infection with *B. coli.* (bar = 10 μm)

(Romaña's sign: **420**). It spreads, via the bloodstream, to the liver and spleen where it may be eliminated. If not, it develops intracellularly (as an amastigote) in cardiac muscle and other tissues. Distribution is in the Americas (south of the Tropic of Cancer) but infection is commonest in Brazil. Animal reservoirs are cats, dogs and armadillos. Diagnosis is by demonstration of the amastigote in tissues and an IgM response can be measured. Treatment is with the nitrofurfurylidine derivative Nifurtimox.

Leishmania spp.

Oriental sore (**421**) is due to *L. tropica* and is transmitted by phlebotomine flies (sandflies). It occurs in the southern and eastern Mediterranean regions, southern former-USSR states (Armenia, Azerbaijan), Afghanistan and India. Man is the reservoir. Diagnosis is primarily clinical but can also be by demonstration of amastigotes in monocytic inflammatory cells in the lesion or by culture. Treatment is with pentestam.

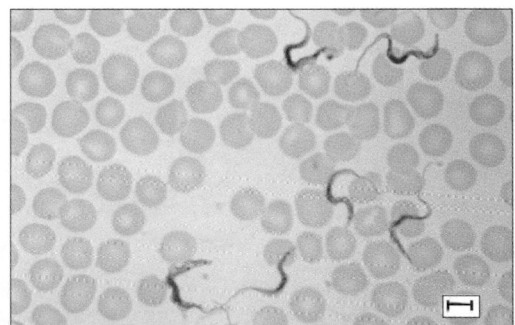

419 *Trypanosoma brucei* found in blood film. A blood film from a patient with sleeping sickness. The trypomastigotes of *T. brucei* are clearly visible. (bar = 5 μm)

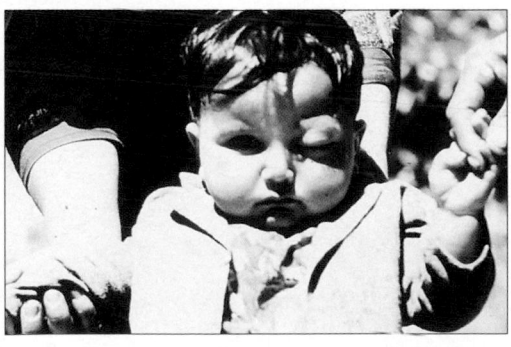

420 A child infected with *Trypanosoma cruzi* showing Romaña's sign.

Muco-cutaneous leishmaniasis is due to *L. brasiliensis* and is endemic in South America where it is called espundia. Forest rodents and dogs are the reservoirs and infection is spread by sandflies.

Visceral leishmaniasis is due to *L. donovani* and is also known as kala-azar. It occurs in many parts of Africa and Asia and in southern Europe. Transmission is by phlebotomine flies and the reservoir appears to be dogs. It produces fever, malaise, anaemia and hepatosplenomegaly. Diagnosis is by demonstration of the organism in macrophages (**422**) obtained by splenic, bone marrow or hepatic puncture. Treatment is with pentestam.

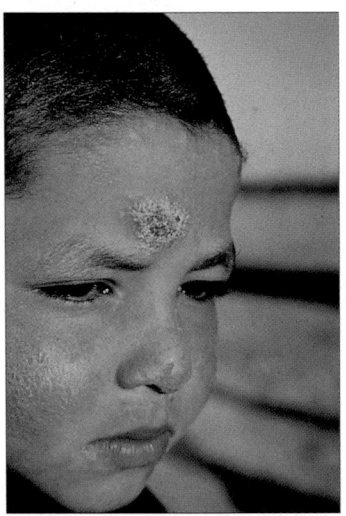

421 A child with oriental sore due to *Leishmania tropica*.

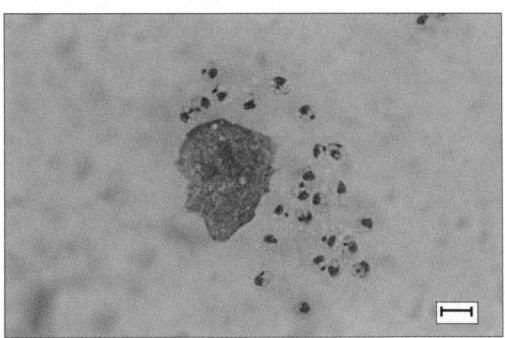

422 Macrophage containing amastigotes. A bone marrow aspirate stained by Giemsa from a child with kala-azar. A macrophage containing numerous amastigotes is visible. *(bar = 10 μm)*

Plasmodium spp.

These protozoa have a complex life cycle in the mosquito and in man. They grow in the anopheline mosquito's intestine. Sporozoites are transferred from the female mosquito to man when she next feeds. In man there are erythrocytic and extra-erythrocytic phases. *Plasmodium falciparum* causes malignant falciparum malaria after an incubation period of 8–11 days.

Fever occurs every 36–48 h and an untreated primary attack lasts 2–3 weeks. Infection can persist for 6–11 months. The major problems are cerebral malaria (**423**) and anaemia.

P. vivax causes vivax or benign tertian malaria after an incubation period of 10-17 days. Fever occurs every 48 h and an untreated primary attack lasts 3–8 weeks or more. Infection can last for 5–7 years. Anaemia is the major complication. Mortality is low.

P. malariae causes quartan malaria after an incubation period of 18–40 days. Fever occurs every 72 h and an untreated primary attack lasts 3–24 weeks. Infection persists for over 20 years with recrudescences. Proteinuria and even frank nephrotic syndrome can be a complication.

P. ovale causes ovale malaria after an incubation period of 10–17 days. Fever occurs every 48 h and a primary untreated attack lasts 2–3 weeks. Infection persists for up to 12 months. It is usually a mild disease.

Diagnosis is by examination of thick and thin blood films stained by Leishman's or Field's stains (**424–427**).

Treatment and prophylaxis depend upon the location of the patient, since resistance to chloroquine is increasing in prevalence. Therapeutic options include quinine, artemether, Fansidar or halofantrine. Prophylactic drugs include chloroquine, proguanil or mefloquine.

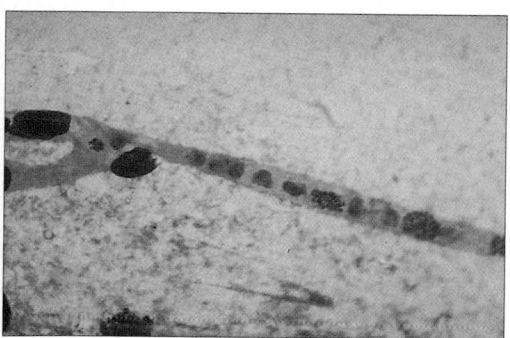

423 Cerebral vessel in cerebral malaria. A cerebral vessel from a child who had died from cerebral malaria. Erythrocytes are adherent to the capillary endothelium.

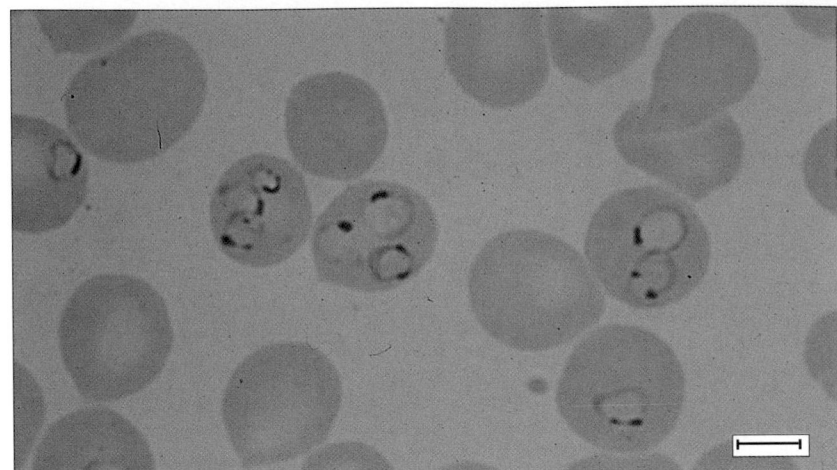

424   *Plasmodium falciparum* trophozoites. A thin blood film from a patient with falciparum malaria. Ring forms of trophozoites of *P. falciparum* are present. *(bar = 5 μm)* *(Copyright Liverpool School of Tropical Medicine)*

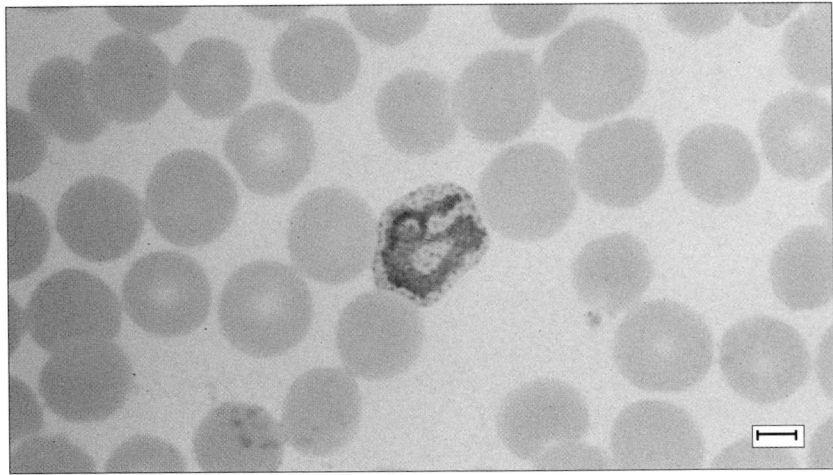

425   *Plasmodium vivax* ring-form trophozoites. A thin blood film from a patient with benign tertian malaria. Both the large amoeboid (centre) and ring-form trophozoites of *Plasmodium vivax* are visible. *(bar = 5 μm)* *(Copyright Liverpool School of Tropical Medicine)*

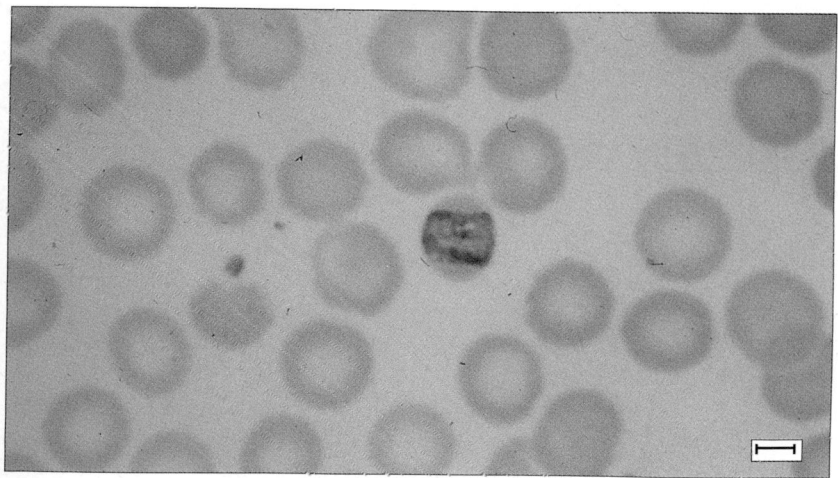

426   Intra-erythrocytic *Plasmodium malariae*. A thin blood film from a patient with quartan malaria. An intra-erythrocytic band form of *P. malariae* is visible. *(bar = 5 μm) (Copyright Liverpool School of Tropical Medicine)*

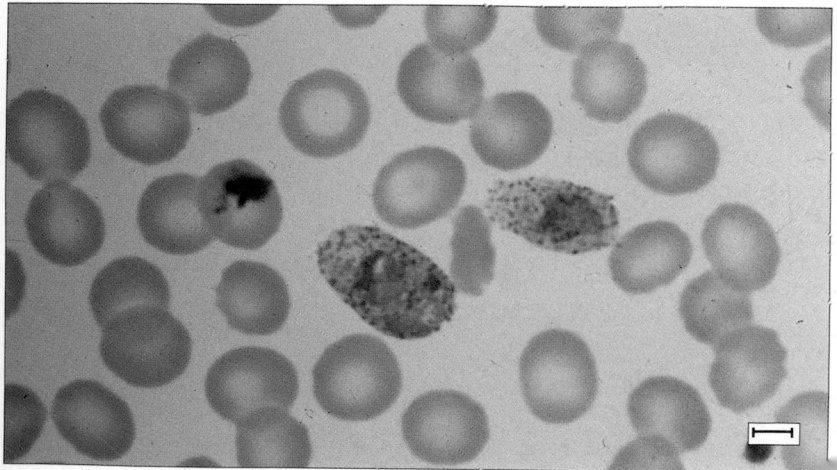

427   Erythrocytes infected with *Plasmodium ovale*. A thin blood film from a patient with ovale malaria. The infected erythrocytes are oval in shape and contain Schüffner's dots and trophozoites of *P. ovale*. *(bar = 5 μm) (Copyright Liverpool School of Tropical Medicine)*

Toxoplasma gondii

This coccidian parasite is found world-wide and its definitive host is the cat. The cat persistently excretes large numbers of oocysts in faeces which, following maturation, can infect other species including man. There are two forms of trophozoites, tachyzoites (**428**) which are rapidly growing and bradyzoites which grow very slowly and form cysts. Man may also become infected by eating under-cooked meat containing bradyzoites.

Infection is asymptomatic in over 50% of cases. When clinically apparent it causes a glandular fever-like illness and, more rarely, encephalomyelitis. In immunocompromised patients it is more likely to produce encephalomyelitis. *T.*

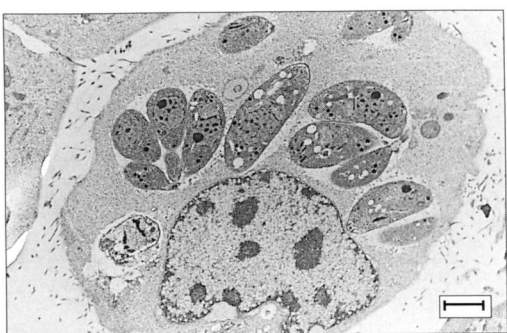

428 *Toxoplasma gondii* tachyzoites. A thin-section electron micrograph of *T. gondii* tachyzoites. *(bar = 5 μm)*

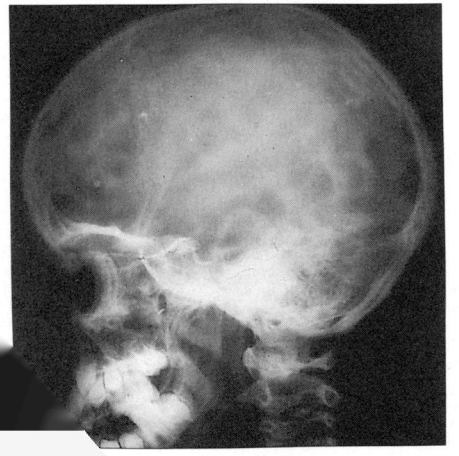

429 Congenital toxoplasmosis. An X-ray of the skull of a child with congenital toxoplasmosis showing intracerebral calcification.

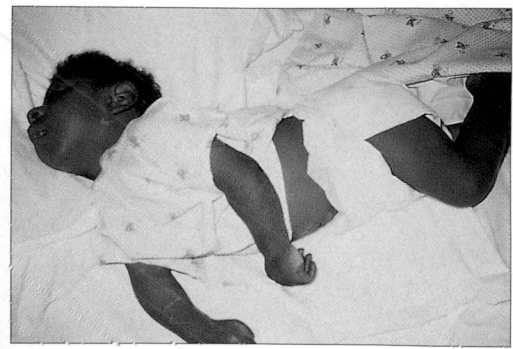

430 Congenital toxoplasmosis. A child with microcephaly and opisthotonos due to congenital toxoplasmosis.

gondii can also cross the placenta to infect the fetus. The major problem in the child is of chorioretinitis and subsequent blindness. This may develop in up to 60% of those infected in utero but only in a minority of infections present at birth. Cerebral damage with intracerebral calcification (**429**) and microcephaly (**430**) can also occur.

Diagnosis is usually serological (IgM or rising titres) but genome amplification by PCR is also available. Treatment is with pyrimethamine-sulfadoxine.

HELMINTHS

The multicellular parasites comprise the Platyhelminthes (flat worms) which contain two classes parasitic on man (Trematodesand Cestodes) and the Aschelminthes in which the class Nematoda contains human pathogens (**431**).

TREMATODES

Trematodes, or flukes, have a complex life cycle involving a mollusc (usually a snail) as an intermediate host. The adult develops in man, who excretes ova in which a larva develops. The larva or miracidium infects the mollusc. In the mollusc, the trematode goes through a series of generations finally liberating more larvae this time called cercariae. These then infect man by penetrating through the skin (e.g. *Schistosoma* spp.), by being eaten in a second intermediate host such as fish (e.g. *Clonorchis sinensis*) or by attaching to vegetable matter, such as watercress, that is then eaten (e.g. *Fasciola hepatica*).

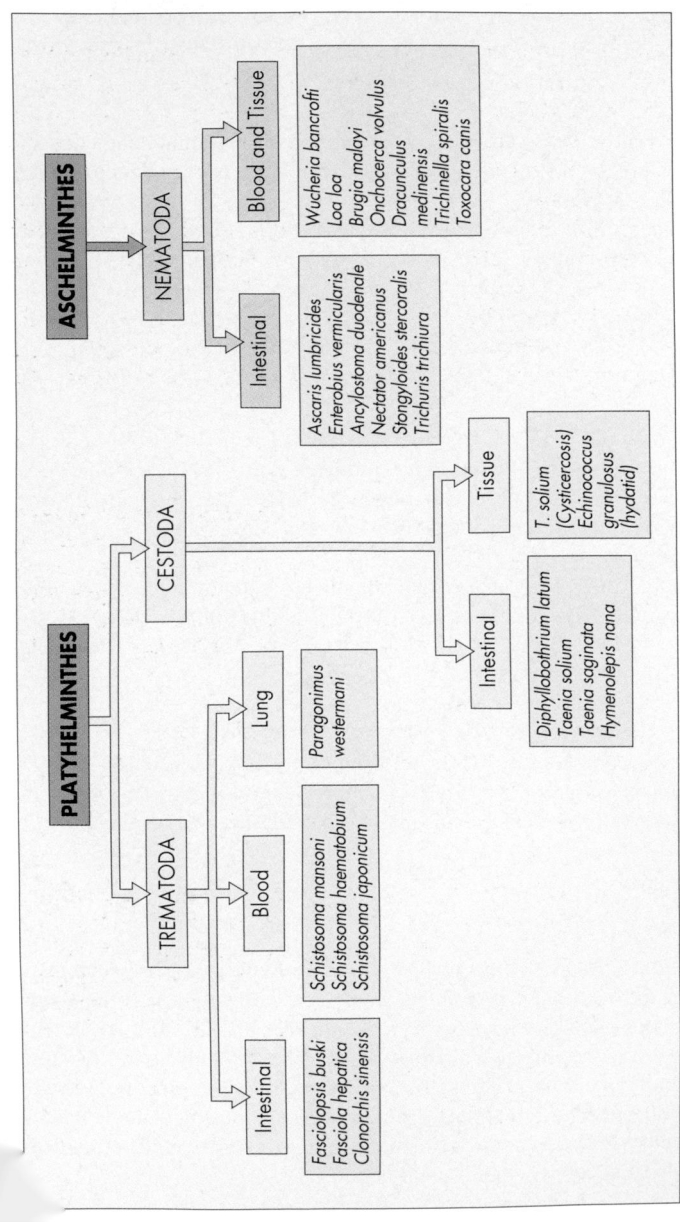

431   Multi-cellular parasites of man.

Intestinal flukes

Fasciolopsis buski is the giant intestinal fluke (2–7.5 cm long) found in the Far East. Infection is acquired by eating contaminated water vegetables (e.g. bamboo shoots, water chestnut). Heavy infestation (>500 worms) results in disease characterized by yellow greasy stool (malabsorption) with vitamin deficiency and hypoalbuminaemia. Diagnosis is by demonstration of ova in faeces (**432**). Treatment is with praziquantel.

Fasciola hepatica (**433**) is the sheep liver fluke and is found in Europe, Latin America and many other areas. Infection is passed to man by ingestion of watercress to which herbivores, especially sheep, have access. The metacercariae enter the liver not via the biliary tree but by burrowing through the duodenal wall. Because of this, infection is frequently symptomatic with fever, chills and signs of cholangitis. Diagnosis is by detection of ova in stools. Treatment is with praziquantel.

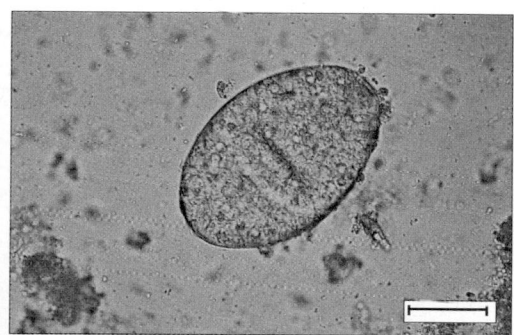

432 Fasciolopsis buski ovum. An iodine-stained wet preparation of faeces showing an ovum of *F. buski*. *(bar = 40 μm) (Copyright Liverpool School of Tropical Medicine)*

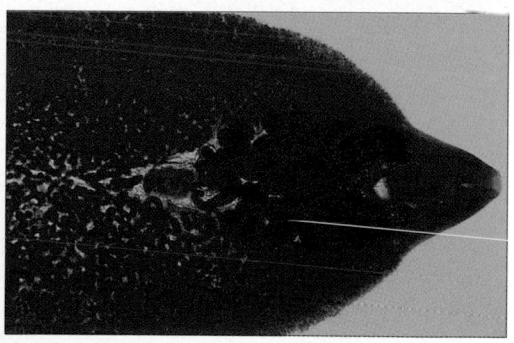

433 Fasciola hepatica anterior portion. The anterior portion of the liver fluke, *F. hepatica*. *(Copyright Liverpool School of Tropical Medicine)*

Blood flukes

Schistosoma mansoni is present in Africa, Arabia and Madagascar and is thought to have been transported to the West Indies and South America by the slave trade. *Schistosoma japonicum* is found in the Far East and *S. haematobium* has spread from the Nile Valley throughout Africa and to Cyprus, Portugal and the Middle East. Schistosomes, unlike other trematodes, are not hermaphrodites. Miracidia hatch from eggs, are excreted in stool (*S. mansoni, S. japonicum*) or urine (*S. haematobium*) and infect freshwater snails where they reproduce to release cercariae. The cercariae penetrate intact skin and enter the circulation. *S. mansoni* lives in the branches of the inferior mesenteric vein (draining lower colon), *S. japonicum* in the superior mesenteric vein (small intestine) and *S. haematobium*

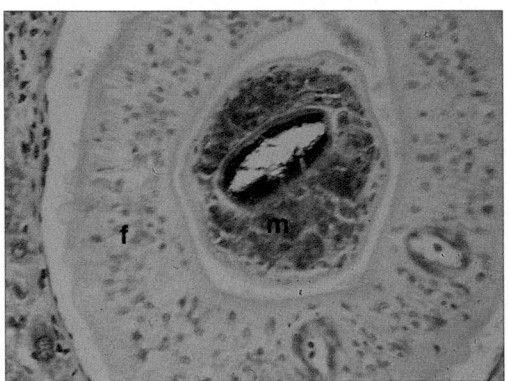

434 *Schistosoma mansoni* in liver section. A section of liver showing adult male (m) and female (f) *Schistosoma mansoni* mating. *(Copyright Liverpool School of Tropical Medicine)*

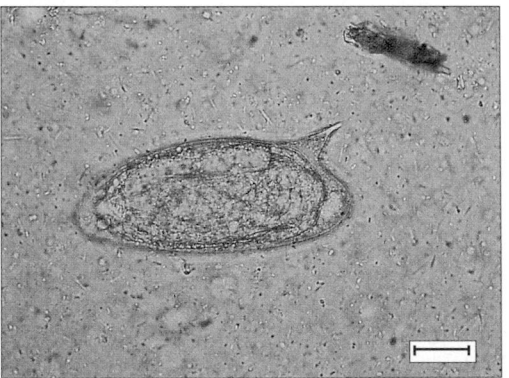

435 *Schistosoma mansoni* ovum. An iodine-stained, wet preparation of faeces showing an ovum of *S. mansoni* with a well-demarcated lateral spine. *(bar = 20 μm) (Copyright Liverpool School of Tropical Medicine)*

in vesical, uterine and prostatic plexuses. Adult males and females (**434**) mate in the respective veins, and eggs are deposited there. They penetrate into the intestine or bladder and are thence excreted. Disease results from the intense inflammation induced by this process. In addition the initial penetration of cercaria can cause an intense skin rash and fever (Katayama fever) which can progress to transverse myelitis. Infection is acquired by bathing or paddling in shallow water containing the host snails.

Diagnosis is by demonstration of eggs in faeces, urine, or tissues. *S. mansoni* has ovoid eggs (150 × 60 μm) with a lateral spine near one pole (**435**), *S. japonicum* has smaller eggs (60 × 50 μm) with a small lateral spine (**436**) and *S. haematobium*, eggs with a terminal spine (**437**).

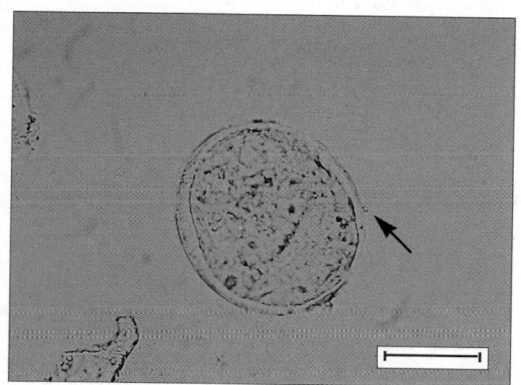

436 *Schistosoma japonicum* ovum. An iodine-stained, wet preparation of faeces showing an ovum of *S. japonicum* with a small spine (arrow). *(bar = 20 μm) (Copyright Liverpool School of Tropical Medicine)*

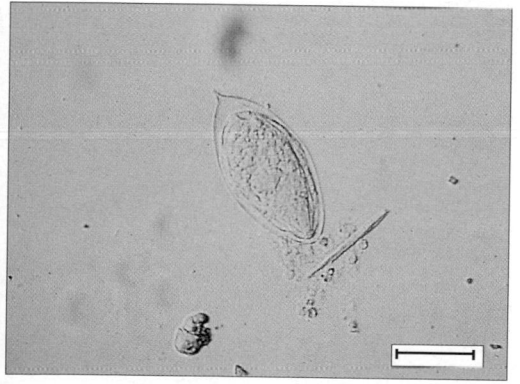

437 *Schistosoma haematobium* ovum. An iodine-stained sample of urine showing an ovum of *S. haematobium* with a terminal spine. *(bar = 50 μm) (Copyright Liverpool School of Tropical Medicine)*

CESTODES

The cestodes are tapeworms that are acquired by ingestion of larvae present in fish (*Diphyllobothrium latum*), beef (*Taenia saginata*) or pork (*T. solium*) which is then inadequately cooked. The beef and pork tapeworms can achieve lengths of 25 metres (**438**). Infection is noticed usually only when segments are excreted in faeces. Treatment is with niclosamide or praziquantel. If the eggs of *T. solium* (excreted in human faeces) are ingested, the larvae invade the intestinal wall, enter the bloodstream and lodge in various tissues including muscle, brain and retina. Here they grow to produce cysts which, if in vital areas, lead to cysticercosis. For example, in the brain they may lead to focal fits, focal neurological deficit,

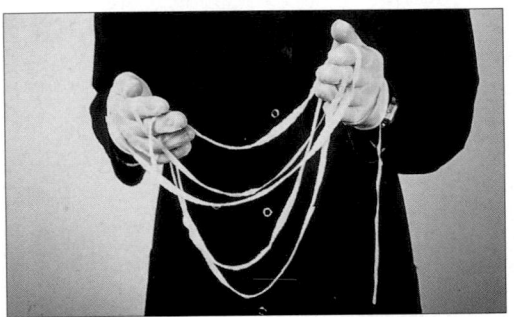

438 Beef tapeworm. A beef tapeworm wrapped around the hands of its host. *(Copyright Liverpool School of Tropical Medicine)*

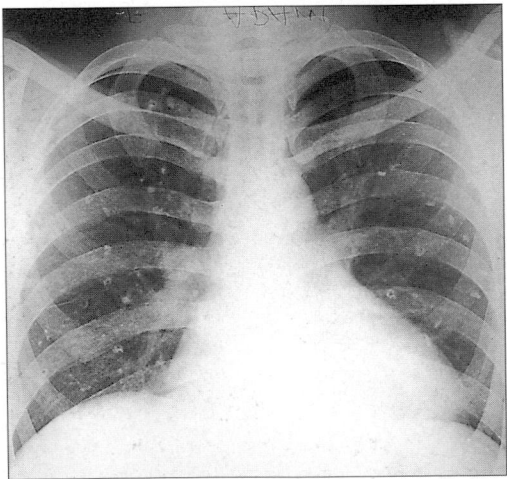

439 Chest X-ray showing calcified cysts. A chest X-ray showing numerous calcified cysticerci.

hydrocephalus or chronic meningitis. Diagnosis is by X-ray (**439**) and demonstration of cysticerci in tissues. Treatment is with praziquantel (except for intraocular disease) with dexamethasone to suppress inflammation around dying cysts.

The dog tapeworm (*Echinococcus granulosus*) is found, in particular, in sheep rearing areas (e.g. New Zealand, Australia, the Balkans, South America). Ingestion of eggs leads to hydatid disease in man. The larvae penetrate the intestinal mucosae and lodge principally in the liver or lungs. The embryo produces a cyst which continues to grow and may achieve a volume of several litres (**440**). The cyst contains protoscolices, daughter cysts and amorphous debris 'hydatid sand' (**441**). Cysts are usually first noticed on radiological examination (**442**). Careful aspiration of the cyst will allow demonstration of hydatid sand. Serological

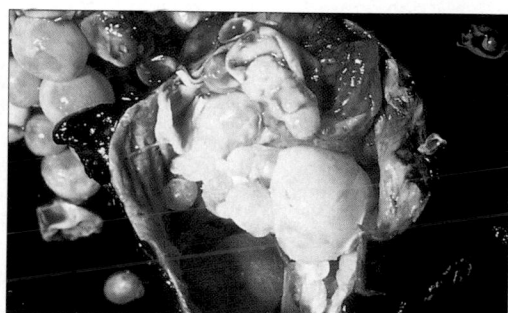

440 Lung showing hydatid cysts. A lung showing several hydatid cysts. (*Copyright Liverpool School of Tropical Medicine*)

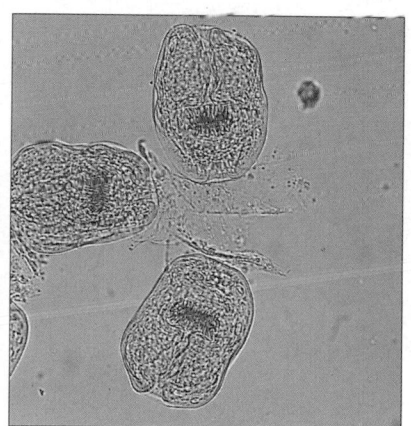

441 Hydatid sand.

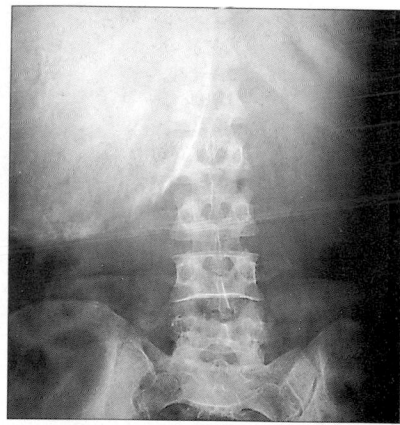

442 Hydatid cysts on liver. An X-ray showing large hydatid cysts on the liver.

diagnosis is also available. Treatment is surgical removal and, when the case is inoperable, with mebendazole.

NEMATODES

Nematodes are non-segmented roundworms, most of which have a free-living stage.

Intestinal worms

Ascaris lumbricoides is a large (20–35 cm) intestinal worm (**443**). Infection is acquired by ingestion of mature embryonated eggs (**444**). Eggs are excreted in faeces. (It was estimated in 1947 that 18,000 tons of *Ascaris* eggs were produced per annum in China.) The eggs hatch in the duodenum and the larvae penetrate

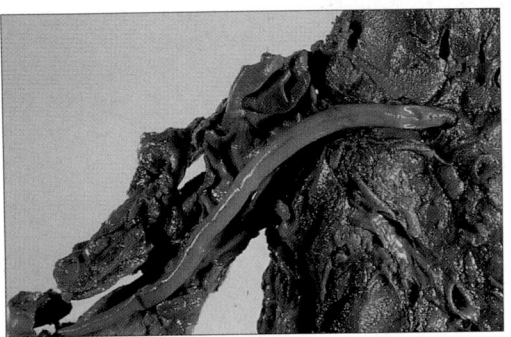

443 *Ascaris lumbricoides* in renal vein. The roundworm *A. lumbricoides*. It escaped from the intestine following a knife wound and has lodged in the renal vein.

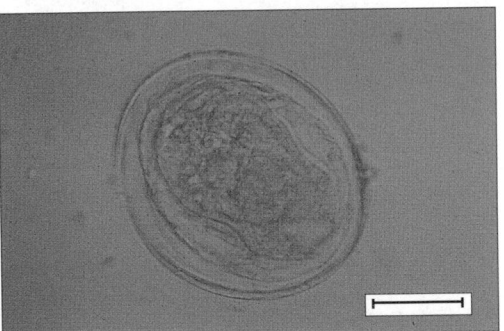

444 *Ascaris lumbricoides* ovum. An ovum of *A. lumbricoides* in faeces. The larva is visible inside the egg. (bar = 20 μm) (Copyright Liverpool School of Tropical Medicine)

the intestinal wall, enter blood or lymphatic vessels and pass to the liver. Thence they pass to the pulmonary circulation, break into the alveoli, ascend to the pharynx and descend the oesophagus to the intestine. There they mate and release eggs (about 200 000 per day). Most often the infection is asymptomatic except during the migratory phase when asthmatic disease may occur or worms may take a wrong turn and emerge through the nose or mouth. Heavy intestinal infestation may cause obstruction or failure to thrive. *Ascaris* is found world-wide, especially in areas of poor sanitation. Diagnosis is by detection of eggs in faeces (**444**). Treatment is with mebendazole.

Enterobius vermicularis, the threadworm, is a common infection of children world-wide. The adult worm resides in the caecum and adjoining areas. Gravid females (**445**) migrate to the anus where they deposit eggs on the anal verge (**446**). This is intensely irritant and causes the child to scratch; the eggs are then transferred to fingers and thence to the mouth to autoinfect or infect others. The

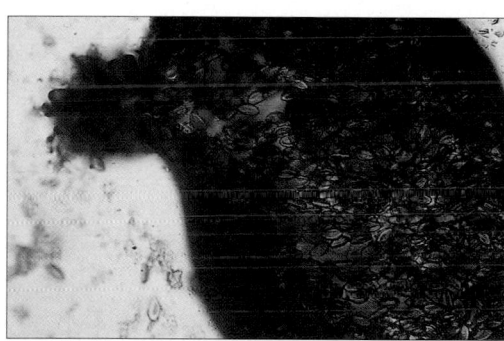

445 Female *Enterobius vermicularis*. A gravid female threadworm, *E. vermicularis*, full of ova.

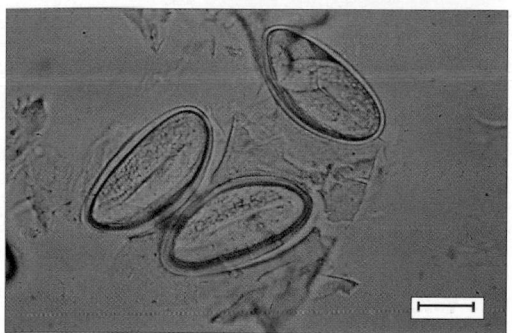

446 *Enterobius vermicularis* ova. Eggs of *E. vermicularis*. (bar = 20 μm)

clinical features vary according to the amount of irritation but the condition often interferes with sleep since the worms come out at night. They may also migrate to the vagina causing vulvovaginitis. Diagnosis is by the cellophane tape method. The tape is applied to the anal verge early in the morning and picks up eggs. The tape is then stuck to a microscope slide and examined using a ×10 objective, rendering the eggs clearly visible (**446**). Treatment is with mebendazole or pyrantel pamote. The whole family will need to be treated.

The hookworms, *Ancylostoma duodenale* and *Necator americanus* both infect man by penetrating the intact skin, usually of the feet. Man appears to be the only host of *A. duodenale* but rabbits, lambs and calves can be experimentally infected with *N. americanus*. *A. duodenale* is found in Europe, South America, India, China and the Pacific Islands. *N. americanus* is found in sub-Saharan Africa and was probably taken to America (North and South) by the slave trade. Hookworm eggs (**447**) are excreted in faeces and hatch, preferably on moist sandy soil, to produce larvae (rhabditiform). They then moult to become filariform or infective larvae which wait until a suitable area of human skin is available. They are carried to the lungs by the bloodstream where they burrow into the alveoli. They then ascend

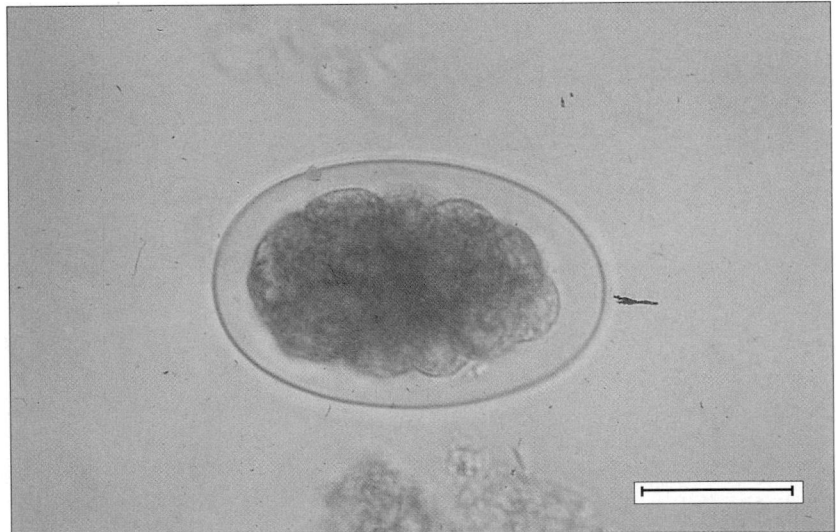

447 ***Ancylostoma duodenale* ovum.** An ovum of the hookworm, *A. duodenale*, in faeces. *(bar = 20 μm)*

to the pharynx and descend the oesophagus to the small intestine. Here they attach to the wall by means of teeth, or cutting plates. Penetration of the skin is accompanied by pruritus (ground itch), and when they enter the lung they may cause pneumonitis. Once in the intestine they may cause abdominal pain. With persistent heavy infestation the major problem is of severe iron deficiency anaemia. Diagnosis is by demonstration of eggs in faeces (**447**). Treatment is with mebendazole.

Strongyloides stercoralis has a similar geographic distribution to hookworm. Cats and dogs may also be infected. Under optimal environmental conditions (moist and warm) the free-living rhabditiform larvae can go through several generations. Eventually, they transform into the infective filariform larvae which congregate together (**448**) and enter man by penetrating the skin. Thereafter the path is similar to that of hookworm. Unlike hookworm, *S. stercoralis* is usually excreted as rhabditiform larvae rather than eggs and these larvae may transform to filariform infective larvae in the intestine, setting up repeated cycles of infection in the same host. Thus infection persists for decades. For example, there are numbers of British soldiers who were kept in Japanese prisoner of war camps

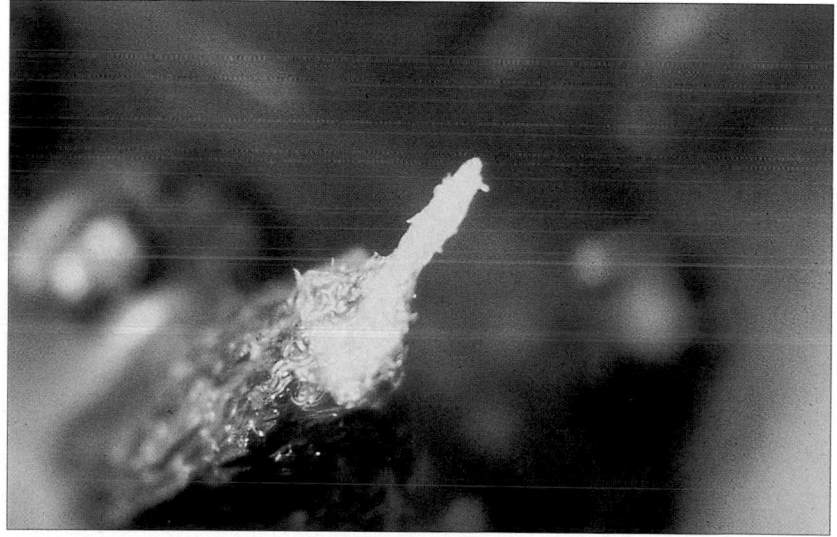

448 *Strongyloides stercoralis* **larvae.** Infective filariform larvae of *S. stercoralis* on soil ready to penetrate the exposed skin of the unwary. *(Copyright Dr R. Ashford)*

who are still infected 50 years later. Patients may develop pulmonary symptoms as worms pass through the lung, or malabsorption with heavy intestinal parasitism. Worms may lose their way occasionally and produce cutaneous larva migrans (**449**). When infection is very heavy, or the immune system is suppressed, a life-threatening hyperinfection of disseminated strongyloidiasis occurs, with Gram-negative septicaemia and penetration of worms into the heart, liver, lungs, kidneys and central nervous system. Diagnosis is by demonstration of larvae in stool (**450**) or by duodenal aspiration. Serologic tests are available in specialized

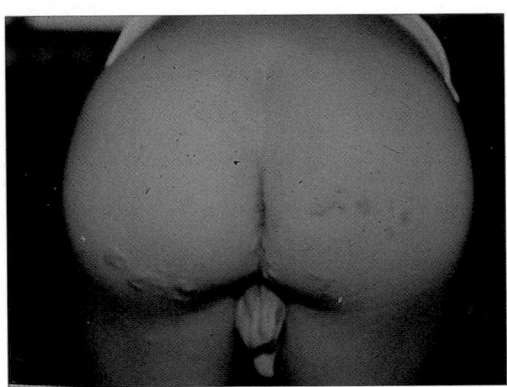

449 *Strongyloides stercoralis* **cutaneous larva migrans.** A patient with cutaneous larva migrans due to *S. stercoralis*. *(Copyright Dr R. Ashford)*

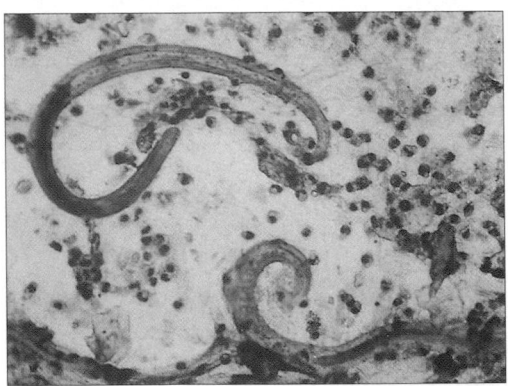

450 *Strongyloides stercoralis* **larvae.** Rhabditiform larvae of *S. stercoralis* in faeces. *(Copyright Dr C. Parry)*

centres. Thiabendazole is the drug of choice but is compromised by a high incidence of side effects and incomplete efficacy.

Trichuris trichiura, the whipworm (**451**), has a world-wide distribution and is acquired faeco-orally. Most often it produces asymptomatic infection but may rarely give abdominal distension, bloody mucoid diarrhoea, weight loss and anaemia, if infection is heavy. Diagnosis is by demonstration of the characteristic barrel-shaped eggs in stool (**452**). Treatment, if necessary, is with mebendazole.

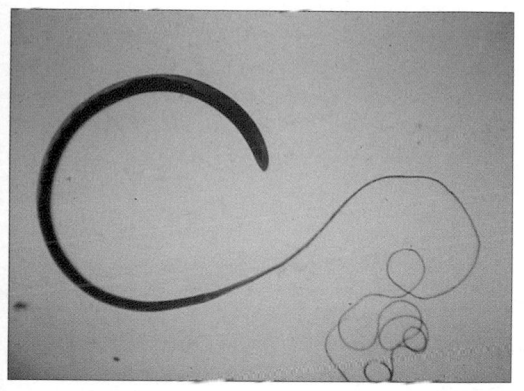

451 Trichuris trichiura.
The whipworm *T. trichiura.*
(Copyright Liverpool School of
Tropical Medicine)

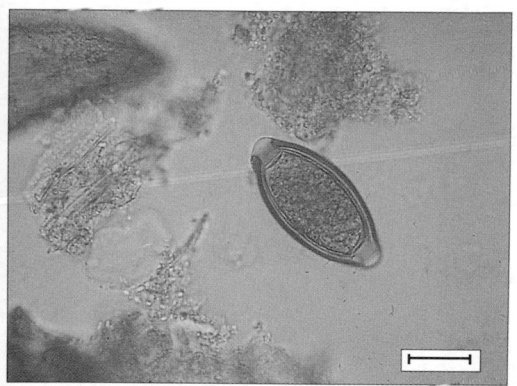

**452 Trichuris trichiura
wet preparation.** An ovum
of *T. trichiura* in a wet
preparation of faeces stained
with iodine. (bar = 20 μm)

Blood and tissue nematodes

The filaria (*Wuchereria bancrofti, Loa loa, Onchocerca volvulus, Brugia malayi*) are widely distributed in the tropics and subtropics. They all have an insect (mosquito, mango fly or black-fly) as an intermediate host and are deposited on humans when they are bitten. They produce lymphatic blockage leading to lymphoedema (**453**), cutaneous larva migrans or ocular damage, depending on the particular worm.

The guinea worm (*Dracunculus medinensis*) is found in Africa, in the Nile Valley and in Asia, as far east as Pakistan and central India. The adult female can grow to 1.5 metres (**454**) but the male is far less impressive at a mere 2 cm long. The gravid female is present in the subcutaneous tissue and at the head-end produces a skin blister (**455**) which, when put in warm water, bursts releasing large numbers of larvae. These are then ingested by *Cyclops* spp. where they mature. If the *Cyclops* spp. are ingested by humans, the larvae penetrate the intestinal wall entering deep connective tissue where they mature and mate. Infection becomes apparent when the gravid female emerges (**455**). Treatment is with mebendazole or niridazole. Elimination of guinea worm is a WHO goal and can be achieved by proper control of drinking water.

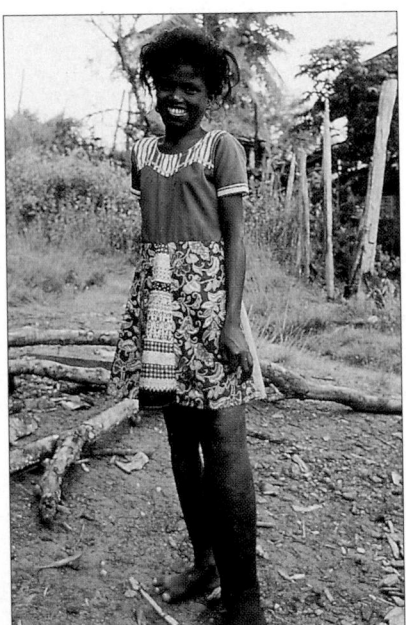

453 Elephantiasis due to *Loa loa*.
An African child with elephantiasis (lymphoedema) due to *L. loa*. (Copyright *Liverpool School of Tropical Medicine*)

Trichinella spiralis is transmitted to man by consumption of undercooked contaminated pork or other meat. In the intestine male and female worms mate to produce larvae. These burrow through the intestinal wall to the lymphatics and thence to the bloodstream. They then penetrate the sheaths of striated muscle where they encyst (**456**). Muscle invasion is characterized by fever, eosinophilia

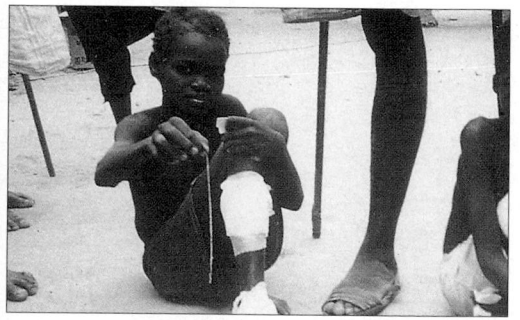

454 Dracunculus medinensis. A Sudanese boy displaying the guinea worm (*D. medinensis*) that has been removed from his leg.

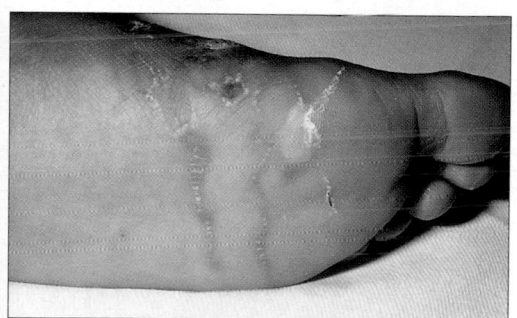

455 Dracunculus medinensis blister with larvae. A blister due to *D. medinensis* on the foot of a Nigerian child . The blister is full of larvae. The worm can be seen winding subcutaneously across the sole of the fool.

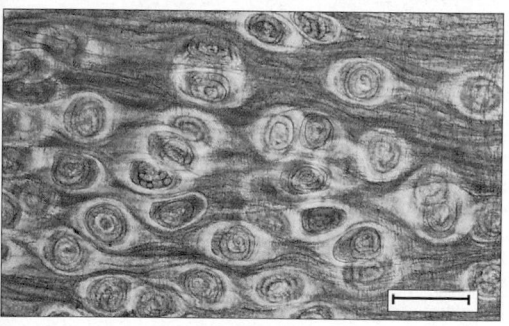

456 Trichinella spiralis larvae. A section of muscle full of *T. spiralis* larvae. (bar = 10 µm) (Copyright Liverpool School of Tropical Medicine)

and muscular pain and tenderness, and circumorbital oedema is a pathognomonic sign. They may also invade the brain causing encephalitis. Diagnosis is by serology or demonstration of encysted organisms in muscle. Treatment is primarily to damp down inflammation (dexamethasone). The role of thiabendazole or mebendazole is unclear.

Visceral larva migrans in temperature countries is principally due to *Toxocara canis* or *T. cati*. As their names imply, the adult worms are present in the intestine of dogs and cats (**457**). The ova are excreted in faeces and mature outside the host. Man (in particular the child) becomes infected by ingestion of cat or dog faeces. In the human intestine the eggs hatch and penetrate through the intestinal wall and enter the tissue (viscera). Here they encyst. The clinical features can vary from none with eosinophilia, to hepatomegaly with eosinophilia, to retinitis (**458**) through to severe pulmonary disease and death. The latter is fortunately very rare. Diagnosis is on clinical grounds. Serology and laparoscopy are adjuncts to diagnosis. Treatment is usually not given but if necessary thiabendazole can be used.

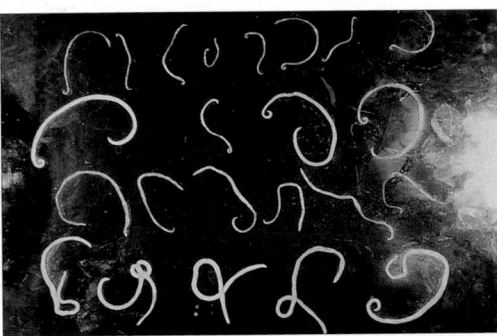

457 Adult *Toxocara canis*. Adult *T. canis* worms from dog faeces. *(Copyright Dr R. Ashford)*

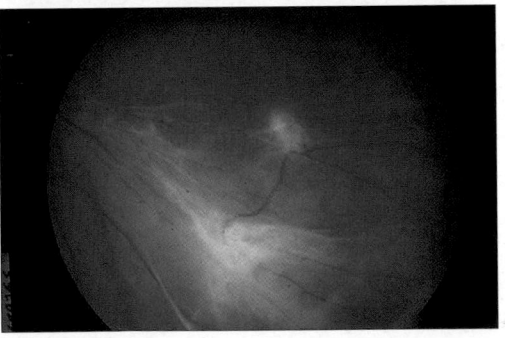

458 *Toxocara canis* retinitis.

7.
Medically Important Insects and Other Ectoparasites

The phylum Arthropoda (from Greek *arthron* - joint, *pous* - foot) contains numerous genera (over 800,000) and species, most of which are not harmful to man. The medically important arthropods fall into six classes (**459**). It is, however, more useful to classify them into agents that directly cause disease (**460**) and those that act as vectors for other diseases (**461**). From this it can be seen that some arthropods fall into both classes.

The medically important arthropods	
Insecta or Hexapoda	True insects with a head, thorax and abdomen. The only class in which some members possess wings (e.g. flies, fleas, lice, mosquitoes, bugs).
Arachnida	Possess a fused head and thorax (cephalothorax) and abdomen but no feelers or antennae (e.g. ticks, mites, spiders, scorpions).
Crustacea	Possess a head, thorax and abdomen, distinguished from all other arthropods by having two pairs of antennae (e.g. crabs, lobsters, water fleas).
Chilipoda	Possess a head and a long dorsoventrally flattened fused thoraco-abdomen made up of numerous similar segments. Each segment has a pair of walking legs. The first pair of legs is modified to form poison claws (e.g. centipedes).
Diplopoda	Possess head bearing mouthparts and antennae. The cylindrical thoraco-abdomen is made up of numerous identical segments most of which have a pair of legs. The anterior genital opening differentiates millipede from centipede (e.g. millipedes).
Pentastomida	Were previously classified as nematodes but the larvae of some possess appendages. The pathogens are highly specialized endoparasites of man (e.g. *Armillifer* and tongue-worm, *Linguatula*).

459 The medically important arthropods.

AGENTS DIRECTLY CAUSING DISEASE

LEECHES

Land leeches are found in India, S.E. Asia and parts of Oceania and South America. Aquatic leeches have a world-wide distribution. They are annelid worms with specialized chitinous mouthparts and secrete an anticoagulant, hirudin. Land

Arthropods and other ectoparasites which induce diseases directly by trauma, poison or hypersensitivity	
Annelida	Land leeches (e.g. *Haemadipsa* spp.) Aquatic leeches (e.g. *Limnatis* spp.)
Insecta	Myiasis – cutaneous or body cavity maggots (e.g. *Cordylobia anthropophaga*) Jiggers (e.g. *Tunga penetrans*) Lice (pubic lice, *Phthirus pubis*; head (body) louse, *Pediculus (corporis) capitis*) Hymenoptera* (e.g. bees, wasps, hornets, ants) Fleas* (e.g. *Pulex irritans*) Mosquitoes* (e.g. *Aedes* or *Anopheles* spp.) Midges* (e.g. *Culicoides* spp.) Tabanidae (e.g. horse-fly: *Tabanus* or *Chrysops* spp.) Bugs (e.g. bed bugs, *Cimex*; reduviid, *Triatoma* or *Panstrongylus* spp.)
Arachnida	Spiders (e.g. black widow, *Lactrodectus mactans* or funnel web, *Atrax robustus*) Scorpions (e.g. *Antroctonus crassicauda*) Ticks (e.g. *Dermacentor andersoni*) Mites (e.g. *Sarcoptes scabiei*; house dust mite*, *Dermatophagoides pteronyssinus*)
Chilipoda	Centipedes (e.g. *Scolopendra* spp.)
Diplopoda	Millipedes (e.g. *Rhinocricus*, *Spirobolus* and *Spirastreptus* spp.)
Pentastomida	Tongue worm (*Linguatula* spp.)

*Some or all of the damage is due to hypersensitivity.

460 Diseases due to arthropods and other ectoparasites induced directly by trauma, poison or hypersensitivity.

leeches have strong jaws that can penetrate external skin (**462**), whereas aquatic leeches are weaker and attack mucous surfaces.

Leeches can cause severe loss of blood and, if pulled off, the jaws may remain in the skin and lead to secondary infection. They can be induced to release themselves by heat (a lighted match or cigarette), hypertonic salt solutions, alcohol or vinegar. Leeches are also used for medical purposes, for example to remove subcutaneous collections of blood. Although leeches suck blood they are not known to be disease vectors.

Arthropods as vectors of disease

	Vector	Diseases
Insecta	Sandflies (Phlebotominae)	leishmaniasis, Oroya fever (bartonellosis), phlebovirus
	Mosquitoes (*Aedes, Anopheles, Culex*)	alphaviruses, flaviviruses, bunyaviruses, malaria, filariasis
	Blackfly (*Simulium*)	onchocerciasis
	Tabanidae (*Chrysops*)	loiasis (Calabar swelling)
	Tsetse fly (*Glossina*)	African trypanosomiasis (sleeping sickness)
	Flies	diarrhoeal disease, trachoma
	Lice (*Pediculus*)	typhus, trench fever, relapsing fever
	Bugs (*Cimex*)	?hepatitis B
	Bugs (Reduviidae)	Chagas' disease (South American trypanosomiasis)
	Fleas	plague (*Yersinia pestis*), typhus
Arachnida	Ticks (*Ixodes, Ornithodoros*)	Lyme disease (*Borrelia burgdorferi*), relapsing fever (*B. hermsi, B. duttoni*), Rickettsiae, flaviviruses, alphaviruses, bunyaviruses, babesiosis
	Mites (Trombiculidae)	Scrub typhus
Crustacea	Water flea (*Cyclops*)	Guinea worm (*Dracunculus medinensis*), *Diphyllobothrium latum.*
	Crabs, crayfish	*Paragonimus westermani*

461 Arthropods as vectors of disease.

DIPTEROUS FLIES

The condition myiasis is when the larvae of dipterous flies invade tissue and develop into maggots. This can occur on skin or within body cavities. The larvae of some flies are opportunistic invaders of pre-existing wounds (e.g. *Lucilla* spp.) but some invade intact skin. The larva of the tumbu fly (*Cordylobia*

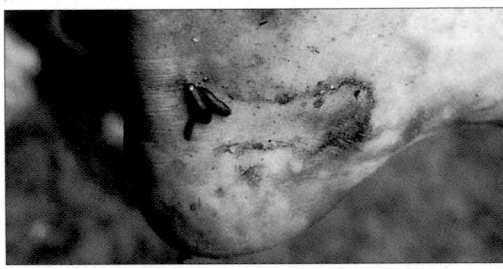

462 Land leeches. Land leeches in Papua New Guinea. *(Copyright Dr R. Ashford)*

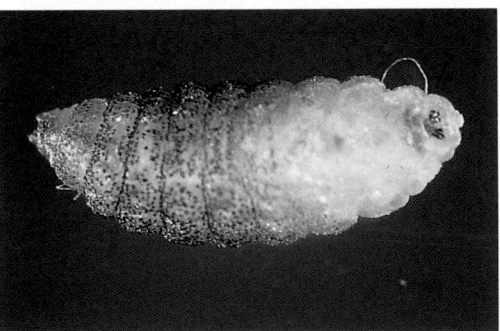

463 *Cordylobia anthropophaga* maggot. The maggot of the tumbu fly (*C. anthropophaga*). *(Copyright Liverpool School of Tropical Medicine)*

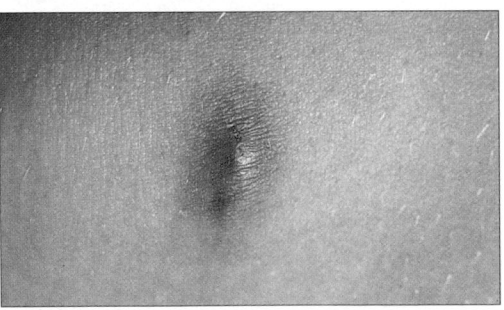

464 *Cordylobia anthropophaga* lesion. A carbuncle-like lesion of the tumbu fly maggot. *(Copyright Liverpool School of Tropical Medicine)*

anthropophaga) (**463**) develops from eggs deposited in clothing and invades skin to produce a carbuncle-like lesion (**164**). The lesion is less painful than a boil. Close inspection reveals not pus but the respiratory spiracles of the maggot. To remove the maggot from the mature lesion, it should be covered with vaseline or paraffin oil (**465**) to asphyxiate it. It will then wriggle partly out and can be gently squeezed from its burrow. Prevention is by hanging clothes to dry in a place where the fly cannot reach and by ironing clothing seams carefully to destroy eggs. Other maggots, such as *Dermatobia hominis,* have large spines and must be removed surgically. Myiasis of body cavities, such as sinus or middle ear, is due, for example, to the screw fly (*Chrysomyia bezziana*) and is much more damaging, with a measurable mortality (up to 8%). Some maggots (e.g. *Lucilla*) have been used therapeutically to debride wounds.

JIGGERS AND OTHER FLEAS

Jiggers are burrowing fleas (*Tunga penetrans*) that can produce painful and even crippling lesions (**466**). Adults are free-living but, when fertilized, the female flea

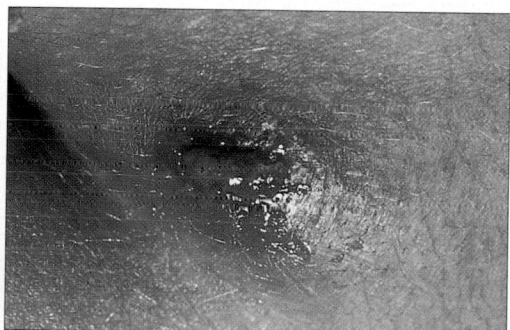

465 *Cordylobia anthropophaga* maggot emerging. The same lesion treated with vaseline to cause the maggot to emerge. *(Copyright Liverpool School of Tropical Medicine)*

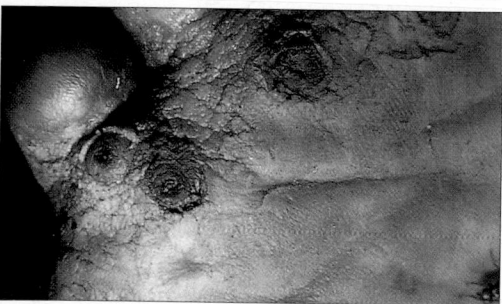

466 *Tunga penetrans* lesions. A case of jiggers. The circular lesions are due to the burrowing flea *T. penetrans.* *(Copyright Dr R. Ashford)*

attaches to a suitable host (poultry, pigs, man or other animals) and penetrates cracks or crevices in the skin. Inside the crevice, the gravid female flea grips firmly and swells, often to the size of a pea (**467**). After 8–12 days the swelling is large enough to cause irritation. Severe inflammation is followed by ulceration and expulsion of large numbers of eggs. Secondary infection and even tetanus may follow.

Treatment is to remove the jigger with a sterile needle (without it bursting), and to cover the lesion with sterile dressings and antiseptics. Prevention is by wearing appropriate foot covering, since this flea cannot jump well, and using a 'scorched earth' policy.

Other fleas produce localized irritation or allergy. The human flea, *Pulex irritans*, is diminishing in importance. Most human flea bites are due to cat and dog fleas (*Ctenocephalides felis* and *C. canis*)(**468**). The rat flea (*Xenopsylla cheopis*) is the classic vector of plague (*Yersinia pestis*) and murine typhus

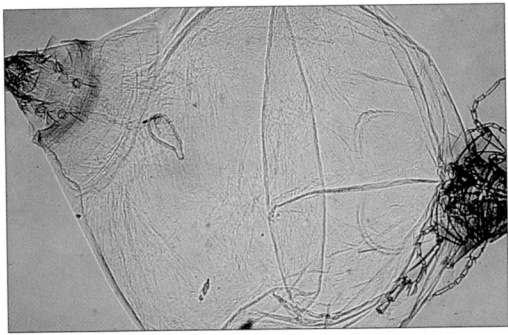

467 The gravid female *Tunga penetrans.*

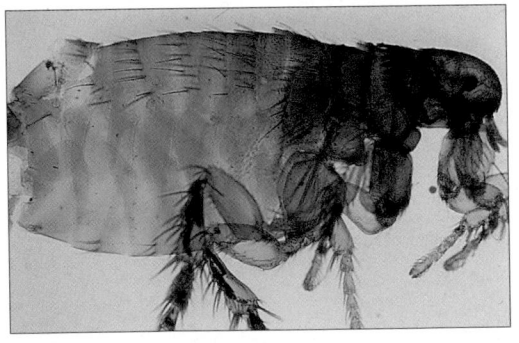

468 *Ctenocephalides canis.* The dog flea.

(*Rickettsia mooseri*). This and other fleas may transmit dwarf tapeworms (*Hymenolepis* spp.) if accidentally ingested. Increasing resistance to DDT is being observed and malathion may be more effective.

LICE

Three species of lice infest man, namely *Phthirus pubis* (the pubic or crab louse), *Pediculus corporis* (the body louse) and *Pediculus capitis* (the head louse). In fact the latter two are very similar, differing only in minor anatomic details, and are often grouped as *Pediculus humanus*.

Head lice infect the hair-covered areas of the head (**469**). The adults roam over the scalp. They feed by grasping the skin with a sucking mouth, the haustellum, and penetrate it with two stylets, to draw blood. After fertilization, the female grasps a hair and cements an egg to the shaft, leaving the characteristic nit (**470**).

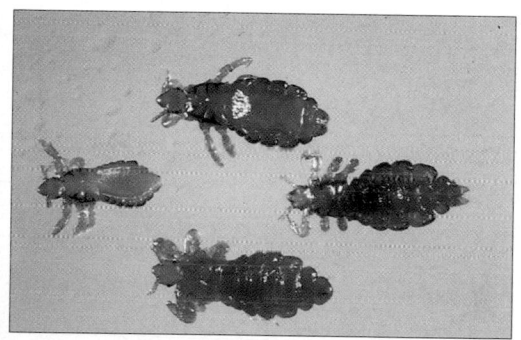

469   *Pediculus capitis.*
Head lice.

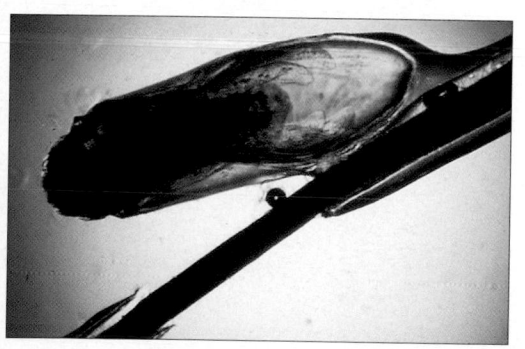

470   Nit with emerging louse. A nit with a louse about to emerge. *(Copyright Liverpool School of Tropical Medicine)*

Nits are deposited at a rate of 7–10 per day and the female is reproductively active for about a month. The total cycle from egg to egg is about 16 days. Head lice are spread by close contact and are endemic in many schools. They are not usually vectors of disease and can be managed by removing nits with a fine comb and treatment with an appropriate insecticide (e.g. malathion). It is not necessary to shave the head.

Body lice flourish under conditions of poor hygiene. They infest areas of the body that are covered by hairs, but prefer areas that are also covered by clothes. They are found world-wide but tend to be most prevalent in conditions of relative cold. They are spread by close contact and shared clothes or bedding. The female

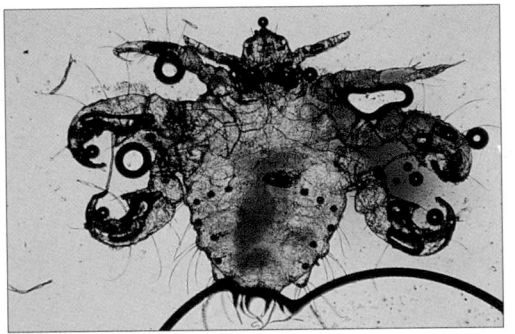

471 *Phthirus pubis.* The crab or pubic louse.

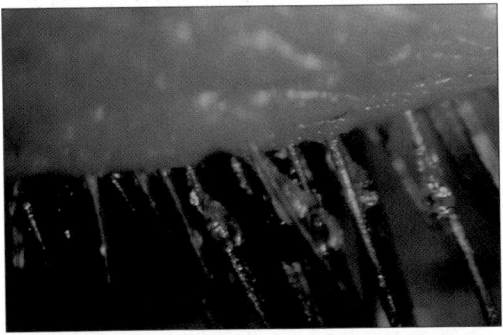

472 Pediculosis. Lice infestation can even involve the eyelashes.

lays eggs on body hairs but more frequently (70% of eggs) on fibres in clothes or bedding. Body lice are the sole vector of louse-borne typhus (*Rickettsia prowazeki*), louse-borne relapsing fever (*Borrelia recurrentis*) and trench fever (*Bartonella quintana*). Malathion is used to control body lice on humans. Lice cannot survive without feeding on humans for more than 10 days; thus they do not persist in houses. The nits will survive on clothing for up to 4 weeks. Nits are destroyed by heating at 70°C for 30 min.

Pubic lice (**471**) have crab-like claws on their second and third legs with which they grasp pubic hairs. They are rather sluggish and usually confined to the pubic region although they can infest beards, eyebrows and eyelashes (**472**). *Phthirus pubis* is still killed by DDT. However, DDT is not active against nits and malathion is preferred.

HYMENOPTERA

There are over 4000 species of stinging bees, wasps and hornets. The direct damage induced by the sting is usually local (redness, pain, swelling) and short-lived. The venom is injected through a barbed sting and contains a variety of bioactive amines (e.g. histamine), enzymes (e.g. phospholipase A) and toxic peptides (e.g. mellitin). Deaths occur due to hypersensitivity to the venom (present in 0.5% of the population) resulting in anaphylaxis. The commonest stings are due to wasps (**473**) and honey bees (*Apis mellifera*). Local treatment involves removal of the sting (it continues to inject venom) and perhaps local antiseptics. Management of anaphylaxis requires subcutaneous adrenaline (0.5–1 ml of 0.5% solution), maintenance of airways and urgent hospitalization.

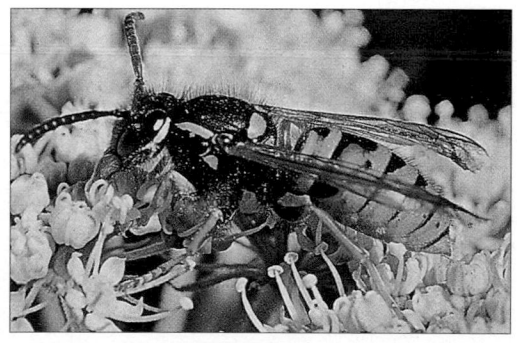

473 A wasp. *(Copyright Liverpool School of Tropical Medicine)*

MOSQUITOES

There are at least 35 genera of mosquito. They are found world-wide from above the Arctic circle to well below the equator. Adults of both sexes feed on nectar, but some also suck the blood of a variety of animal and bird species. Hypersensitivity to the saliva of the mosquito results in the appearance of mosquito bites. However, female mosquitoes are also important vectors of disease. *Anopheles* spp. (**474**) are important biological vectors (i.e. the agent replicates in the mosquito) of malaria, filariasis, alphaviruses (e.g. Venezuelan equine encephalitis), flavivirus (e.g. St Louis encephalitis) and bunyaviruses (e.g. Tahyna) although they are not the principal vector of the latter three. *Aedes* spp. (**475**) also transmit filariasis and are major vectors of alphaviruses (e.g. chikungunya), flaviviruses (e.g. dengue and yellow fever) and some bunyaviruses (e.g. Californian encephalitis).

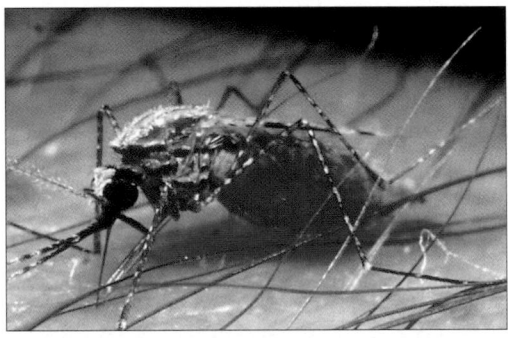

474 Anopheles mosquito. An anopheles mosquito close to the end of a meal. *(Copyright Liverpool School of Tropical Medicine)*

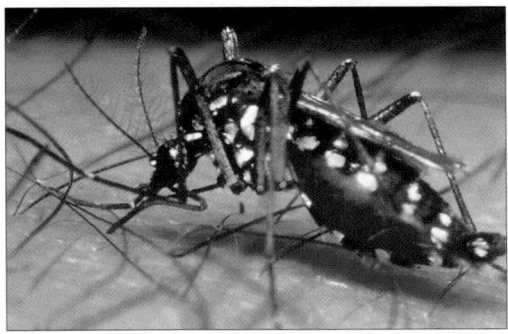

475 *Aedes aegypti.* *A. aegypti* feeding. *(Copyright Liverpool School of Tropical Medicine)*

TABANIDAE

This family includes several flies that pose a biting nuisance and are the largest blood-sucking files with a wingspan of over 6 cm. Only the females bite and they can take a large blood meal (20–200 mg). In addition *Chrysops* spp. (**476**) are biological vectors of loaiasis (Calabar swelling due to *Loa loa*). Other Tabanidae may also be mechanical vectors of anthrax, tularaemia and, perhaps, Lyme disease.

BUGS

Bed bugs have a world-wide distribution. The major parasites of man are *Cimex lectularius* (**477**) and *C. hemipterus* (principally in the tropics). Females lay up to 100 eggs in a lifetime. They are deposited in cracks and crevices in walls, behind

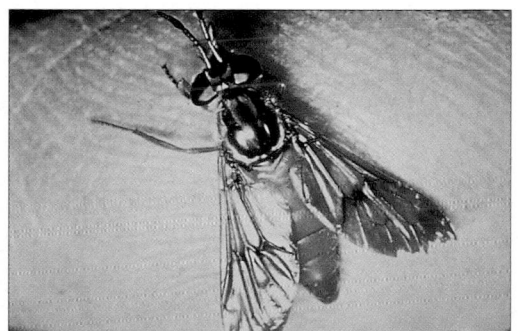

476   Chrysops dimidiata. A mango fly. *(Copyright Liverpool School of Tropical Medicine)*

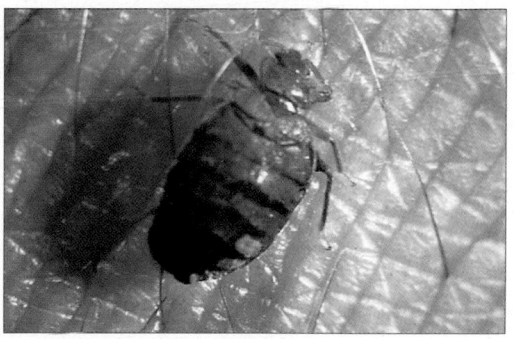

477   Cimex lectularius. A bed bug.

pictures and wallpaper and in beds and mattresses. They produce irritating bites and may be a vector of hepatitis B virus.

SPIDERS

There are numerous genera of spiders, most of which cause no harm. Most often the large hairy spiders are harmless, and relatively small, insignificant-looking spiders are the most poisonous.

In general, the venoms are necrotizing or neurotoxic. The black widow spider (*Lactrodectus mactans*) (**478**) produces a powerful neurotoxin and was responsible for 63 deaths in the USA over a 10-year period in the 1950s. Funnel web spiders include *Atrax robustus* which is found in and around Sydney, Australia.

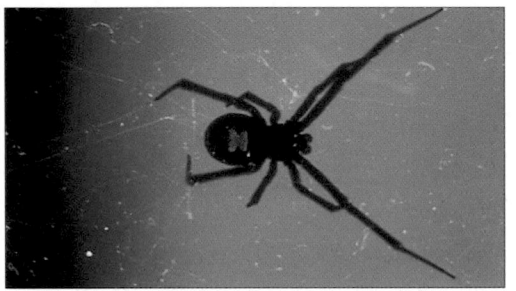

478 *Lactrodectus mactans.* The black widow spider. *(Copyright Liverpool School of Tropical Medicine)*

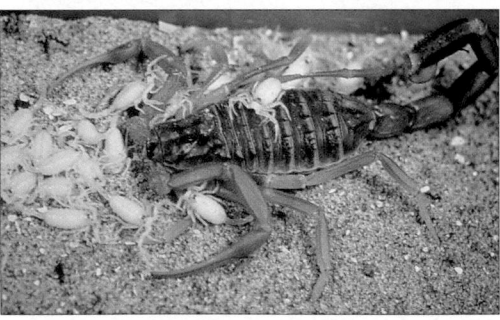

479 A scorpion. *(Copyright Liverpool School of Tropical Medicine)*

SCORPIONS

Scorpions (**479**) are widely distributed in the tropics and subtropics. They deliver venom by a comma-shaped sting at the top of the tail. Following stinging, mortality rates can be as high as 55%, especially in young children. In Mexico there is an incidence of death of 84 per 100,000 per year in Colima state. The venoms produce both local necrosis and neurotoxic features.

MITES

Mites and ticks are in the subclass *Acari* in which there are over 30,000 species. Although there are over 200 families of mites, only a few affect man. *Sarcoptes scabiei* causes scabies (**480**) and is found world-wide. Its incidence increases

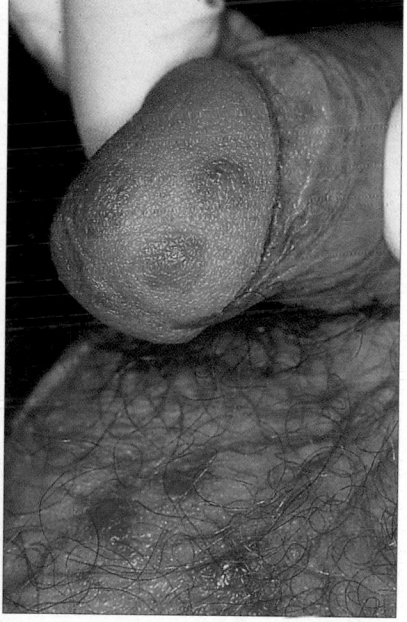

480 Genital scabies. A patient with genital scabies. Each lesion is a burrow containing *Sarcoptes scabiei*.

greatly in times of war, famine or other disasters. It is spread person-to-person by close contact in families and can be spread by sexual contact. It is estimated that in the British Army in the second World War as many as 6000 new cases were diagnosed per month. The adult form of the scabies mite (**481**) is a small (250–350 µm) flattened disk with eight short squat legs. The fertilized female burrows into the skin for several millimetres to centimetres (never below the stratum corneum). The sites chosen are where the skin is thin and wrinkled, e.g. wrists, exterior surfaces of elbow, axillae, penis, scrotum and under the breasts. As she is burrowing she lays 20–30 eggs, which hatch into larvae within 4–5 days. In the burrow, the larvae moult into nymphs and then again to become adults. The life-span from egg to egg takes 2–3 weeks. Treatment is of all the family with benzyl benzoate, Eurax, or γ-benzene hexachloride. Scabies is only transmitted by close contact, thus there is no absolute need to disinfect bedding.

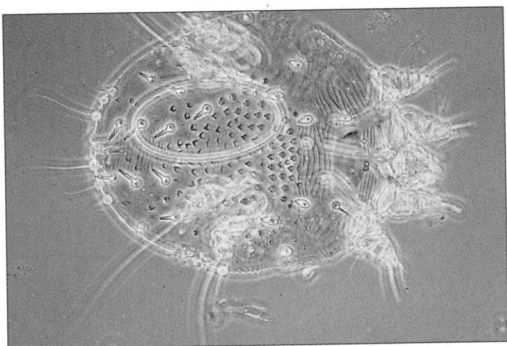

481 Sarcoptes scabiei.
The scabies mite (*Sarcoptes scabiei*). (*Copyright Liverpool School of Tropical Medicine*)

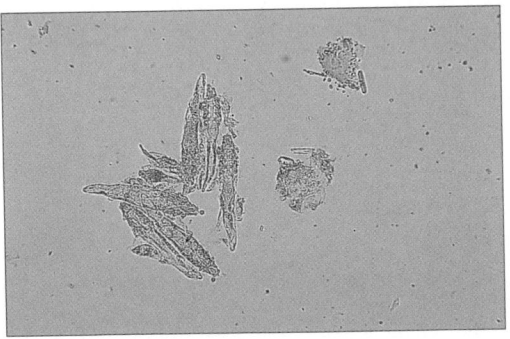

482 Demodex folliculorum
The follicle mite.

Follicle mites, *Demodex folliculorum* (**482**) cause no disease apart from, perhaps, neurosis. They are normal inhabitants of skin follicles of the eyelids, nose or face.

Dermatophagoides pteronyssinus, the house dust mite (**483**), as its name implies, feeds on desquamated skin. It can reach very high population densities in pillows, mattresses and settees. The faeces of the mite are a potent allergen inducing asthma and allergic rhinitis. Control is by treating infected sites with insecticides and regular vacuum-cleaning.

CENTIPEDES

Centipedes (**484**) also have a world-wide distribution but it is only the large, tropical and subtropical varieties that can inflict harmful bites. The venom which is delivered by claws adapted from its first pair of legs, produces localized necrotic lesions.

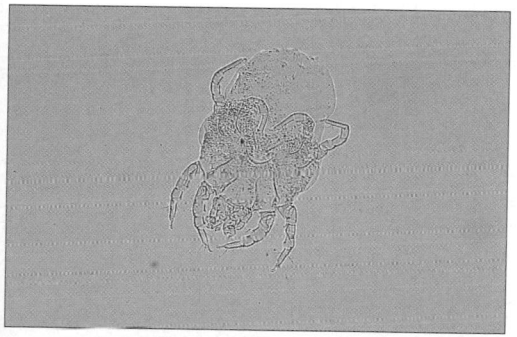

483 The house dust mite. *Dermatophagoides pteronyssinus.*

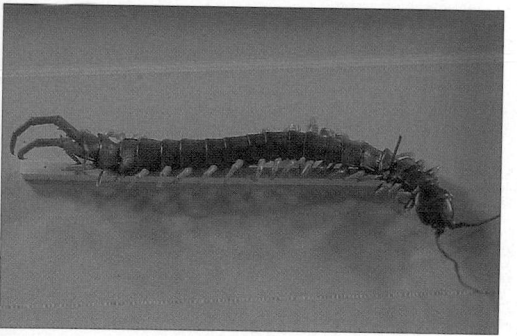

484 A centipede. (*Scolopendra* spp.).

MILLIPEDES

Millipedes (*mille* thousand, *ped* foot) (**485**) differ from centipedes in having a cylindrical body and many more segments and legs. They either secrete or forcibly eject a toxic fluid from specialized glands. It is very irritant to skin, conjunctivae and other mucous membranes.

PENTASTOMIDA

This comprises two genera, *Linguatula* (**486**) and *Armillifer* (**487**). Adult *Linguatula* live in the nasal passages of dogs, wolves and foxes. Man can become infected by either ingestion of eggs (visceral liguatulosis) or larvae. In the latter, the larvae

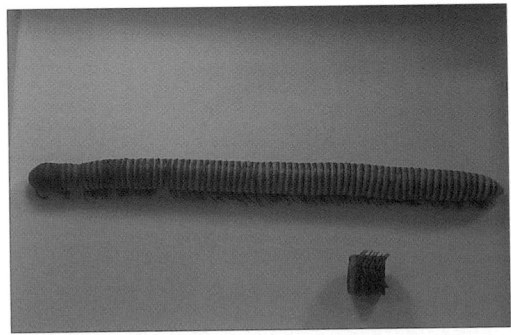

485　A millipede.

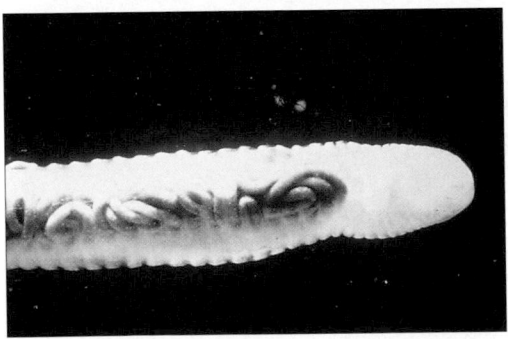

486　*Linguatula serrata.*
The tongue worm. *(Copyright Liverpool School of Tropical Medicine)*

become established in the nasal passages producing halzoun (hoarseness, dysphagia, dyspnoea and vomiting). *Armillifer* is acquired by eating raw python, or other snakes, or drinking water contaminated by snakes. Most often, the disease is asymptomatic, though it can produce liver damage (**488**).

VECTORS OF DISEASE

PHLEBOTOMINE SANDFLIES

The sandflies are *Phlebotomus* (**489**) in the Old World and *Lutzomyia* in the New World. Only the females feed on blood.

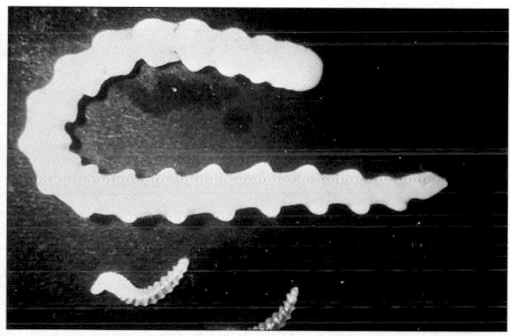

487   Armillifer armillatus.
(Copyright Liverpool School of Tropical Medicine)

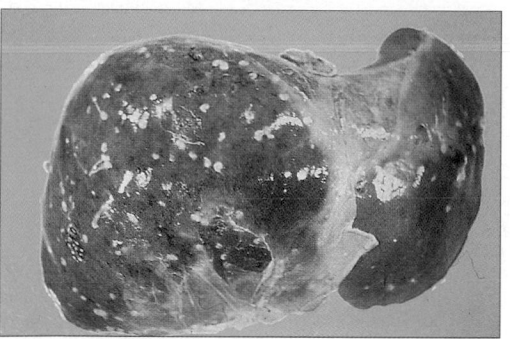

488   Liver granulomas and calcification due to Armillifer armillatus.
(Copyright Liverpool School of Tropical Medicine)

Bites may result in an urticarial reaction but their most important role is as vectors of cutaneous and visceral leishmaniasis, Oroya fever (in the Andes) and phleboviruses (Sandfly or pappataci fever). The adult flies are small and difficult to find. They fly only at night.

BLACKFLY

It is the females of *Simulium* spp. (**490**) that feed on blood. They transmit the filarial parasite *Onchocerca volvulus* causing onchocerciasis both in Africa and South and Central America.

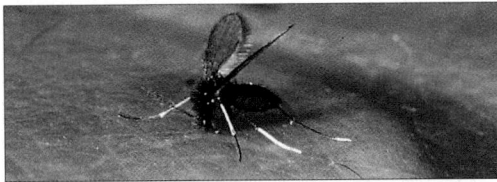

489 A sandfly (*Phlebotomus papatasi*) feeding. *(Copyright Liverpool School of Tropical Medicine)*

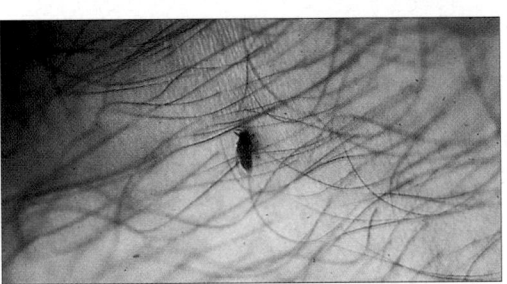

490 A blackfly (*Simulium damnosum*) feeding. *(Copyright Liverpool School of Tropical Medicine)*

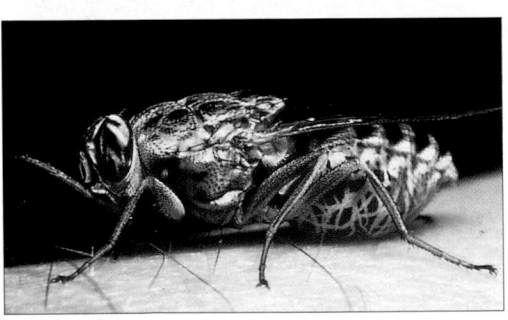

491 A tsetse fly (*Glossina morsitans*). *(Copyright Liverpool School of Tropical Medicine)*

TSETSE FLY

Tsetse flies, *Glossina* spp. (**491**) are confined to tropical Africa. They are attracted by bright colours and powerful odours. They produce painful bites. More importantly they are the vector of sleeping sickness (*Trypanosoma brucei*).

BLUEBOTTLE

Bluebottles (**492**) and house-flies can act as mechanical vectors of diarrhoeal pathogens and of trachoma (*Chlamydia trachomatis*).

BUGS

Triatomite or reduviid bugs (**493**) defecate as they bite the skin and thus release *Trypanosma cruzi* which enter the bite. This results in a local chagoma (Romaña's sign) and subsequently Chagas' disease (South American trypanosomiasis).

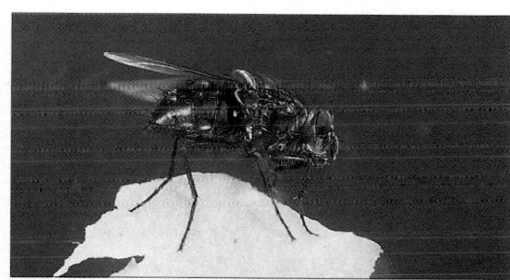

492   A bluebottle (*Calliphora* spp.) feeding.
(Copyright Liverpool School of Tropical Medicine)

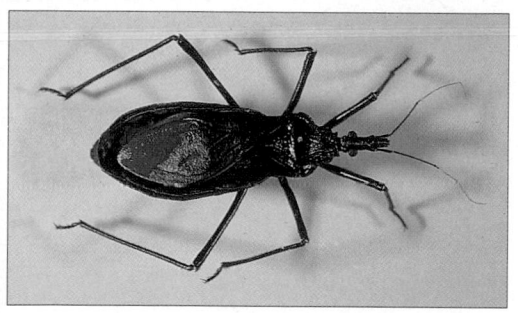

493   A reduviid bug (*Triatoma dimidiata*).
(Copyright Liverpool School of Tropical Medicine)

TICKS

All ticks are obligate blood-sucking parasites (**494** and **495**). There are two basic forms: soft, or argasid ticks and hard, or ixodid ticks. The hard ticks are slow feeders and remain attached for days, whereas the soft ticks feed quickly, often overnight. Most feed on domestic or other animals and only feed on man by chance. The soft tick of southern Africa (*Ornithodorus moubata*) is the only one to specialize in man and poultry. Soft ticks transmit tick-borne relapsing fever (*Borrelia duttoni, B. hermsii, B. persica*) to man in Africa, Asia, America and Mediterranean Europe. The hard ticks transmit Lyme disease (*B. burgdorferi*), rickettsioses (fièvre boutonneuse, Rocky Mountain spotted fever, Siberian tick typhus), babesiosis, flaviviruses (Kyasanur Forest and Omsk haemorrhagic fever) and bunyaviruses (Crimean-Congo haemorrhagic fever).

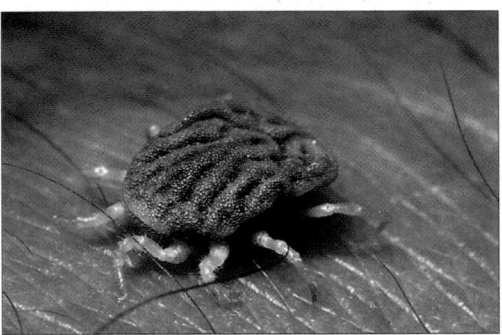

494 A soft tick (*Ornithodorus moubata*) about to feed. *(Copyright Liverpool School of Tropical Medicine)*

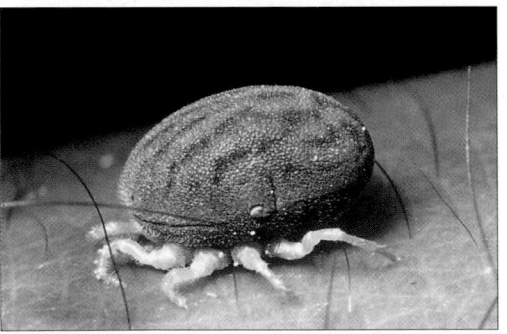

495 *Ornithodorus moubata* engorged with blood. The same tick engorged with blood. *(Copyright Liverpool School of Tropical Medicine)*

Appendices

Nervous system infections

	Most important	Less common	Tropical or geographically limited
Encephalo-myelitis	Enteroviruses (including polio) Human herpesviruses (HHV) 1 and 2, Human immunodeficiency virus (HIV), Mumps	HHV-3*, 4* and 5, Influenza A and B*, Lymphocytic choriomeningitis virus, Measles*, Rubella**, Borrelia burgdorferi, Leptospira spp., Listeria monocytogenes, Mycobacterium tuberculosis, Mycoplasma pneumoniae, Cryptococcus neoformans, Naegleria fowleri, Toxoplasma gondii	Bunyaviruses, Rabies, Togaviruses, Borrelia recurrentis, Brucella spp., Rickettsia spp., Trophyrema whippelii, Histoplasma capsulatum, Plasmodium falciparum
Acute meningitis			
a) Neonate	HHV-1 and 2, Enteroviruses, Escherichia coli, Group B streptococci, Listeria monocytogenes	Enterobacter spp., Haemophilus influenzae (b), Klebsiella spp., Neisseria meningitidis, Salmonella spp., Streptococcus pneumoniae, Candida albicans	
b) Older Individuals	Enteroviruses, Mumps, H. influenzae (b), N. meningitidis, S. pneumoniae	Adenovirus, HIV, HHV-2, Lymphocytic choriomeningitis virus, Measles, Borrelia burgdorferi, Enterobacteriaceae, Leptospira spp., Listeria monocytogenes, M. tuberculosis, Treponema pallidum	Togaviruses
Chronic meningitis	M. tuberculosis Cryptococcus neoformans	Borrelia burgdorferi, Brucella spp., Leptospira spp., L. monocytogenes, N. meningitidis, T. pallidum, C. albicans	Francisella tularensis, Blastomyces dermatitidis, Coccidioides immitis, Histoplasma capsulatum

(continued on page 300)

Appendix 1 Nervous system infections.

Nervous system infections (*cont.*)		
	Most important	Less common	Tropical or geographically limited

	Most important	Less common	Tropical or geographically limited
Intracranial suppuration **Local spread** from mucosal surfaces	Polymicrobial: anaerobes, *Streptococcus* spp., Enterobacteriaceae	—	—
by trauma or surgery	Mono- or polymicrobial: *Staphylococcus aureus*, Enterobacteriaceae, *Pseudomonas* spp.	—	—
from meningitis	*H. influenzae* (b), *L. monocytogenes*, *Citrobacter diversus*	—	—
Bacteraemic spread	Enterobacteriaceae, *Salmonella* spp., *S. aureus*, Viridans streptococci, *Candida* and *Aspergillus* spp.	*Burkholderia pseudomallei*	—
Spinal cord and peripheral nerves Toxins	*Clostridium botulinum*, *C. tetani*, *Corynebacterium diphtheriae*	—	—
Infections a) Cord	Polioviruses 1, 2, 3, *Treponema pallidum*	Enteroviruses (70, 71), Coxsackie A, B, *Borrelia burgdorferi*, *Brucella* spp.	*Schistosoma* spp.
b) Peripheral nerves	Varicella zoster (HHV-3)	—	*Mycobacterium leprae*
Post infectious or vaccination			
Guillain–Barré	Epstein–Barr virus and Cytomegalovirus (HHV-4 and 5), HIV, Rubella	*Borrelia burgdorferi*, *Campylobacter jejuni*, *Salmonella typhi*	Human T-cell lymphotropic Virus I (HTLV-1) *Trophyrema whippelii*

* Infective and post infective encephalomyelitis.
** Only post infective or post vaccination.

Appendix 1 Nervous system infections (*cont.*).

Head and neck infections

Mouth
Caries
Gingivitis

Periodontitis
Thrush
Dental abscess

Streptococcus mutans
HHV-1
Spirochaetes and *Prevotella intermedia* (acute necrotizing ulcerative gingivitis)
Spirochaetes, *Porphyromonas gingivalis*, *Actinobacillus actinomycetemcomitans*,
Candida albicans
Polymicrobial; anaerobes.

Rhinitis

Adenovirus, coronaviruses, influenza virus, parainfluenza virus,
respiratory syncytial virus, rhinoviruses.

**Tonsils and
pharynx**

Adenoviruses, coronaviruses, enteroviruses, HHV-4, influenza virus,
parainfluenza, respiratory syncytial virus (RSV), *Arcanobacterium
haemolyticum*, *Chlamydia pneumoniae*, *Corynebacterium diphtheriae*,
C. ulcerans, *Mycoplasma pneumoniae*, *Neisseria gonorrhoeae*, *Streptococcus
pyogenes* (Gp.A), *C. albicans*.

Vincent's angina

Bacteroides spp., *Fusobacterium* spp.

Peritonsillar abscess
(Quinsy)

S. pyogenes, anaerobes.

Ludwig's angina

Polymicrobial, anaerobic streptococci, *Bacteroides* spp., *Fusobacterium* spp.

**Retropharyngeal
abscess**

Polymicrobial, anaerobes, staphylococci, streptococci.

Sinuses and middle ear
Acute

Respiratory viruses
Haemophilus influenzae, *Moraxella catarrhalis*, *Staphylococcus aureus*,
Streptococcus pneumoniae, *S. pyogenes*.

Chronic

Anaerobes, Enterobacteriaceae, *Pseudomonas* spp.,

**Parameningeal
structures**
(Subdural abscess,
Epidural abscess)

Polymicrobial, anaerobes, Enterobacteriaceae, *Pseudomonas* spp., *S. aureus*,
streptococci.

Appendix 2 Head and neck infections.

Respiratory tract infections

Laryngo-tracheo-bronchitis	Adenovirus, Enterovirus, Influenza virus, Parainfluenza virus, Respiratory syncytial virus (RSV), Rhinovirus. *Haemophilus influenzae* (secondary infection), *Staphylococcus aureus, Streptococcus pneumoniae.*
Laryngeal papillomata	Human papillomavirus.
Epiglottitis	*H. influenzae* (b), (*S. pneumoniae, S. aureus*; rare).
Bronchiolitis	*RSV,* Adenovirus 7.
Whooping cough	*Bordetella pertussis, B. parapertussis,* adenovirus.
Community-acquired pneumonia	Adenovirus, Influenza virus, Measles, Parainfluenza virus, RSV. *Chlamydia pneumoniae, C. psittaci, Fusobacterium necrophorum, H. influenzae, Legionella pneumophila, Moraxella catarrhalis, Mycobacterium tuberculosis, Mycoplasma pneumoniae, S. aureus, S. pneumoniae* and other anaerobes (aspiration). In tropics: *Bacillus anthracis, Francisella tularensis, Yersinia pestis.*
Pneumonia in the Immunocompromised	HHV-1, HHV-3, HHV-5, Measles. Enterobacteriaceae, *H. influenzae, L. pneumophila, Mycobacterium avium/intracellulare, M. tuberculosis,* Nocardia spp., Pseudomonas spp., *S. aureus, S. pneumoniae.* Aspergillus spp., *Cryptococcus neoformans,* Mucor spp., *Pneumocystis carinii, Strongyloides stercoralis, Toxoplasma gondii.*
Bronchiectasis and chronic obstructive airways disease	*Burkholderia cepacia* (in cystic fibrosis), *H. influenzae, Pseudomonas aeruginosa, S. aureus, Stenotrophomonas maltophilia, S. pneumoniae.* Aspergillus spp., Candida spp.
Lung abscess and empyema	*Klebsiella pneumoniae,* Anaerobes (e.g. *Fusobacterium necrophorum*), *S. aureus, Streptococcus milleri, S. pneumoniae.* *Entamoeba histolytica.*

Appendix 3 Respiratory tract infections.

Exanthems

Maculopapular erythematous	Enteroviruses, HHV-4 (glandular fever), HHV-6 and 7 (exanthem subitum), HIV, Measles, Parvovirus (erythema infectiosum, 5th Disease), Rubella. *Neisseria meningitidis* (septicaemia), *Salmonella typhi,* *Staphylococcus aureus* (toxic shock syndrome), *Streptococcus pyogenes* (scarlet fever), *Treponema pallidum* (secondary syphilis).
Petechial purpuric	Arboviruses, Adenoviruses, Enteroviruses, Measles (in immunocompromised). *N. meningitidis* Other Gram-negative bacterial septicaemia *Rickettsia* spp.
Haemorrhagic	Alphaviruses, Arenaviruses, Filoviruses, Hantavirus, Nairovirus, Phlebovirus, Togaviruses. *Rickettsia* spp., *N. meningitidis, Pseudomonas aeruginosa.*
Vesicular/pustular	Enteroviruses (hand, foot and mouth disease), HHV-1 (cold sores), HHV-2 (genital herpes), HHV-3 (chickenpox and shingles), *S. aureus, S. pyogenes* (impetigo).
Nodules	
Multiple	Molluscum contagiosum, Monkey pox, Papillomaviruses (warts).
Usually single	Orthopoxvirus (cowpox, tanapox), Parapoxviruses (Orf).
Kaposi's sarcoma	Kaposi's sarcoma associated herpes virus (HHV-8).

Appendix 4 Exanthems.

Gastrointestinal infections

	Most important	Less common	Tropical or geographically limited
Gastritis	Helicobacter pylori		
Peptic ulceration	Helicobacter pylori		
Hepatitis	Hepatitis A, Hepatitis B, Hepatitis C, Hepatitis D	HHV-4, HHV-5, Rubella (congenital) Brucella spp. Leptospira spp. Mycobacterium tuberculosis Treponema pallidum Yersinia enterocolitica	Hepatitis E Yellow Fever Histoplasma capsulatum Entamoeba histolytica Schistosoma mansoni
Vomiting	Norwalk agent Bacillus cereus (toxin) Staphylococcus aureus (toxin)		—
Diarrhoeal disease			
Non-inflammatory	Adenovirus 40/41, Astrovirus, Calicivirus Norwalk agent, Rotavirus. Aeromonas spp., Campylobacter spp., Enterotoxigenic E. coli, Salmonella spp., Cryptosporidium parvum, Giardia lamblia.	Bredavirus, Coronavirus, Pestivirus, SRV, Torovirus. B. cereus, Clostridium perfringens (food poisoning toxin), Enteropathogenic E. coli, Plesiomonas spp., Vibrio parahaemolyticus, Blastocystis hominis, Enterocytozoon bieneusi (in AIDS), Isospora belli.	Trophyrema whippelii Vibrio cholerae Cyclospora cayetanensis
Inflammatory	Aeromonas spp., Campylobacter spp., Clostridium difficile, Enteroaggregative E. coli, Enterohaemorrhagic E. coli, Salmonella spp., Shigella spp.	Enteroinvasive E. coli, Y. enterocolitica.	Clostridium perfringens (pig bel), Entamoeba histolytica

Appendix 5 Gastrointestinal tract infections.

Genito-urinary tract infection

Urinary tract

Urethritis *Chlamydia trachomatis, Neisseria gonorrhoeae, HHV-2.*

Cystitis *Escherichia coli* (>90%), *Staphylococcus saprophyticus,* HHV-2 (trigonitis). (rarely *Proteus, Klebsiella, Enterococcus* spp.).

Acute pyelonephritis *F. coli* (>90%), (rarely *Proteus, Klebsiella* spp.).

Complicated urinary tract infection (by congenital defect, surgery, calculi and catheterization) *E. coli* (30%), *Proteus* spp., *Klebsiella* spp., *Pseudomonas* spp., *Enterococcus* spp., *Candida albicans.*

Genital tract

Vulvo-vaginitis (discharge) *Neisseria gonorrhoeae, Chlamydia trachomatis,* HHV-2, *Candida albicans, Trichomonas vaginalis , Enterobius vermicularis.*

Bacterial vaginosis ?*Gardnerella vaginalis,* ?*Mobiluncus* spp., ?Anaerobes.

Genital ulcers HHV-2, HHV-1, *Treponema pallidum, Haemophilus ducreyi, C. trachomatis* (LGV), *Calymmatobacterium granulomatis.*

Genital nodules Human papillomaviruses, Molluscum contagiosum.

Ectoparasites *Phthirius pubis, Sarcoptes scabiei.*

Epididymitis *C. trachomatis, N. gonorrhoeae, Mycobacterium tuberculosis.*

Orchitis/oophoritis Mumps.

Pelvic inflammatory disease *C. trachomatis, N. gonorrhoeae,* Anaerobes. *Mycoplasma hominis, Ureaplasma urealyticum. M. tuberculosis, Actinomyces israelii.*

Carcinoma of the cervix Human papillomaviruses 16, 18, 33.

Appendix 6 Genito-urinary tract infections.

Skin and soft tissue infections

Eyes

Blepharitis

HHV-1, HPV, Molluscum contagiosum, *S. aureus*, *Moraxella lacunata*,

Conjunctivitis

Adenovirus (3,7,8,19), Enterovirus (70), Coxsackie (A24), HHV-1. *Haemophilus influenzae*, *H. aegyptius*, *Streptococcus pneumoniae*, *Neisseria meningitidis*, *N. gonorrhoeae*, *Chlamydia trachomatis* (A-C: trachoma), *C. trachomatis* (D-K: ophthalmia neonatorum).

Keratitis

HHV-1, *Staphylococcus aureus*, *Streptococcus pyogenes*, *Pseudomonas* spp., *Fusarium solani*, *Candida albicans*, *Acanthamoeba* spp.

Retinitis

Toxocara canis, HHV-5 and *Toxoplasma gondii*.

Orbital cellulitis

H. influenzae (b), *S. aureus*, *S. pyogenes*, *S. pneumoniae*, *Trichinella spiralis*, *Taenia solium*.

Skin

Carbuncle, furuncle

S. aureus

Vesicles

HHV-1, HHV-2, HHV-3, Enteroviruses.

Impetigo

S. aureus, *S. pyogenes*.

Nodules

Molluscum contagiosum, Human papillomavirus, Cowpox, Orf.

Granulomas

Mycobacterium tuberculosis, *Mycobacterium marinum*.

Ringworm

Microsporum, *Trichophyton*, *Epidermophyton* spp.

Intertrigo

Candida albicans.

Tinea versicolor

Malassezia furfur.

Infected bites

Human

Anaerobes, *Eikenella corrodens*, *S. aureus*, *S. pyogenes*.

Animal

Capnocytophaga canimorsus, *Pasteurella multocida*, anaerobes.

Insect

S. aureus, *S. pyogenes*.

Soft tissue

Erysipelas

S. pyogenes (Group A; rarely C and B).

Acute cellulitis

S. pyogenes, *H. influenzae* (b), *Vibrio vulnificus*, *Clostridium perfringens*, *Bacillus anthracis*, *Erysipelothrix* spp., *Aeromonas hydrophila*.

Necrotizing fasciitis

S. pyogenes. Synergistic infection with *S. aureus* and anaerobes.

Lymphadenitis

Brucella spp., *M. avium/intracellulare*, *M. tuberculosis*, *Bartonella henselae* (cat scratch disease), *S. pyogenes*, *Treponema pallidum*.

Appendix 7   Skin and soft tissue infections.

Bone, joint and muscle infections

Bone
Acute osteomyelitis

Staphylococcus aureus (95%), *Haemophilus influenzae* (b), *Salmonella* spp., *Streptococcus agalactiae* (in neonates).

Chronic osteomyelitis

Anaerobes, *Brucella* spp., Enterobacteriaceae, *Mycobacterium tuberculosis*, *Pseudomonas aeruginosa*, *Staphylococcus epidermidis* (implant infection).

Joints
Septic arthritis

S. aureus, *H. influenzae* (b), *Streptococcus pneumoniae*, *Neisseria gonorrhoeae*, *N. meningitidis*, Enterobacteriaceae (in immunocompromised), *Brucella* spp., Parvovirus, Rubellavirus.

Reactive arthritis
(reaction to infection
elsewhere)

Campylobacter spp., *Chlamydia trachomatis*, *N. gonorrhoeae*, *N. meningitidis*, *Salmonella* spp., *Yersinia enterocolitica*.

Muscle
Pyomyositis
Gas gangrene
Parasitic disease

S. aureus, *Streptococcus pyogenes*
Clostridium perfringens
Toxoplasma gondii, *Cysticercosis*
Hydatid disease, *Trichinella spiralis*,
Toxocara canis, *T. cati*.

Bornholm disease

Enterovirus.

Appendix 8 Bone, joint and muscle infections.

Cardiovascular infection

Infective endocarditis	Viridans streptococci, *Staphylococcus epidermidis, Cardiobacterium hominis, Coxiella burnetii, Haemophilus aphrophilus, Enterococcus* spp., *Candida albicans, Aspergillus* spp., *Staphylococcus aureus* (acute).
Prosthetic valves	*S. epidermidis* in particular.
I.V. Drug abusers	Enterobacteriaceae, *Pseudomonas aeruginosa, Candida* spp., in particular.
Pericarditis	Coxsackie B virus *Haemophilus influenzae* (b), *Streptococcus pneumoniae, Streptococcus pyogenes, S. aureus, Neisseria meningitidis, Mycobacterium tuberculosis.*
Myocarditis	Coxsackie A and B; ECHO, Mumps viruses. *N. meningitidis, S. aureus, S. pyogenes.*

Appendix 9 Cardiovascular infection.

Fever of unknown origin*

	Most important	Less common
Infections (up to 40% of cases)		
Localized	Intra-abdominal abscess Subphrenic abscess Pelvic abscess Tuberculous meningitis	Perinephric abscess, Splenic abscess, Dental abscess, Brain abscess, Chronic sinusitis, Chronic meningitis, Chronic osteomyelitis, Cholangitis, Bacterial endocarditis, Mastoiditis, Pyelonephritis, Lung abscess, Hepatitis, LGV, Psittacosis, Lyme disease (*Borrelia burgdorferi*).
Disseminated	HHV-4, HHV-5, HIV Miliary tuberculosis Typhoid fever Malaria	Brucellosis, Relapsing fever (*Borrelia recurrentis*), Rat-bite fever (*Spirillum minus*), Leptospirosis, Q-fever (*Coxiella burnetii*), Cat scratch disease (*Bartonella henselae*), Erlichosis, *Rickettsia* spp., *Cryptococcus neoformans, Histoplasma capsulatum, Toxoplasmosis, Toxocariasis, Trypanosomiasis*, Katayama fever (*Schistosomiasis*).
Neoplasia (about 15%)	Lymphomas, Hypernephroma Metastases to liver or CNS	Hepatoma, Carcinoma of pancreas, Atrial myxoma, Neuroblastoma.
Autoimmune (about 15%)	Still's disease, Giant cell arthritis	Rheumatoid arthritis, Polyarteritis nodosa, SLE, Felty's syndrome, Rheumatic fever.
Other (10–20%)	Drug fever, Kawasaki's disease	Anhidrotic octodermal dysplasia Diabetes insipidus Fabry's disease Factitious fever Familial dysautonomia Familial Mediterranean fever Pancreatitis Periodic fever Pulmonary embolism Serum sickness Thyrotoxicosis
Undiagnosed (10–20%)		

* Petersdorf suggests, as a definition, a minimum temperature of 38.8°C for 3 weeks with at least 1 week of intensive hospital investigation. In paediatric practice a shorter period of fever of 1 week is often used.

Appendix 10 Fever of unknown origin.

Index